DYNAMICS OF NURSING

DYNAMICS OF NURSING

LILLIAN DeYOUNG, R.N., B.S.N.E., M.S., Ph.D.

Dean and Professor of Nursing, University of Akron
College of Nursing, Akron, Ohio

FIFTH EDITION

Illustrated

The C. V. Mosby Company

ST. LOUIS • TORONTO • PRINCETON   1985

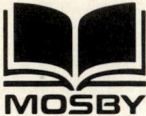

MOSBY

A TRADITION OF PUBLISHING EXCELLENCE

Editor: Julie Cardamon
Assistant editor: Bess Arends
Editing supervisor: Elaine Steinborn
Manuscript editor: Mary Wright
Design: Gail Morey Hudson
Production: Susan Trail

FIFTH EDITION

Previous editions copyrighted 1966, 1972, 1976, 1981
Printed in the United States of America

The C.V. Mosby Company
11830 Westline Industrial Drive, St. Louis, Missouri 63146

Library of Congress Cataloging in Publication Data

DeYoung, Lillian.
    Dynamics of nursing.

    Includes bibliographies and index.
    1. Nursing. I. Title. [DNLM: 1. Nursing. WY 16 D529f]
RT82.D48 1985   610.73'0692   84-14678
ISBN 0-8016-1284-5

GW/VH/VH 9 8 7 6 5 4 3   03/D/307

Contributors

MARIANNE CRAWFORD, R.N., M.S.N.

Director of Nursing, Akron General Medical Center, Akron, Ohio

LEAH CURTIN, R.N., F.A.A.N.

Editor, *Nursing Management*, Cincinnati, Ohio

MARY FISHER, R.N., M.S.N.

Director of Nursing Education and Inquiry, Akron General Medical Center, Akron, Ohio

JOANN HOLT, R.N., M.S.N.

Vice President, Nursing, Akron General Medical Center, Akron, Ohio

NANCY KILBANE, R.N., M.S.N.

Director of Nursing, Akron General Medical Center, Akron, Ohio

JANICE K. LANIER, R.N., B.S.N.

Assistant Executive Director, Lobbyist, Ohio Nurses Association, Columbus, Ohio

JOANNE MARCHIONE, R.N., M.A.

Associate Professor, University of Akron College of Nursing, Akron, Ohio

SHIRLEY MOWDOOD, R.N., J.D.

Attorney-at-law, Akron, Ohio

VIRGINIA NEWBERN, R.N., Ph.D.

Associate Professor and Director, Continuing Education, University of Southern Mississippi, Hattiesburg, Mississippi

To students past and present
who have contributed to my belief
in nursing as a dynamic profession

Preface

When *The Foundations of Nursing: As Conceived, Learned, and Practiced in Professional Nursing* was published in 1966, its success was evidence of a need well met. The world of nursing was drastically changed in 1981; with that in mind the fourth edition became basically a different text. *Dynamics of Nursing,* a text of the 1980s, was written to capture the spirit of the past and the movement of nursing from a vocation to a profession.

This fifth edition, like previous ones, offers undergraduate students a historical perspective to help them understand today's issues in nursing. Brevity continues to be a positive aspect of the text; faculty knowledge and additional student reading can effectively augment content. It is my hope that students will be stimulated sufficiently by the content to accept the challenge of past and present nurse leaders and advance nursing to greater accomplishments.

The text is a valuable source book for faculty who teach history, issues, or trends courses; recruiters or counselors of prospective students; and graduate faculty and students. Content is intended to extend beyond an introductory course in nursing throughout the undergraduate educational program.

In the fifth edition, each chapter begins with an objective to guide the student in study and ends with discussion questions to assist in developing dialogue about the content.

Part One, Evolution of and Trends in Nursing, discusses the historical perspective of service, education, theories, and changing patterns of nursing. Each of these chapters is important, but Chapter 4, Evolution of Theories of Nursing, is perhaps the most significant for tomorrow's practitioner. Joanne Marchione guides the student through theory development to the theories of nursing now influencing practice. All chapters were revised and updated.

Part Two, Contemporary Perspectives, discusses nursing practice, leadership, entry into practice, research, and issues in nursing. This entire section provides the student with a perspective on where nursing is today and the leadership role nurses are assuming. The chapters on research, collective bargaining, and politics in nursing discuss areas that will have the most significant impact on the future of nursing.

In this part, five completely new chapters were prepared. They are Professional Nursing Practice, Nursing Leadership, Ethical Aspects of Nursing, Collective Bargaining in Nursing, and Power, Politics, and the Nurse. All other chapters were revised and updated.

Part Three, Professional Perspectives, discusses professional nursing, legal aspects, opportunities in nursing, continuing education, and dynamic nursing. The section is written primarily for the senior who is about to move from student to practitioner. Shirley Mowdood, in the chapter on legal aspects, addresses a neglected issue: the consequences of becoming a professional, while I end the text with thoughts about dynamic forces in nursing.

I am grateful to the following persons for contributing new chapters to this edition: Marianne Crawford, Mary Fisher, Nancy Kilbane, and Joann

Holt wrote Chapters 7, 8, and 10. This was a collaborative effort from nursing service administrators to share what they believed to be important in nursing practice, nursing leadership, and collective bargaining. Janice K. Lanier, lobbyist for the Ohio Nurses Association, willingly shares her knowledge of power, politics, and the nurse in Chapter 11. Leah Curtin provides insight into ethical aspects of nursing in Chapter 9.

I continue to be grateful to the following for their contribution to whole or parts of chapters: Marilyn Burkhart for the section on diploma nurse education, Gay Lindsay for the section on practical nurse education, Joanne Marchione for the chapter on theories of nursing, Shirley Mowdood for sections in the chapter on legal aspects, and Virginia Newbern for the chapter on continuing education.

Leah McPherron, graduate assistant at the University of Akron, was valuable in doing the library research for several chapters. Other colleagues read the fourth edition and offered constructive criticism that served as a guide in discarding much of the old material and adding the new. No author is without someone who is technically skilled in typing and professionally astute in editing. I am therefore grateful to Brenda Freiberg, who provided this expertise.

Revision is not an easy task, nor is writing a book. However, if *Dynamics of Nursing* is read by students and used by faculty to promote the growth of nursing as a responsible, accountable profession, then the painful task of writing becomes a satisfying one.

Lillian DeYoung

Contents

PART ONE
EVOLUTION OF AND TRENDS IN NURSING

Florence Nightingale   Nursing is an art; and if it is to be made an art, it requires as exclusive a devotion, as hard a preparation, as any painter's or sculptor's work; for what is the having to do with dead canvas or cold marble, compared with having to do with the living body—the temple of God's spirit? It is one of the Fine Arts; I had almost said, the finest of the Fine Arts.

History offers an opportunity to trace cause and effect in the social achievement or failure of nursing from precivilization to the present. It is the spectacle of human nature and social organization in a process of struggle, of challenge and response. The history of nursing must be viewed from the total picture of the times, since most of nursing history is interwoven with general history. Almost any incident, influence, progress, or change that has affected general history is reflected in nursing history. Drawing from the past helps in understanding the present and anticipating the future, making history become an endless cycle.

Nursing as a profession is comparatively young; it has been considered a respectable profession for the past 100 years. Because nursing has a great tradition, the following chapters are designed to give to the student an understanding of how nursing evolved to its present status and what the future holds for the profession of nursing. A knowledge of nursing history will help the student to acquire an appreciation of the relationships of nursing to religious, cultural, sociological, and economic phases of human progress and will give to nurses a feeling of belonging to, identification with, and pride in their chosen profession.

Of necessity the following chapters must be an overview of the history of nursing. There are many other sources available to give the student a broader picture of nursing. Students may continue to reinforce their knowledge of nursing by reading the reference material suggested at the end of each chapter.

CHAPTER 1
Evolution of nursing—service

OBJECTIVE: On completion of this chapter, the student of nursing will have an understanding
of the historical perspective of nursing and the impact our society has had
on nursing.

To understand the problems of nursing today, an overview of how nursing services have been given through the ages is invaluable. Nursing has not always been an organized effort based on scientific principles; its history has been one of frustration, ignorance, and lack of sympathy toward the ill.

NURSING SERVICE BEFORE THE FLORENCE NIGHTINGALE ERA
Nursing service before ancient civilizations

The evolution of nursing service has been extremely uneven in the world, probably because of the basic differences in the cultures of East and West. History actually tells us little of how the service of nursing was performed or what methods were used until the pre-Nightingale period. Most of nursing history is interwoven with general history.

Nursing itself is as old as humankind. Primitive people lived in tribes primarily for mutual protection. Each individual was expected to serve to his or her utmost capacity. Nursing of the sick seems to have been one of the assignments designated for the women of the tribes. Women learned to meet the emergencies created by the illness of a member of the tribe and also learned methods for prevention of sickness. The ill and helpless became the special charge of the tribal women. The beliefs of the pre-civilization tribes had tremendous influence on how

the ''nurse'' cared for the ill. Innumerable superstitions, beliefs, and practices developed.

The comforting effects of water were learned early, and the invention of fire making made primitive people cognizant of the value of heat. In their experimenting with certain herbs and plants, they probably discovered which ones could cause them to vomit and which ones would act as laxatives. Because these people attributed illness to an evil spirit within the body of the person who was ill, these concoctions were used to rid the person's body of the evil spirit. Pummeling was also used to pound the evil spirit out of the body. Trephining, or boring holes in the patient's skull, was introduced to allow the evil spirits to be released from the head.

In their journeys afield, the men brought back new remedies for curing illness. Some of the men became expert in curing and were called medicine men. These medicine men lived apart from the group and attempted to keep many of their practices secret. The medicine man became a person with high standing in the tribe. He dressed fantastically, conceived wild dances, and made strange noises. This ancient practitioner used both ''black'' and ''white'' magic to cure ills and impress the rest of the community with his abilities and powers. The medicine man was required to demonstrate his ability to get the assistance of the good spirits to drive off evil ones, and he had to prove he could bring disaster or disease on the enemies of his tribe. He was actually invested with a social power comparable to that of the chief of the tribe.

White magic practices were for helpful purposes, whereas black magic was more destructive in its goals and was aimed at enemies rather than members of the community. The cure of illness gradually took on a ritualistic religious tone, and the medicine man was set apart from the rest of the community as a "holy person."

As nursing of the ill became associated with religion, the medicine man was replaced by the priest-physician, whose practice had a strange mixture of superstition and fact. Often the priest and the physician were not the same person, but both dealt with problems of life and death and were authorities on the folklore of the community they served.

Both the medicine man and the priest-physician performed those rituals of the particular tribe or culture that were believed to drive out the evil spirits and cure the patient. Potions, pummeling, rubbing, applications of hot and cold, purging, and trephining all became a part of the repertoire of these "sages" of precivilization time.

Primitive people endowed natural objects with the same qualities that they possessed. The belief that grew up around this basic concept is called animism. The influence of the basic belief caused primitive people to explain disaster or disease on the basis of supersition and a system of empirical medicine, which to some extent still influences people today.

Nursing service at the beginning of civilization

With the establishment of complex social systems and institutions of the ancient civilizations came primitive medicine (naturalistic) in combination with religion and magic. The cultures that developed along the Indus, Euphrates, Tigris, and Nile Rivers all had some form of naturalistic medicine. In the history of these early civilizations is

found no counterpart for the nurse of the twentieth century.

Ancient nurses were probably domestic servants who gave instinctive care to the sick and needy. Whether these nurses were male or female is not clear, but whatever their sex and whatever their duties, they lived in a civilization of people skilled in calculation and observation.

Hammurabi of Babylonia formulated a code of laws that established for the first time legal and civil measures that regulated the practice of physicians and protected the safety of the patient. The concepts of both hygiene and social medicine were at a high level in ancient Babylonia.

In Egypt the people were skilled mathematicians and architects. They also made great progress in sanitation. The Egyptians were probably the healthiest of all ancient peoples. According to Egyptian mythology, the control of health was in the hands of gods. Imhotep was the most famous of all these gods and was called the first priest-physician and the god of medicine. He was noted for his great wisdom and learning in the field of health, magic, and religious rituals.

Diagnosis seems to have been important in the Egyptian culture. The Ebers Papyrus lists approximately 1000 prescriptions. Some of the remedies used by the Egyptians are known to us today. There were no hospitals, but undoubtedly the temples had some kind of housing for the sick. But who cared for the sick in these temples remains a historical mystery.

In all probability much of the knowledge of the Hebrew people was borrowed from the Egyptians, since Moses, the adopted son of Pharaoh's daughter, most likely was educated at the University of Heliopolis (now Cairo). Undoubtedly Moses was well versed in the wisdom of the Egyptians.

The Hebrews believed that all persons were entitled to the same medical treatment. They provided a house for travelers called the xenodochium. Attached to the xenodochium was a "sick house" where the ill and infirm were given care.

The Hebrew people attained a high level of hygiene and sanitation. Bathing was an important part of the purification and sanitation process. Probably some of the nursing duties in the sick houses of the Hebrew people were done by women, but the only specific person to be mentioned as a nurse at this time is Deborah, who was actually a child's nurse and companion. Deborah was the first nurse to have her name come down in history.

Hebraic medicine provided a basis of social hygiene for all other civilizations. Historically, Moses has been regarded as the father of sanitation because many of his concepts of isolation, quarantine, and disposal of wastes are pertinent in preventive medicine and nursing today. In the regulations now known as the Mosaic Code, Moses organized a method of prevention of disease that included personal hygiene, rest, sleep, cleanliness, hours of work, selection and inspection of food, regulation of diet, public hygiene, diagnosis, and the reporting of communicable disease. The priest-physician was the health inspector, and every person who became ill reported to him and could not return to the tribe without the permission of this authority.

In Greece, treatment of diseases was primarily in the hands of priests. Hippocrates (Father of Medicine) is the most outstanding individual in the medical history of Greece. In 400 BC Hippocrates admonished his students to "treat the whole patient." Today both nursing and medical students are taught to think in terms of the total or whole patient and not just the affected physical area when planning the nursing or medical care of patients.

In addition, nursing has fostered the philosophy that a person is greater than the sum of all of his or her parts, thus taking on the concept of holistic nursing. This concept will be further explored in Chapter 2.

Hippocrates does not mention nurses in his writings, but it can be inferred that nurses were present, since he refers to cold sponging, hot gargles, cool drinks, fluid diet, and warm baths. Someone would have had to perform these functions and initiate the physician's orders. What nursing care was ac-

tually like must of necessity be left to the imagination of the reader.

In the ancient Roman civilization, medical advancement was considerably less than in Greece. The citizens of Rome appreciated hygiene. Their system of sewers, drains, and street paving tended to make their cities cleaner than those of any of the other ancient civilizations. Great aqueducts brought pure drinking water to the citizens of Rome. Bathing eventually developed into a cult, involving the use of hot and cold water, inunctions, and massage. Rome had many epidemics of disease, probably because of the influx of conquered people, the rapidity of growth, and the malaria-infested marshes that surrounded Rome.

The Romans clung to their gods, superstition, and herbs to cure the ills of their people. After 200 BC the Greek physicians who were slaves of the Romans did the medical work. Army hospitals were well conducted, and the Roman soldiers received good nursing care wherever they were fighting. Who gave them this care besides the Greek slave-physicians is not known.

Many hospitals were built along the frontiers of the Rhine and the Danube Rivers. Some of these hospitals could house 200 sick or wounded soldiers. These hospitals contained wards, baths, rooms for attendants, recreation areas, pharmacies, and even convalescent centers for war-weary officials. The physicians were nocombatants in the army. The auxiliary medical personnel who accompanied the physicians probably acted as the nurses. These ancient physicians always avoided near-dead persons and pregnant women. The nurse-midwife was still the attendant at childbirth.

Civilizations also appeared early in China and India. In China, dissection was permitted before 2000 BC. Studies of the circulation of the blood were carried out, and diagnosis of illness was made on the basis of a complicated pulse theory. The Chinese classified 200 types of pulse beat. There is no reference to nurses in the literature of the ancient Chinese. If there were professional nurses, they were probably not women, since Confucius clearly defined woman's position as inferior to that of man. The woman's only place was in the home, and her value was greatest when she produced a son.

India was the first country to record the use of a nurse in the care of the sick. The sacred books of the Hindus outlined the duties of the nurse. Four qualifications seem to be the most significant for the attending nurse of ancient India: "The Nurse (usually male, or in rare cases, old women) must have knowledge of the manner in which drugs should be prepared or compounded for administration, cleverness, devotedness to the patient waited upon, and purity (both of mind and body).''*

King Asoka (250 BC) established hospitals throughout India and was the first to require the licensing of physicians. Trustworthiness and skill were demanded of physicians, as well as nurses and midwives. They were admonished to have short fingernails, to maintain high moral standards, and to consider the prevention of disease their prime objective. All operations were preceded by religious ceremonies and prayer.

Nurses were employed in the hospitals of India. Requirements for the nurses, who were always men, were similar to those for practical nurses today. The public hospitals in India were also schools of medicine.

In the precivilization and ancient history of the world, little mention is made of nurses or nursing as separate entities. From the earliest times the midwife has probably been accepted in her role during childbirth, as has the child's nurse. Priestesses probably assisted the priest-physicians in the various temples built by the people of these ancient civilizations. During the eras discussed, religion, nursing, medicine, superstition, and education all centered around the temples, and the beliefs, mores, and culture of each civilization influenced the way in which the nursing care was given, who gave it, and what was given.

---

*Vyas, K.C.: India through the ages (translated by F.A. Steele), New York, 1963, E.P. Dutton & Co., Inc., p. 10.

Nursing service at the beginning of the Christian era

Nursing as an organized service to society began in the early Christian era. Unselfishness and the responsibility of each individual for the general welfare were emphasized. The world was one in which a minority was wealthy and the majority of humanity was either poverty stricken or in a state of slavery. Christianity taught a better way of living built on kindliness and brotherly love. Since this period in history, the service of nursing has been recognized as one of the tenets of the Christian way of life. The women in the early Christian church shared the activities with the men in caring for the ill and infirm. Considerable carry-over of the magic, empirical remedies, and home treatments of the earlier periods of history is apparent in the nursing care given by the early Christian nursing orders.

Phoebe, the bearer of St. Paul's Epistle to the Romans, is considered the first deaconess and first visiting nurse because of her interest in the welfare of people and her nursing of the poor in their homes.

Before the rise of the monasteries, three nursing orders developed—the Virgins, Deaconesses, and Widows. Their main responsibility was the nursing care of the sick. Women in these orders concentrated on social work and nursing, which is suggestive of the present role of the public health nurse.

Many of these orders flourished because they were an outlet for the philanthropic aspirations of some of the women as well as a form of security for women made destitute by wars. They were required to be devoted in hospitality, have a reputation for piety, and be anxious to relieve the afflicted. The Virgins' chief duty seems to have been distributing alms, but they were awarded great honor by the church and ranked in equality with clergy.

One of the great social contributions of early Christianity was the establishment of hospitals for the poor. In these institutions were places for orphans, old persons, persons with contagious diseases such as leprosy, the ill, the maimed, and the deformed, and there were hospitality centers for strangers. One of the most famous of these hospitals is the one founded by St. Basil the Great, often referred to as the "Basilias." According to Walsh (1929), there were both resident physicians and resident nurses, carriers of the sick, and also working men and women to do the menial or artisan work connected with the establishment. Nearly everything used in the hospital had to be made on the grounds, since there were no industries or manufacturing plants from which the administrators of the institution might order the necessary supplies.

In Rome one of the ways the wealthy matrons made their contribution to society and the culture of the time was through helping the poor and the ill. Three of the most famous of these matrons were Marcella, Fabiola, and Paula. Each contributed to the care of the sick in a different way. Their friendship with St. Jerome inspired them to become advocates and teachers of the Christian way of life.

Marcella converted her home into a monastery for women, thus establishing the first Christian monastery in Rome. Marcella devoted her time to the instruction of other women, charitable work, and prayer. She was also a highly educated woman for that time and was able to help St. Jerome in the translation of writings of the Hebrew prophets.

The first Christian hospital in Rome was founded by Fabiola in her own palace. It is said that Fabiola did much of the nursing care of the poor herself and was particularly proficient in the dressing of wounds and sores.

Paula established hospitals for the pilgrims on the way to Palestine and Bethlehem. St. Jerome has described the nursing duties of Paula and her followers in his letters, *Nicene and Post-Nicene, Fathers of the Christian Church*. Besides doing the bathing, treatments, and other duties connected with the nursing care of patients of this period, Paula and her nurses trimmed lamps, lighted fires, swept floors, cleaned vegetables, washed dishes, and waited on others. Perhaps this is the beginning of the tradition in nursing service that a nurse must do hard manual work to be an efficient or good nurse.

The care of the sick became a function of many religious orders. Monasteries assumed prominence in the social structure of the early Middle Ages.

Among the more influential groups to take the responsibility of giving nursing service to the sick and wounded were the religious communities organized by St. Benedict of Nursia in the sixth century. His monastic organizational pattern consisting of the novice and three groups of monks within the order—seniors ("wise-folk"), middle class, and juniors—can be seen reflected in the patterns of nursing service and education of the twentieth century.

Privileges and duties were arranged by the Benedictine rule in accordance with the preceding four divisions. The hardest work and strictest rule fell to the lot of the novitiate. The "pecking order" was later adapted by both Catholic and Protestant nursing orders and in parts of Europe by the Red Cross.

The period of being a novitiate was not easy in St. Benedict's order because it was a time of probation to determine the person's fitness for monastic life. The fledgling was under constant supervision, restrictions, and isolation. No one spoke to him without permission from the master in charge, and the novice was required to rise to receive reproof. The restrictions and supervision placed on the beginning student nurse in the late 1890s and early 1900s compare closely to Benedictine rules of conduct and promotion.

Monastic houses for women grew in number in the sixth and seventh centuries because of the prevailing need for protection. Many of these women were wealthy and had great influence. Some even became heads of monasteries and were called abbesses. One of the most renowned of these was St. Radegonde. She founded a hospital for lepers and nursed them herself. She advocated bathing to maintain good health.

One of the most famous of the abbesses was St. Hildegarde. She belonged to the Benedictines in Germany. Hildegarde was well educated and devoted her time to the study of medicine, nursing, and natural science. She became skillful in the practice of medicine; people all over the world sought her advice, and her cures became famous. She believed in fresh air and free use of water. In her writings she described such things as jaundice, lung diseases, and dysentery.

During the period of feudalism, nursing service was performed by the lady of the manor. Her knowledge of home remedies for all kinds of illness had to be all-encompassing, since she was called on to provide nursing care for family, guests, serfs, and villagers. She was doctor and nurse combined.

Guilds were first mentioned in the eighth century. Many historians believe that the first references to guilds came from England. The religious guilds seem to have been the most concerned with giving service to their members in case of illness. In the craft guilds, help was given to families of the workers if need arose.

In England the religious guilds were used as eleemosynary institutions in the twelfth and thirteenth centuries and did play an important part in English social life.

The apprenticeship type of nursing, which is prevalent in the European countries today and was the pattern for nursing education in the United States until the 1940s, was probably influenced by the pattern set up by the craft guilds to train men and boys for their chosen craft or vocation.

About the middle of the seventh century Mohammed and his followers were gathering converts in the Byzantine Empire, Egypt, Africa, Spain, and France. The Islamic beliefs united many tribes in common ways of thinking and living. The works of Hippocrates and Galen were translated into Arabic. The Islamic interest in medicine brought about the building of great hospitals. The most famous of these were in Baghdad and Cordova. Evidently women did the simple nursing care of patients in these hospitals, but the care of women during childbirth remained in the hands of uneducated midwives. Both physiology and hygiene were studied by the Moslems. They developed an extensive materia medica and learned to use *Hyoscy-*

amus, Cannabis indica, and opium as anesthetics. They excelled in surgery and are credited with the use of catgut. Rhazes was considered their greatest physician.

Military nursing orders such as the Knights Hospitallers of St. John of Jerusalem developed during the crusades. A female branch of the order established hospitals in Spain, Portugal, France, England, and Malta. Nursing service has inherited a tradition of rigorous discipline, strict supervision, unquestioned obedience, efficiency of hospital management, hierarchy of nursing organization, and wearing of a uniform from these military monastic orders. The men fought on the battlefield during the day; when the fighting was over, they carried the wounded from the battlefield and cared for them in the hospitals or first aid stations.

Two other military nursing orders achieved renown during the seven major crusades, which continued over a period of 200 years. These are the Knights Templars and the Teutonic Knights. Lazarettos were built all along the routes of the crusades for the people who contracted leprosy. The disease was early recognized as communicable, and the people realized that isolation of the afflicted was a must. Although there was no system of nursing education during the period of the crusades, certainly there were many men and women who heroically and with dedication gave nursing service to the sick and wounded.

One of these dedicated individuals was St. Francis of Assisi, who was the founder of the Franciscans and principal patron of Italy. St. Francis embraced a life of poverty and formed one of the most famous of the mendicant orders of the twelfth century. The second order formed by St. Francis was for women, with St. Clara as the head of the order. St. Francis formed the third order for those who could not leave their families and homes. The people in this order were called tertiaries. St. Elizabeth of Hungary was a member of the third order. Her influence was felt in the nursing service of the time through her interest in visiting the ill in hospitals and homes. She gave baths, changed surgical dressings, fed patients, and cared for children. St. Elizabeth of Hungary has earned a place in history as the forerunner of the visiting and public health nurses of the twentieth century.

A different type of nursing order of this era was that of the Beguines, who still carry on the same devoted service that has characterized the order for the past 8 centuries. The order of the Beguines was founded outside Liege in Flanders as a model community of laywomen who were organized for religious purposes. Cottage communities were built around the church at Liege, and the women lived in these cottages. Many of the women were married; others were widows who were pathetic vagabonds because their husbands had joined the crusades and never returned. The women who belonged to the order seem to have come from all levels of society and were particularly interested in an avenue of useful service to the community.

All kinds of tasks associated with feminine industry were undertaken by these women. Visiting nursing in the neighborhood homes was started, and fees were charged for the service if the families were able to pay. If a hospital was a part of the community "Beguinage," nursing of the hospitalized patient became a responsibility of the women of the order. By the end of the thirteenth century there were about 200,000 of these lay workers scattered over the communities of Belgium. The people of Belgium learned to depend on these orders in time of emergency much as Americans learned to depend on the Red Cross Nursing Service of the United States in time of disaster or war.

Society's awakening to social service

The beginning development of social service and a greater awakening of a social obligation to improve the nursing care given to the people were stimulated by St. Vincent de Paul and his order, the Sisters of Charity. A trend toward the modernization of nursing began when St. Vincent de Paul with the help of St. Louise de Marillac laid down the principles for the guidance of the Sisters of Charity. Today the Sisters of Charity form one of the largest and most widely distributed nursing orders in the world. This was the only nursing order not suppressed during the French Revolution. Mother Elizabeth Seton founded a branch of the Sisters of Charity in the United States in 1812. The nursing order is interested in the improvement of patient care as well as the education of women and men for the nursing profession.

Florence Nightingale spent a period of time at the Sisters of Charity Hospital in France observing their system of nursing service and care of the patient.

The order of the Augustinian Sisters was the first one devoted entirely to nursing. These sisters have been in charge of the nursing service of the Hotel Dieu in Paris since the twelfth century. The Sisters of Charity supplemented the nursing service of the Augustinian nuns at the Hotel Dieu in Paris. Probably the greatest contribution of the Augustinian nuns to nursing service was their preservation of the known nursing procedures of the era during what is often termed the "dark period of nursing."

Another woman, St. Catherine of Siena, insisted that nurses should have some education. St. Catherine was a deeply religious woman and, when 16 years of age, joined the Dominican Tertiaries. She was the first person to start an ambulance service. St. Catherine started the service during the plagues of the fourteenth century. Her great devotion to the care of the sick during the plagues is often used as an example of devotion to duty and the service of nursing.

The plagues affected mainly the lower class elements in society. Members of the upper class would leave the plague-stricken city, but their servants often remained. To make a living, the ex-servants worked as nurses, caring for the people who were ill with the plague. Outstanding nursing service was done by both men and women during this period. For example, during the bubonic plague of the seventeenth century the nurses in the various London hospitals remained at their posts to give care to the ill, even though the physicians fled the city.

Influences of the Reformation

Religious unrest was prevalent during the thirteenth and fourteenth centuries and into the fifteenth and sixteenth centuries, when Martin Luther became the leader of the group of dissatisfied people who broke away from the Roman Catholic Church and formed what was called the Protestant Church. The forming of these two religious camps caused many nursing orders to dissolve. Many kings, hungry for power, seized monasteries for revenue, and monastic nursing declined.

Nursing and the care of the sick were in a changing and stressful situation. Almost all men were removed from the ranks of nursing. The Protestant camp urged that care of the sick be taken up by the state. The Catholics attempted to preserve some of their nursing orders, with the Augustinian nuns probably being the most successful.

Many of the religious groups as well as communities established hospitals and tried to bring about practical reform and better management of hospitals. There were no nurses outside of the religious orders who had experience or education in the care of the ill.

Henry VIII of England granted endowments for some hospitals because he had closed most of the monastic hospitals. From these endowments came St. Bartholomew's and St. Thomas' Hospitals, as well as a hospital for the mentally ill (the hospital of Bethlehem, or Bedlam).

Nurses in St. Bartholomew's Hospital made beds, cooked the food, fed the patients, and washed the patients' linen and clothes. Bathing and attending the patient were important functions. In their spare time the nurses did the mending, hemmed the sheets, and made other supplies needed in the hospital. These nurses were provided with room and board, and as many as 13 slept in a single large room. Roaches, bugs, and vermin plagued the nurses in the hospitals of the period.

The term *sister* was used for these nurses and still is in Europe and other parts of the Western world (except the United States) for referring to a graduate nurse, especially one in charge of a unit or ward of a hospital. The title has no connection with the religious affiliations of the nurse.

St. Bartholomew's had an outpatient ward connected with the hospital, to which a nurse was assigned and in which she helped with the care of people who came to the hospital for medical attention but did not remain overnight.

Hospitals were for the poor. Most of the influential people remained indifferent to the deplorable conditions and kind of nursing care given in the hospitals. Several people did attempt to reform the nursing practices and conditions in prisons, hospitals, and mental institutions. Probably the best known of these people are John Howard, Elizabeth Frye, Phillippe Pinel, William Tuke, and Mother Mary Catherine McAuley; later in the nineteenth century Dorothea Linde Dix began similar reforms in America.

In the eighteenth century John Howard of England advocated cleanliness in hospitals, fresh air, white walls, and plain furnishings. Elizabeth Frye carried on John Howard's cause after his death. In 1840 Mrs. Frye established the Institute of Nursing Sisters. Her students had little training, but they were devoted and respectable women. They visited and cared for the poor in their homes. They also gave nursing care to people who were able to pay.

Phillippe Pinel earned fame for his modern, open-door treatment of the mentally ill. He was able to prove that the insane were sick and not immoral or possessed of devils. He insisted that these persons suffered from sick minds in the same way that other patients suffered from diseases in other parts of the body.

In England, William Tuke raised money to establish a home in which mental patients would be treated as human beings. The home, which was called "The Retreat," provided good nursing care inexpensively. The philosophy of this home was to provide understanding, tender loving care, an atmosphere conducive to convalescence, and the motivation for the patient to again face life as a contributing citizen of the community. William Tuke was the beginning of a long line of Tuke gentlemen who concerned themselves with improving nursing care for the mentally ill.

Mother Mary Catherine McAuley of Ireland formed a group of women who visited and cared for the sick in Dublin. The nursing done by these women consisted of providing comfort and nutrition for the patient. In 1831 this group of women became the Sisters of Mercy and served along with Florence Nightingale in the nursing care of the soldiers during the Crimean War. Today the Sisters of Mercy are the second largest Roman Catholic order in the world and have hospitals all over the world.

In America, Dorothea Linde Dix exerted a strong influence on the improvement of nursing care. Her constructive work in surveying the needs of the mental patients and prisoners in Massachusetts led to the establishment of more than 30 psychiatric hospitals in the United States.

Most of the nurses in the eighteenth century gave good nursing care, were conscientious about their occupation, and helped their patients in every way they knew. Evidently much undeserved criticism was leveled at the nurses of this century because of the unsavory activities of a few. Two centuries later the same statement could be made about professional nurses and their critics.

At the end of the eighteenth century, nursing was changing even though many hospital administrators brought in untrained people and women of the street to do the nursing to reduce hospital expenses. Nursing service was recognized as important to the welfare of the patient, but it was not considered a respectable occupation for women in the middle class or the upper strata of society.

Influences on nursing service before Florence Nightingale's time

Much of the nursing reform pertaining to the care of the patient was carried over into the nineteenth century. One of the important developments in nursing that probably exerted a tremendous influence on the improvement of nursing service came from Kaiserswerth, Germany. Pastor Theo-

dore Fliedner (1800-1864) founded a hospital for the indigent and revived an early order of deaconesses to do the nursing. Fredericke Fliedner, the pastor's wife, was in sympathy with her husband's reforms. Both of them recognized the lack of facilities and good nursing for the sick.

Fredricke Fliedner became the superintendent of the order. The would-be nurses were given 1 to 3 years of theory and practice as a preliminary to becoming consecrated as deaconesses. The nursing care of patients was relatively simple when compared to the many complex nursing care procedures of today. The deaconesses' duties consisted primarily of bed making, bathing and dressing patients, serving food, feeding patients, and giving medications. The sisters were not allowed to enter the men's wards after 8 PM.

Nursing service had no distinctive part in the colonial development of the United States. Nursing of the sick was done by the women in the home. Colonial medicine was in the hands of any man who possessed an education. Measles, scarlet fever, smallpox, and diphtheria were often epidemic. The Catholic communities fared better than the Protestant groups, since many priests and nuns came to America with the French and Spanish settlers and supplied a minimum of nursing care to these communities.

Boards of health were unknown. Garbage was thrown in the streets. There were no city sewers, and city water supplies were drawn from dirty rivers or exposed wells. Rich and poor, educated and uneducated were alike in their filth and lack of cleanliness. There were no public baths as in the Roman days. Fleas, mice, rats, and lice were permanent inhabitants of all classes of society.

Hospitals were built in Latin America long before any public hospitals were established in the United States. In most of these hospitals the nursing service was conducted by one of the Catholic nursing orders of the period. The Ursuline Nuns, Augustinian Nuns, and Sisters of Charity are most often mentioned in the history of nursing service in the hospitals of North and South America.

In the early part of the eighteenth century the hospitals of the North American continent became so crowded and the beds in the wards were so close together that cleaning was impossible. The nursing procedures became even simpler than before. Bed baths were not attempted. Nursing in the secular hospitals was done by women too old or ugly to be prostitutes or too incompetent to be housemaids. When there was an insufficient number of nurses, the city authorities ordered the female prisoners to serve their sentences working on the wards of the municipal hospitals. The Sairey Gamp and Betsy Prig of Charles Dickens' *Martin Chuzzlewit* typified the general duty and private duty nurses of the period just before Florence Nightingale's time.

Charles Dickens and his pen were forceful weapons for reform. He was able to portray vividly the startling social evils of the early nineteenth century. He had social observational powers that enabled him to focus on the many ills of the times and stimulate the interest of his reader as well as give motivation to influential members of society to attempt to improve conditions.

The order of the St. Augustine nuns, devoted to nursing alone, preserved the few nursing methods that had been developed in the past 3 centuries.

The status of nursing service was at a low ebb. Educated women and those of the upper class disapproved of manual labor; they no longer considered it one of their social responsibilities to care for the sick and needy. In the home the actual care of the sick was still the responsibility of the mother. Tender loving care was given to friends as well as members of the family. Every bride received a cookbook containing a section on first aid and care of the sick. Most families kept sick members at home, and the family physician was held in high esteem. Respectable people considered it a disgrace to send one of their relatives to the hospital.

Nurses' wages were so low that only those who could get no other work resorted to nursing. There was practically no nursing from 8 PM until 6 AM except for a woman in childbirth or a dying patient.

Medicine had withdrawn from the monasteries and had become a part of the university community. Thus medical advance was assured, whereas nursing remained unchanged and was not yet respectable.

NURSING SERVICE IN THE FLORENCE NIGHTINGALE ERA

The service of nursing began its slow climb up the ladder of respectability when Florence Nightingale undertook the superintendency of the Sick Governesses' Home at 1 Upper Harlem Street in London. Here, Miss Nightingale insisted on fresh air for patients and raised the pay of the nurses. Still, most of the nursing was of a domestic type. Bathing the patients, scrubbing floors, and laundering were all part of the nurse's duties.

Miss Nightingale did expand the service of the institution to include the finding of convalescent homes or jobs for the governesses when they left the hospital.

A war proved to be the catalyst that enabled Florence Nightingale to pursue her interest in nursing. She had become associated with a committee to provide an ''establishment for gentlewomen during illness'' and was serving as superintendent of this nursing home at the time of the Crimean War. She had continued to maintain her interest in hospital reform and was regarded by many as an authority in this area. It is easy to see why her name was mentioned early in connection with reforms needed in the care of sick and wounded soldiers of the Crimean War. Newspaper reports of poor care of the wounded had aroused the interest and support of the British public. Included in these reports was a comparison of the adequate care given to the French soldiers by a religious nursing order and the lack of care of the British soldiers. The interest of the public was pointed toward the provision of more adequate nursing for the Crimean wounded.

Nursing service during the Crimean War

When the Crimean War (1854-1856) broke out, there were no nurses to care for the English soldiers. Through the recommendation of Sir Sydney Herbert, England's Secretary of War, Florence Nightingale was given the job of recruiting nurses.

Miss Nightingale organized a group of 38 nurses, attempting to choose those most adequately prepared in nursing. Members of several nursing orders were included in this group. The party sailed for Scutari in the Crimea in 1854. There were many problems to overcome before the nurses could provide the needed care measures. They were not accepted by the medical staff for many reasons. The arrival of the group of outsiders indicated that the care for which the medical personnel were responsible was inadequate. They were not accustomed to working with a nurse with training, and the idea of accepting female nurses in a military hospital was rejected completely. In addition to receiving opposition and hostility, Miss Nightingale found that resources for the care of the ill and wounded were practically nonexistent. In spite of the evidence of the need for her services, she decided to wait until the cooperation of the medical staff was evidenced by a request for the assistance of the nurses. A person less aware of the implications might have initiated actions that would have resulted in the failure of this mission. Her action was opposed by her own nurses.

Gradually she and her nurses won acceptance, and they could begin their work with the wounded. The results of this work are well known and proved the value of prepared individuals in the care of the ill. Perhaps less well known are Miss Nightingale's efforts in meeting needs of the soldier other than nursing care. She established reading and recreation rooms, implemented measures to care for the wives of soldiers who accompanied their husbands to Crimea, and wrote to the families of sick and dying soldiers. The efforts of this amazing woman completely changed the image of the nurse in the mind of the British public and paved the way for her later achievements.

Miss Nightingale spent nearly 2 years in the Crimea. She was exhausted and ill when she returned to England. Her illness and perhaps her awareness of the inability of a woman to participate directly in affairs of government or the community initiated her "retirement." She remained in this retirement for the remainder of her life. In light of the social standards of today it is difficult to understand Miss Nightingale's retreat from society. But, when standards of today are compared with those of mid-Victorian England, it is evident her actions were probably essential to the accomplishment of her goals. Her retirement removed the need to participate in superficial social activities, and she could devote her time and energies to other endeavors in a manner that would be acceptable to her society. This period of retirement was probably the most active and productive period of Miss Nightingale's life; her interest in nursing and nursing reform was not diminished.

Miss Nightingale had definite ideas of what nursing service was. In her *Notes on Nursing* she depicts nursing as signifying "the proper use of fresh air, light, warmth, cleanliness, quiet, and the proper selection and administration of diet—all at least expense to the patient."*

She argued that a nurse was not a housemaid and that laundering clothes, scouring, and scrubbing were a waste of nursing resources. She emphasized that good nursing was important to a swift recovery and that the nurse should pay attention to the idiosyncrasies of the patients. Further, she stressed how vital it was for the nurse to make sound observations, for the sake of saving life, increasing health, and bringing comfort to the patient.

She advocated nursing for the healthy as well as for the ill. But she did not want what she called the handicraft of nursing to be neglected. Turning the patient, keeping the patient dry, bathing the patient, and keeping clean sheets on the sick bed were all a part of her philosophy of what nursing should be.

When William Rathbone called on her to help

---

*Nightingale, F.: Notes on nursing, New York, 1946, Appleton-Century-Crofts, Inc., p. 8.

him establish a home nursing service in Liverpool, England, she was able to give him counsel and assistance. Rathbone's interest spread to the improvement of the workhouse infirmaries of Liverpool. Agnes Jones, a Nightingale graduate, became the superintendent of the program. *It was soon apparent to the founders of the program that the condition of the sick improved when educated nurses were there to care for the people.* Even more important to the public, the new program cost less than the system it replaced. Rathbone's work in Liverpool has often been called the beginning of modern visiting nursing.

In establishing nursing as a profession, Miss Nightingale opened up a whole new field of endeavor to women. More women became trained nurses. Miss Nightingale became an advisor on nursing service and hospital matters to the whole world.

Over the years little or nothing was known about nurses, other than Miss Nightingale, who served in the Crimean War. Jamaica's national heroine in that war was Mary Seacole, who died in London in 1881. Mrs. Seacole is honored by the Jamaican Nurses Association as one who with her own funds went to the Crimea to serve. Florence Nightingale kept her waiting 40 minutes, so Mary Seacole went about visiting the sick and wounded. Miss Nightingale rebuked her as one who was "interfering." A historian of the war wrote in 1902, "Even in an enlightened century Mother Seacole stands out preeminent, and cannot be passed over" (Briefing—one hundred years on, 1982).

Mary Seacole was of mixed heritage and suspected she was deprived of services because of color. However, because of her heritage she was able to "respond to the prejudice" and moved forward in her service to the sick.

Nursing service during the Civil War

The Sanitary Commission of the United States asked for Miss Nightingale's advice at the beginning of the Civil War because there were no organized nursing groups, no ambulances, and no field hospital service. Hundreds of devoted Catholic nursing sisters came to the battlefields to give nursing care, but there were not enough of them to care for the wounded and sick. Many lay men and women volunteered as nurses. The most famous of these are Clara Barton, Walt Whitman, Louisa May Alcott, Louise Schuyler, Mary Ann Bickerdyke, and Dorothea Linde Dix. All these people gave devoted service to the soldiers in time of need, but none of them had been educated as a nurse.

Dorothea Linde Dix was appointed Superintendent of the Female Nurses of the Army. Women from all parts of the country offered their services. The army nurses were required to be over 30 years of age, plain looking, and dressed in black or brown with no frills on the clothes. Louisa May Alcott described the job of the nurse during the Civil War in her *Hospital Sketches,* published in 1863:

Up at six, dress by gaslight, run through my ward and throw up the windows, though the men grumble and shiver. But the air is bad enough to breed a pestilence. . . . Til noon I trot, trot, trot giving out rations, cutting up food for helpless "boys," washing faces, teaching my attendants how beds are made or floors are swept, dressing wounds. . . . At twelve comes dinner for patients and afterwards letter writing for them or reading aloud. . . . Supper at five sets everyone running who can run . . . evening amusement . . . final doses for the night.

Probably the greatest nurse-heroine of the Civil War was Mary Ann Bickerdyke. She organized diet kitchens, laundries, and an ambulance service, supervised the nursing staff, and distributed supplies for the North. At night she often walked through the abandoned battlefields looking for survivors among the bodies.

Louise Schuyler's experience as a nurse in the Civil War probably stimulated her interest in Bellevue Hospital when she returned to New York. Miss Schuyler organized the New York Charities Aid Association. This organization made a study of conditions at Bellevue. The women found squalor, degradation, and almost complete lack of nursing for patients at Bellevue. Patients who were able to be ambulatory helped with the care and feeding of the more seriously ill people. Usually there was only one untrained attendant to a ward. This so-called nurse slept in an adjoining room at night. The beds in the ward were so close that it was impossible to care adequately for any patient. Stench, rodents, lice, and bugs of all kinds were everywhere. The public regarded the hospitals as "pest houses," and the prevalent public opinion was that "you only go to the hospital to die."

Miss Schuyler's committee recommended good standards of nursing education as one means of correcting the deplorable nursing service given to the sick in the hospitals. Bellevue Hospital has been used as an example of the conditions in nursing service after the Civil War. Almost all hospitals were in the same condition.

On the Confederate side, Miss Sally Tompkins gave nursing care to the soldiers during the Civil War. She had many dedicated women who worked with her. But despite all efforts of these self-sacrificing women and the religious sisters, many soldiers had inadequate care and many died from neglect rather than battle wounds.

Progress of nursing in the late nineteenth century

The women leaders of the late nineteenth century concentrated their efforts on the improvement of nursing care since there was medical opposition to women physicans. But nursing was regarded by most as an important responsibility of women. The goals of the women leaders were twofold: the improvement of nursing service and the widening of opportunities of women for respectable positions in the social order of the times. These women were influential in establishing many of the early schools of nursing in the United States and in other parts of the world.

Once the reform of nursing service was initiated, the expansion was explosive. Hospital authorities soon discovered not only that nursing students improved the nursing service to patients, but also that the cost to the hospital for the improved service was less. This led to exploitation of the student, who worked long hours and did hard physical labor in payment for the apprentice-type education received. Many hospitals had schools of nursing for the sole purpose of using the nursing service contributed by the students for the care of patients.

Primarily, the nursing service done in the late nineteenth century was of the housekeeping type. Scrubbing floors, laundering, and cooking were still part of nursing service. Students were sent to care for patients in their homes. The fees collected for this care went into the coffers of the hospital conducting the school of nursing.

America's first trained nurse

Linda Richards, a graduate of The New England Hospital for Women and Children in Boston, Massachusetts, in her book, *Reminiscences of America's First Trained Nurse*, points out that nurses were not allowed to take temperatures or pour medications. These procedures were done by the physicians. Nurses were allowed to carry the medication to the patient and administer it. They did not know what the medicine was, what it was supposed to do for the patient, or what side effects could be expected.

Each student was responsible for the six patients in the ward both day and night. The student nurses wore no uniforms, but the clothes they wore on duty had to be washable.

Public health nursing as a service

During the last 25 years of the nineteenth century, countries all over the world became aware of the need for improved care of the sick in both the hospital and the home. Another pioneer field of nursing service, which began in England in 1863 and in the United States 30 years later, was visiting nursing. Jane Addams at Hull House in Chicago and Lillian Wald with her friend Mary Brewster at the Henry Street Settlement in New York began what was the forerunner of the fast-growing public health nursing field of today.

For the first time since the Middle Ages, women of the better classes left their homes to care for the sick. The lives of these women were regulated by a mixture of the military rule and custom, inherited from the army, military nursing orders, and religious nursing groups of the past centuries. To paraphrase a statement of Rudyard Kipling, the nurse of the late nineteenth century was expected to do or die and not to reason why.

Even though nursing service at the end of the nineteenth century left much to be desired and the nurse did not even perform as many nursing tasks or have an education as good as the modern licensed practical nurse, forward strides had been made that benefited both the practicing nurse and the public.

Reforms in nursing

There were other reforms and discoveries that helped to change the service of nursing after the Civil War.

Clara Barton was finally able to persuade the United States to join the International Red Cross in 1882. She became the first president of the Red Cross Society in the United States. Nurses have been contributing their services to it since the time of the organization of the Red Cross Nursing Service by Jane Delano.

The Salvation Army, YMCA, YWCA, and medical missionaries in India, Africa, China, Japan, and other countries have helped to establish hospitals, schools of nursing, and dispensaries wherever there were people who needed the service. Nurses were a part of these reforms, and many of these leaders helped to establish such institutions in other lands.

Sir Wilfred Grenfell's work in Labrador is an excellent example of the courage and dedication of lay persons, physicians, and nurses in the development of hospitals and nursing service wherever people were in need of care.

In *My Cap and My Cape,* Mary Williams Brinton relates several incidents that give an inkling of the kinds of tasks performed by nurses in the missionary field:

During the years of my training, I never dreamed of meeting a situation like this. The operation took place in a cold corner room under the most extraordinary circumstances. It was the doctor's first experience on his own. I was a novice in giving ether, and we were so short-handed, in desperation the dentist was called upon to help. The patient half Indian and half white, was sure she was going to die, but seemed perfectly resigned to her fate, which made me even more squeamish. To make matters worse, as the surgeon worked it started to rain. The roof leaked and the water dripped so perilously near the patient we had to move the table to keep our field sterile. At the same time the native assistant turned green and had to be led from the room. Harrowing as it was, there was a sense of freedom which we all felt. No one to tell us what to do! We were on our own and it brought out the best in us. Whatever skill and initiative we had, counted. Even the saw from the kitchen proved remarkable for its purpose. . . . When the operation culminated successfully we felt strangely elated. The half-breed patient could not believe she could go home and everything was all right. . . . We gave her a routine sendoff with a pair of new crutches.*

Both medicine and nursing were influenced and stimulated by the revolutionary contributions to scientific knowledge by Louis Pasteur, Robert Koch, Lord Joseph Lister, Pierre and Marie Curie, and many others. The stethoscope, thermometer, microscope, and x-ray film all came into general use during the nineteenth century.

All these reforms, scientific discoveries, and public attitudes made it necessary to devise new techniques in the practice of nursing and the care of the patient. The demand for more and better-prepared nurses became apparent.

The attitude of the government toward nurses in the Spanish-American War (1898) gave support to the idea that adequate nursing care was a must for society. Dr. Anita Newcomb McGee was given the position of director of nurses for the duration of the war. Anna C. Maxwell, chief nurse at the camp hospital of Chickamauga Park, Georgia, provided outstanding service during the war but had many

---

*Brinton, M.W.: My cap and my cape, Philadelphia, 1950, Dorrance & Co., p. 81.

of the same obstacles and problems that had confronted Florence Nightingale at Scutari some 40 years earlier.

Even with government recognition of trained and partly trained nurses, there was no efficient system of recruitment or nursing care once the nurses went on duty. Typhoid fever, malaria, yellow fever, and dysentery threatened the troops in the camps. A total of nearly 1600 graduate nurses served in the Spanish-American War and invariably won the esteem and recognition of the soldiers. Conditions were such that the nurses could not give adequate nursing care or even maintain minimum standards of hygiene in the care of the sick.

At the close of the nineteenth century the nurse stood out as especially feminine and attractive. She was typically a bedside nurse. The skilled service she gave was new to the patients. Much appreciation, praise, and admiration were lavished on this "new nurse." Except for the hospital camps and battlefield stations during wartime, most of the service of nursing was given either in the hospital or in the home. The "trained nurse" brought dedication, a deep devotion, and unaffected enthusiasm to her chosen profession.

NURSING SERVICE IN THE TWENTIETH CENTURY

The rise in the standard of living; the identification of the causes of many diseases; phenomenal scientific and drug discoveries; progress in transportation, communications, and other technological areas; government legislation; public opinion; as well as the lengthening of the life span have influenced the change in nursing services to the patient.

The twentieth century has brought the change from the horse-and-buggy era to the space age. Any social influence that has played a part in the current history of society has also been instrumental in changing the pattern of nursing service.

In the first 35 years of the twentieth century, a world war, problems of social welfare, self-organization of nurses, government and nursing legislation, and the interest of national foundations in the health fields gave impetus to the expanding progress and improvement of nursing service. The complexities of medicine demanded changes in nursing. By the early 1960s the whole concept of nursing had to be reevaluated and changed.

Nursing service during World War I

War began in Europe in 1914, but the United States did not declare war until April 1917. At that time there were about 400 army nurses. The Surgeon General appointed Jane A. Delano (1862-1919) as superintendent of the Army Nurse Corps, and she also became chairman of the Red Cross Nursing Service. Because of her position with the army, the Red Cross, and nursing, she was able to supply about 20,000 nurses for duty with the Army and Navy during World War I. The nurses were assigned to camps, base hospitals, evacuation and mobile hospitals, and hospital trains. Some of the nurses served with surgical teams close to the front lines.

Both the Red Cross and the nursing leaders held the view that nursing no longer consisted of routine care, comfort, and custards; it required a scientific background and skills unknown in any preceding war.

During World War I and until 1947, the relationship between the American Red Cross and professional nursing had no counterpart in any other part of the world. Miss Delano, through her efforts as chairman of the Red Cross Nursing Service, had given a status to nursing in the United States that was not accorded to professional nursing in any other Red Cross society in the world. In addition to providing nurses for disaster and for teaching home nursing and other courses, the Red Cross provided reserve nurses for the armed services.

In the camp hospitals and camp units the nurses worked under the most primitive conditions, but through their own ingenuity they maintained the principles of safe nursing. The care of patients suffering from inhalation of poison gas was a challenge to the nurse's powers of observation and technical skills. Shock, hemorrhage, and infection were not new to the nurse of World War I, since patients with these conditions had been cared for in the homes and hopsitals of the nurse's own community.

The influenza epidemic of 1918 taxed the imagination and abilities of both physicians and nurses. Many nurses and physicians succumbed to the disease, as did over one-half million people in the United States. Both civilian and military personnel suffered a high morbidity and mortality rate.

Probably the nurse-heroine of World War I was English-born Edith Cavell. She was director of a school of nursing in Brussels, Belgium, when the war began in July of 1914. She was offered safe conduct to England, but she chose to remain in Brussels and continue her work at the hospital and school of nursing.

When Brussels was captured by the Germans in August 1914, Miss Cavell began making plans to oppose the enemy:

The German commander in charge of Brussels issued a directive that discharged male patients over eighteen years of age were to report at once to the German military police, which usually meant they would be sent to forced labor camps in Germany. To thwart this plan, Edith Cavell arranged that when a young man was discharged, either she or the nurse in charge would direct him to the police or to the home of Mme. X, leaving the choice to the patient. If he chose to go to the home of Mme. X, she should hide him until some way was found to spirit him out of the city. By late winter of 1914, wounded French and British soldiers were being cared for in the hospital and were helped to escape from there. Soon allied soldiers in disguise began coming to the hospital and were helped to escape. Miss Cavell helped to organize an underground system whereby, when it was time for the soldiers to leave, guides would take them away in late afternoon or at night in groups of four or five, disguised as laborers and carrying forged identification papers. Since the German guards at the border could not speak French, those crossing the border were seldom questioned.*

*Dietz, L.D.: History and modern nursing, Philadelphia, 1963, F.A. Davis Co., p. 147.

Eventually the Germans became suspicious and imprisoned Miss Cavell, who made no effort to defend herself. She was court-martialed on October 5, 1915, and faced a German firing squad at 7 AM 5 days later.

The execution of a woman and a nurse stirred deep feeling throughout the troubled world. Miss Cavell's memory was honored in an impressive ceremony at Westminister Abbey. Her body was finally returned to England in 1919 and buried near the cathedral at Norwich, England.

One of the impressive sights in London is the Edith Cavell Memorial in Trafalgar Square. Her stately figure sculptured by Sir George Frampton, R.S., is a part of the memorial. The artist seems to have caught her dedication, calmness, poise, dignity, and sereneness. Yet there is an aloofness and ethereal quality about the figure that call to mind her last remark before facing the German firing squad on that October 10: ''I now know that patriotism is not enough; I must have no hatred and no bitterness toward anyone.''* Students may learn more about Edith Cavell in *A Whisper of Eternity* by A.A. Hoehling.

The nursing profession emerged from World War I with a deep sense of pride in its accomplishments, having gained increased prestige in the eyes of the public. The nurses themselves were eager for a more liberal and independent status for nurses and women in general.

The public became increasingly aware of the need for the expansion of public health programs, child welfare, school nursing, and industrial or occupational nursing. Private duty nursing became less popular, and more nurses were working in the hospitals.

Problems of social welfare

Before World War I the United States was a rural society, and suddenly after the armistice it became an urban society. Smaller houses were being built

*Cited in Judson, H.: Edith Cavell, New York, 1941, The Macmillan Co., p. 281.

and fewer servants employed. Advances in medicine were rapid, and more hospitals were constructed. Public health nursing continued to make progress, and much of the nursing service given by the visiting nurse or public health nurse was preventive in nature. The fact that the nurse came to the home, gave the necessary care, and then went on to her next patient was one more step in the rise of nursing service to a more acceptable status than ever before.

In 1902 Lillian Wald suggested that nurses be used to supplement the work of physicians in the school systems. Linda Rogers from the Henry Street Settlement was the first nurse to do school nursing in the United States. A few years before, Amy Hughes began doing school nursing in London, England.

Both cancer and tuberculosis nursing became a part of the nursing service given by nurses in the early 1900s.

The first White House Conference on Children and Youth was held in 1909. As a result of this conference, Congress established the United States Children's Bureau. Since the first White House Conference, maternal and child nursing has been a concern of the Children's Bureau and the nursing profession.

One of the notable figures who exemplifies nursing in the early 1900s is Mary Breckenridge, who established the Frontier Nursing Service in the isolated mountains of Kentucky. Miss Breckenridge's nurses were educated as midwives as well as nurses. Until the advent of the ''Nurses on Horseback,'' both nursing and midwifery had been practiced under medieval conditions by ''granny women.''

The first health center set up by Miss Breckenridge and her nurses was in Hyden, Kentucky. The nurse-midwives traveled on horseback to visit their patients and served a population of about 800 people. Today these nurses use jeeps to reach their patients.

Occupational health nursing was given a boost during World War I when various governmental agencies encouraged the hiring of nurses to cut down on absenteeism. Large companies realized the importance of first aid on the job. As this field of nursing service developed, the safety and health of the worker became a part of the nursing service performed in industries.

Self-organization of nursing

In the first third of the twentieth century, nurses began to think of organizing nursing nationally to secure legal standards of education and practice to protect those needing nursing service and those giving the care. National nursing organizations were formed; practice acts and nurse registration were advocated. The nurses realized that in unity there was strength. Group consciousness, which was prevalent in all of society, had permeated the professional boundaries of nursing. See Chapter 13 for information on professional organizations.

Nursing registries were organized by private concerns, schools of nursing, and alumnae groups. These registries helped nurses to be placed on ''cases.'' To a small extent the registries helped nurses to establish in the mind of the public the difference between a graduate nurse and the vast number of untrained or semitrained women who called themselves nurses.

In the first 35 years of nursing organization there was considerably more talk than action in attempting to improve the working conditions, hours, and pay of the graduate nurse.

Private duty nurses worked long hours at very little pay. In 1926, 80% of the nurses worked a 12-hour day, 18% worked a 24-hour day, and 2% had a different schedule. The nurse earned 49 cents an hour. Charwomen were making 50 cents an hour and had more regular employment.

Nursing care in the first third of the twentieth century was done on a one-to-one basis, regardless of whether the nurse worked in a hospital, in a public health agency, in industry, in school, or in the home as a private duty nurse. Such nursing was wasteful and expensive. Few graduate nurses were employed by hospitals since most of the nursing care in hospitals was done by nursing students. The nursing staff was called on to scrub floors, carry trays, clean equipment, repair supplies, and do numerous other nonnursing tasks.

In 1909 there were 4359 hospitals and 1100 schools of nursing in the United States alone; thus in slightly more than one out of every four hospitals the nursing care of patients was carried on almost entirely by student nurses.

Routine care of patients and the strict adherence to the steps in a technical procedure kept these students so busy that there was little time for them to make a constructive contribution to the recovery of the sick or the peace of mind of either patient or family.

During this period in history a report of the Committee on the Grading of Nursing Schools, another report on costs of medical care, and the White House Conference of 1930 provided an extraordinary amount of factual material and recommendations for nurses, planning agencies, and professional organizations.

Eight foundations contributed about $1 million toward the work of the committee studying costs of medical care. Facts made available through these funds were used effectively by the U.S. government to make medical and nursing care available to all people of the United States of America.

The recommendations for nursing that were made by this study committee include the following:

1. Nursing education should be restructured to provide well-educated and well-qualified registered nurses.
2. Education should provide for the preparation of nurse aides, attendants, and midwives.

The depression of the late 1920s and early 1930s had a tremendous effect on nursing service and the employment of nurses. The distribution of nurses was uneven; many nurses in certain areas were without jobs, whereas in other areas there were not enough nurses to care for the people.

Nursing service from 1935 to the 1960s

With the growing advances and complexities of medicine, army physicians were demanding nurses who could administer the new drugs as well as teach patients and families about health routines. Social legislation of the late 1930s effected a sharp turn away from rugged individualism, which had been a national characteristic throughout the first part of the twentieth century. Hospitals were becoming more popular as aseptic technique made them safer. Many of the procedures being done for the sick could be carried out more efficiently in the hospital. Hospitalization insurance and prepayment plans for hospital care became popular. By 1940 about 4.5 million persons were enrolled in some form of health insurance program. By 1937 there were 28,000 graduate nurses doing staff duty in hospitals—seven times as many as 10 years before.

World War II brought the usual exaggerated demand for nurses, and the need to augment the peacetime supply of nurses and other health workers for both civilian and military needs became apparent to nursing leaders and government officials.

Federal legislation developed for nursing in connection with the Social Security Act and in the Nurse Training Acts beginning in 1956 left its imprint on the nursing services of the middle twentieth century.

Change in the function of the nurse

By 1940 the introduction of new drugs and techniques called for radical changes in nursing care. These included sulfa drugs, penicillin, potency liver extract, identification of vitamins, cyclopropane, barbiturates for intravenous use, Wangensteen suction, and other methods of applying the principles of suction and siphonage to the care of surgical and cord-injury patients.

The nurse of the 1940s did blood pressure measurement; aided in transfusions; applied suction to surgical wounds, tracheostomas, and chest cavities; assisted the surgeon in the operating room;

helped in the delivery of babies; and worked in outpatient departments of hospitals. Esther Lucile Brown in her book, *Nursing for the Future,* reported that in an on-the-spot check in a large teaching hospital she found some 100 procedures that were more or less technical in nature. These were exclusive of the operating, obstetrical, and outpatient services. As she points out by quoting Dennison,

[Nurses] managed the apparatus for Wangensteen suction, tidal irrigation, and bladder decompression. They irrigated eyes, cecostomies, colostomies, and draining wounds. They did artificial respiration, applied sterile compresses, and painted lesions. . . . They did catheterizations, sitz baths, and turpentine stupes. They gave insulin and taught the patient or his relatives to give the drug and examine urine. They administered approximately 1500 medications daily, by mouth or hypodermic. They assisted with lumbar punctures, thoracenteses . . . and phlebotomies.*

By this time the nurse was performing many of the duties reserved for physicians in the nineteenth century, and many new services and procedures had been added.

Social legislation

Probably one of the best examples of social legislation is the Social Security Act of 1935, which has been amended many times. The act provided for expanded health programs, which were to be administered by the United States Public Health Service and the Children's Bureau. The evolutionary process within the whole field of nursing service was expedited by the Social Security Act, but probably public health nursing was affected the most.

By 1950 practically all nurses, including self-employed private duty nurses, became eligible for "old-age security." In 1939 the National Health

---

*Dennison, C.: Nursing service in the emergency room, Am. J. Nurs. **42**:777, July 1942.

Conference proposed to Congress a national health program that included the following points:
1. Expansion of public health and maternal and child welfare services
2. Expansion of hospital facilities
3. General program of medical care
4. Medical care for the medically needy
5. Insurance against loss of wages during illness

During the late 1950s and early 1960s Medicare was a controversial subject among professional people and lawmakers. Medicare was opposed by the American Medical Association. This group proposed a plan of Eldercare as a substitute for Medicare. The American Nurses' Association favored a health plan through Social Security as early as 1958.

The general plan of Medicare was to provide limited inpatient and outpatient hospital services and limited nursing home and home health services to all persons 65 years of age or older, regardless of their financial status. Medicare has been financed by increases in the Social Security tax rate and an increase in the taxable Social Security wage base. Medicare was passed by the Senate and the House of Representatives in 1965 and signed by President Lyndon B. Johnson in July 1965.

Medicare is a health insurance for people 65 years and older and some people under age 65 who are disabled. It is a federal program run by the Social Security Administration. Medicare has two parts: medical and hospital insurance. Services paid for by Medicare (the insured person also must pay a designated portion) may be provided by physicians, nurses, physical therapists, and chiropractors. The agencies that provide this care must meet certain licensing requirements. Hospitals, skilled nursing facilities, and home health agencies are eligible to participate in the Medicare program.

The Hill-Burton Act of 1946 (Hospital Survey and Construction) made millions of dollars available for construction of hospitals and health centers under prescribed conditions. The emphasis was on needs of rural areas. Many hospitals and nursing homes were built with the assistance of these funds. More hospitals and nursing homes increased the demand for nurses and nursing service.

Many more social legislation reforms have affected the patterns of nursing care and the demand for nurses. President Johnson's ''War on Poverty'' and his ''Great Society'' legislation left their mark on nursing, much as did the Social Security Act with all its ramifications.

Legislation regarding rehabilitation, assistance to the aging, child abuse care, alcohol and drug abuse, and emphasis on cancer increased the demand for nurses and nursing care.

Nursing during World War II

As World War II spread, the United States started a general registration of all men eligible for military service. Military personnel increased, which brought about a demand for more nurses in the armed services.

The Nursing Council on National Defense changed its name to the National Nursing Council for War Service and pledged itself to meet military nursing needs, to assign nurses widely and economically, to supplement civilian services with subsidiary aid, and to provide for future nursing needs.

One of the measures taken to fulfill this pledge was a bill (the Bolton Bill) to create a Cadet Nurse Corps. The bill was passed by Congress in July 1942. The purpose of the bill was to provide additional nurses for the armed services. Lucille Petry was the chief nurse and director of the Cadet Nurse Program. The greatest single contribution of this program was the assistance it gave to nursing schools in securing students, which prevented a disastrous collapse of nursing service on the home front.

Both the Red Cross and the council were active in providing practical nurses, nurse aides, and orderlies on the home front. Many hospitals organized schools of practical nursing to relieve the registered nurse of many of the more simple and practical tasks that could be done by a well-trained practical nurse. The tasks that did not require the skill and knowledge of registered nurses were taught to the practical nurses. The practical nurses gave bedside care to the patients; thus registered nurses were released to do the more complex tasks and to give medications and treatments.

On the war front, nurses from all countries of the world worked together in front-line aid stations, field hospitals, army and navy base hospitals, hospital ships and trains and in the air, caring for the wounded and ill soldiers. Some 75,000 served in World War II and were assigned to 52 areas throughout the world. All through the war, the work of the nurses received special attention.

There were 1619 nurses decorated with such medals as the Army Commendation Ribbon, the Bronze Star, the Air Medal, the Distinguished Service Medal, the Silver Star, and the Distinguished Flying Cross.

Probably the newest nursing service of World War II was flight nursing. These nurses were especially trained to give nursing care to the wounded who were on stretchers piled three tiers high on either side of the airplane. The airplane was a cargo plane converted into a rough ambulance. This was the most dangerous duty assignment given to nurses. Of the 173,527 sick, injured, and wounded soldiers evacuated by air in 1943, only 11 died in flight.

Other nurses on Corregidor and Guam and in the Philippines and Europe gave equally heroic service. They often gave nursing care or helped with emergencies and operations while bombs were dropping on the area. Eighty-three American women became prisoners when Corregidor fell. Of the 83, 63 were army nurses and 17 were navy nurses. They were prisoners for 2½ years.

In April 1983, 32 of these nurses were honored in Washington, D.C.; 60 of the 83 could be located for the occasion hosted by the U.S. Veterans Administration.

Generals and medical officers gave high praise to the nurses of both the army and the navy for their untiring service and for their professional skill as well as their ability to keep up the morale of the wounded to whom they gave nursing care. The nurses proved themselves the equals of men under combat conditions.

Since World War II, nurses have served in the Korean conflict and the Vietnamese action. The heroines of these three war actions are many, and no one nurse can be singled out as the most outstanding figure of the times. The reader who is interested in knowing more about nursing during World War II and nursing as it is carried on in the armed services today needs only to turn to recruitment brochures of the army, navy, and air force.

In 1947 female nurses in the armed services were given permanent commissions. Male nurses were commissioned in 1955. Nurse corps became responsible for their own recruitment and established their own reserves in 1947. Legislation of the 1970s has made it possible for nurses in the armed service to attain the rank of general.

Nursing service—twentieth century style

The social significance of nursing becomes more and more apparent as one begins to think about what nursing is today.

Patient care today is far removed from the Nightingale style practiced over 100 years ago. Nurses today are expected to perform many tasks that were originally done by physicians. They supervise professional and nonprofessional workers as well as provide care utilizing high technology for the planning and implementing of nursing care that would have baffled Florence Nightingale.

Nursing in the 1960s became patient centered not procedure or test centered. Johnson, a sociologist, described the style of nursing service as having two components: expressive and instrumental functions. Of the two functions of the nurse, this sociologist considered the expressive the most important. She described this function by saying: "Her kindness, her willingness to listen and understand, her comforting care . . . as an expressive specialist she is doing something the doctor cannot do as well as she, and is making a unique and important contribution to the doctor-nurse-patient social system."*

In the estimation of the sociologist, the instrumental function of the nurse included all the physical care, medications, and treatments given to the patient by the nurse in attempting to assist the patient in getting well. Being expressive was the nurse's specialized function as a professional person. If nurses were to become associates of the physician rather then semiskilled assistants, it was seen to be in the capacity of an expressive specialist rather than technical expert.

Jahoda, a psychologist, described the modern nurse as one who was under emotional strain, social pressures, legal responsibility, and self-discipline. The activities of the hospital nurse ranged from taking care of equipment through basic nursing of patients to highly skilled technical tasks such as artificial feeding and included a fair amount of administrative work. At the lower level of skill the nurse's job overlapped with that of domestic staff and at the higher level with that of the physician. This overlap was inevitable and accounted to a great extent for the status stresses in hospitals. Nursing defined its status on an in-between level. This problem was further complicated by the peculiar position of those patients whose illness deprives them of the normal duties and privileges of an adult and makes them dependent on the professional nursing staff.

Jahoda summarized the problem:

As the nursing profession is constituted today, you are facing grave problems in both services to the patients and to self-protection. The problems may yield only to radical thought and radical action. This challenge, I am sure, will not discourage you. For to search for the best balance between these twin tasks of professional organization and to adjust it to the ever-changing needs of the community is in keeping not only with the great ideals

---

*Reprinted, with permission, from Johnson, M.M., and Martin, H.W.: A sociological analysis of the nurse role, Am. J. Nurs. **58**:374, March 1958.

of nursing it is also the most human and most humane goal any profession can embrace.*

In the 1960s social problems became more numerous, and there was a dearth of well-prepared personnel. Many times the nurse was forced to assume the role of the missing specialist. The growth of cities, growth of population, changes in the structure of the population's age groups, and nature of human beings all have had an impact on the pattern of nursing care and will have for the rest of the twentieth century. The importance of care of the total patient became more and more recognized as nurses and the public became more skilled in effective interpersonal relations.

Another drastic change in nursing service occurred in ambulatory care. Nurses provided direct care for individual patients and their families. In this role the nurse took medical histories, performed physical assessments, and did developmental examinations, counseling, and health teaching. In these roles nurses were considered important members of the primary health team. They rendered much of the primary care, freeing the physician to concentrate on the aspects of patient care only physicians were qualified to deliver. These nurses worked in neighborhood health clinics, health maintenance organizations, outpatient clinics, walk-in and street clinics, physician's offices, industrial plants, nursing homes, and rural areas. Sometimes physicians were in the immediate area, but often nurses worked independently through protocols and consultation with physicians, either by radio or telephone. Nurses who gave health care as primary health care nurses could specialize in any one of the specialty nursing areas or have a generalized practice.

The nurses added to their traditional role that of personal and familial confidante, spiritual advisor, and general counselor—and as a result, the profession grew in stature.

Quality care became a concern for nursing in the

1970s. Nursing care was fragmented—patients received care from a variety of prepared workers and no one individual seemed to be responsible for the whole. Nursing services were still responsible for the care, cure, and coordinating functions; however, patient satisfaction with care diminished.

The public became more vocal regarding their care and the cost of that care, which had become economically catastrophic. The U.S. Congress legislated in 1976 a physicians' peer review system that was to respond to quality care. As an outgrowth of the physicians' peer review, nursing audits occurred. Nurses audited nursing notes to determine what kind of nursing care was received.

As a result of nursing audits, problem-oriented charting was introduced. The use of problem-oriented charting compelled the nurse to identify the nursing problem and to prescribe the nursing care to be given. The care given was documented and the outcome recorded. Outcome became more important than simply giving the care.

The demand for quality care prompted the evaluation of the methods of giving care and personnel use. Since the 1940s team nursing had represented the functional style of nursing, and care provided was fragmented. Registered nurses were seldom taking direct care of patients. Lesser prepared nurses were often the ones giving direct care. As quality care diminished and the concept of holistic nursing gained momentum, a different approach to nursing had to take place. Primary nursing was introduced.

Primary nursing fostered the philosophy that one registered nurse assigned to a small group of patients for the length of stay was more beneficial. This nurse was responsible for the patient care for 24 hours. Although not always physically present, this nurse developed and altered the nursing care plan. Patients responded favorably to this care. Primary nursing allows the nurse to utilize and synthesize all the cognitive, psychomotor, and affective skills needed to assess the patient's status and prescribe nursing care.

In the 1970s most nurses were employed in hospitals. Illness orientation was still of the utmost

---

*Reprinted, with permission, from Jahoda, M.: Nursing as a profession, Am. J. Nurs. **61**:54, July 1961.

concern in the early part of the decade. Catastrophic illness demanded different kinds of nursing; more hospital patients received care for acute conditions than in earlier decades.

Late in the 1970s, ''nurse burnout'' was evidenced. Nurses were no longer complacent about the demands on their time and efforts in behalf of patients. Nurses became assertive in voicing concerns about staffing patterns, double shifts, and working in special areas where their knowledge base was limited. Nurses looked to unions to solve their problems when the issues could not be resolved. As a result, nurses were organized through local units of the state professional organization to speak to issues surrounding personnel benefits and, more important, quality care. Nurses began leaving the profession, taking less demanding positions in society and speaking out in disenchantment with the profession.

At the close of the 1970s nurses were finding themselves in conflict with (1) demands from physicians to take on tasks once done only by physicians, (2) the need for quality care in catastrophic illnesses, and (3) the expanded role expectations of the profession of nursing.

New definitions for medical and nursing care that differentiated the two types of care were developed by professional nurses. Medical care was defined as the care of the ill, and nursing care was seen as encompassing care of the well and rehabilitation of the ill person to wellness.

Nurses were impelled to become research workers and seekers of a better and more efficient way of caring for patients. They were expected to think scientifically and logically. In many medical centers nurses and physicians were attempting to emphasize their similar goals instead of their differences; in this way each would gain respect for the contribution of the other, and the patient would benefit.

Nursing service in the 1980s

Several major concerns surfaced in the early 1980s that had an impact on nurses, physicians, health care workers, the consumers of nursing,

health care, and health care facilities. The economic recession of the United States, the extreme shortage of registered nurses, the oversupply of physicians, and the high cost of health care all became apparent with great force in 1980.

The United States experienced a recession that affected millions of people. Industries laid off workers by the thousands, and companies experienced decreased sales of their products. Inflation increased rapidly. The cost of health care rose rapidly and at a greater rate than general consumer costs. The need to cut drastically the cost of health care became apparent by the mid-1980s.

In addressing the shortage of nurses, two major studies were undertaken. The first study was chartered by the American Hospital Association. A commission was appointed to determine if the shortage of nursing was real or perceived. At the same time the U.S. Congress mandated that the Institute of Medicine study the issues of nursing to determine if federal support was still necessary. The two studies occurred simultaneously and were completed in early 1983. Congress received the Institute of Medicine study, and the American Hospital Association received this national commission's study with recommendations.

Was there a real shortage? Yes, in some areas of the United States there was a shortage of nurses who had specific skills and advanced degrees. Both studies revealed that the image of the nurse and the profession was poor, nurses were overburdened with functions that rightfully belonged to other workers, the technology of illness care was such that only registered nurses could be utilized, and research and graduate education in nursing were critical and still needed federal financial support.

Ironically, as the two studies were completed the shortage seemed to disappear. So was there a shortage? Yes. The shortage disappeared because nurse turnover lessened, and nurses who did not need to work returned to work because their husbands were laid off. For the first time in the spring of 1983, newly graduated registered nurses experienced difficulty in securing positions. Practical nurse graduates experienced even more difficulty because nursing management in evaluating staffing patterns had determined it was more cost efficient to utilize a predominantly registered nurse staff.

Another factor influencing the decline of the shortage was that health care benefits were no longer available to laid-off workers. The public simply could not afford health care and therefore did not utilize the facilities. Health care was simply a luxury. Hospital beds became open and unused. Nurses were not needed.

Beatrice Kalisch, a distinguished professor of nursing, and Phillip Kalisch, a historian, undertook the challenge of studying the image of nursing from the Nightingale era up to the 1980s. They utilized novels, movies, radio, and television to examine how nurses were portrayed. An excellent report of the Kalisch studies can be found in several issues of *The American Journal of Nursing* during 1982. The Kalisches reported that nurses were portrayed from very wholesome girls to sexpots. Nurses appeared both as very dumb and as bright, sensitive individuals. Always the nurse appeared as a servant to and taking orders from the physician. Rarely was the nurse seen as an independent practitioner delivering primary care.

The Kalisches (1983) reported that nurses in the 1980s are portrayed in a derogatory light. Further, their premise is that such an image affects (1) the public's opinion of nurses and nursing; (2) the quality and number of persons choosing nursing; (3) the policy makers who make decisions on how to allocate scarce resources; (4) the public, who are deprived of vital knowledge about the service nurses perform; and finally, (5) nurses themselves, who undermine their own image, beliefs, and values.

Nurses throughout the country have been exposed to the Kalisches' research and conclusions. A major concern for the 1980s becomes one of selling nurses as primary care givers in the health care system. It means nurses and the profession need to be more vocal in their demands for portrayal as independent practitioners and givers of primary care.

According to Brooks and Kleine-Kracht (1983), the public is more concerned with personal qualities of nurses rather than their abilities and skills. From their point of view, the definitions of nursing ''show a 'tunneling' of nursing into a highly technical profession with minimal involvement in the human societal issues.''

The National Commission on Nursing (1983) proposed 18 recommendations. Recommendations centered around relationships (1) among nurses, patients, physicians, health care administrators, and trustees; (2) between health care institutions; and (3) between nurses and the nursing profession.

Nursing education was also examined. It was recognized that the transition of nursing education into higher education to meet the increased sophistication of complex, technological patient care was necessary. Recommendations in the area of education included the recognition of nurses in practice, educational mobility, and the need for state and regional planning for types of educational programs needed to meet the needs of individual states.

The Institute of Medicine study revealed much the same thing as did the National Commission on Nursing study. The results of this study are to be used by Congress in determining how to finance nursing and nursing education. One result of the Institute of Medicine study included research in nursing as an absolute. To this end Congress received legislation in late summer of 1983 to form a Center for Nursing Research as a part of the National Institutes of Mental Health.

What will become of these studies? Palmer (1983), in an address given to deans from colleges of nursing said, ''Nursing has never had a 'fixed resolve' as to the purpose or direction pursued.'' Many studies have been made on nursing and nursing education with minimum action plans to promote the findings. The divisiveness that has existed in nursing for the past 20 years has not healed. The vested interests of each specialty group and types of educational programs create many proponents and opponents within the profession. This divisiveness gives the public an unclear picture of what the profession of nursing is all about. If Palmer is correct, one can assume the two previously discussed studies will be read and placed on the shelves of many persons with few trying to implement the findings.

An interesting note of historical significance is that in 1981 the Institute of Medicine announced that by 1985 there would be an oversupply of physicians. Too many medical schools existed, and the number of graduates would exceed the needs. What did this mean for nursing? Physicians became more protective of their turf; nurses who were in independent practice were investigated to determine if they were practicing medicine. The skills taught to nurses by physicians were challenged by medical boards. Where once physical assessment was cheered by physicians as a task that could be assigned to nurses and one that nurses were willing to accept, suddenly in 1983 nurses were expected to desist from this activity.

The high cost of health care became a critical issue for the United States. Physicians, nurses, and health care workers became aware that the economic recession was going to change the delivery of health care.

From 1965 to 1983, consumer costs tripled while costs of health care had risen seven times. In 1981, 287 billion dollars was spent on health care. Medicare, Medicaid, and third-payer parties controlled the cost. Payment for care was based on retrospective payments. Late in the 1970s, hospital administrators began promoting shorter hospital stays as one way to decrease health care costs.

Discharge planning began on admission in an effort to maximize the care in the shortest period of time. Studies showed, for example, that the average patient with gallbladder surgery recovered in "x" number of days; therefore every effort was made to make certain discharge occurred within that established time. If it did not, one had to answer as to why not. With early discharge, patients' recovery period was at home rather than the hospital. Early discharge decreased hospital care costs;

however, costs were then incurred for the patient through intermediary care facilities or home care.

Another effort to cut costs was to provide 1-day surgery, and by 1983 a new type of health care facility was available to patients. Freestanding surgicenters, medicenters, and emergicenters were opened. All were "for profit" organizations providing care outside the traditional hospital. These centers were easily accessible to the public. Nursing care was needed in the home and in the new centers. Changes in the need for nursing care became more evident.

With the Reagan administration came a new mandate. Health care costs for the federal government would be reduced. The spending for Medicare and Medicaid would decrease. New Jersey had been exploring and utilizing a prospective plan of pay rather than a retrospective one. This was based on diagnostic related groups. Congress introduced this concept into legislation early in 1982. By September 1982 legislation was passed known as The Tax Equity and Fiscal Responsibility Act (TEFRA). Included was the diagnostic related grouping (DRG). Prospective payment became law and was to be fully implemented in a 3-year period.

In New Jersey, directors of nursing found the system could work but only if nursing did not do the work of housekeeping, maintenance, and others. They also found that the registered nurse was the most valuable worker. Nurse aides (assistants) had too much "downtime." Therefore staffing patterns were adjusted to provide a greater number of registered nurses to nonprofessionals. Registered nurses who were not used to doing direct patient care were thrust into doing "tasks" commonly performed by aides. Primary care given by registered nurses became the conceptual model of care. Fagin (1982) states that "studies have proved that quality and quantity of care is improved with primary nursing."

Nursing in the late 1980s will include a greater use of computers. Computers will be utilized in planning care, providing both medical and nursing diagnoses, preparing for the admission of the patient, evaluating care, and patient and staff education. Technology will not be limited to monitors and equipment for patient care; it will be utilized in providing service not even imagined today. It is because of technology that registered nurses will have to make a more conscious effort to return to the bedside. Comfort, physical, and psychosocial measures cannot be offered through technology; nursing's nurturing measures will become even more important.

Nursing service in the community, home health services, and centers for nursing will need to become more aware of patients who are discharged early. Planning of care for the early discharged patient needs to be done to assure a return to health.

Family health nursing, a young specialty, will become more in demand. Leone in 1962 predicted that in the 1980s hospitals will be acute care centers with families responsible for the care of early discharged patients. She was right on target. The family health nurse helps families to anticipate the noramal and predictable situations. This specialist provides knowledge about healthy behaviors that will allow a quality of life to be maintained. The hospital nurse will be a highly skilled specialist in illness-oriented care.

SUMMARY

The evolution of nursing service has been extremely uneven in the world, probably because of the basic differences in the cultures of East and West. Nursing itself is as old as the human race. There has always been someone to take care of the ill. Both men and women have always cared for patients. The men became involved primarily because they participated in wars. During the day they fought in battle; during the night they cared for the wounded. In India, nursing was usually done by men.

Nursing, like the practice of medicine, was based on superstition. Comfort measures have always been a part of nurse ministrations.

Hippocrates taught his students the value of treating the whole patient, and today nurses believe in treating the whole patient.

St. Vincent de Paul stimulated the social obligation of the people to improve nursing care. The Augustinian Sisters were the first purely nursing order of the Hotel Dieu in France. They preserved the known nursing measures during the "dark period of nursing."

Nursing underwent many changes and a stressful period during the Reformation. Men were removed from nursing. Hospitals were for the poor. Influential people were indifferent to the kind of care given.

The reforms of nursing began in the eighteenth century and were carried over into the nineteenth century. Nursing services continued to be poor. Medicine was advancing, but nursing was still not a respectable vocation.

During the twentieth century many sociological forces have had an impact on nursing services. Two world wars drew many nurses to the war front to care for the wounded. Permanent commissions in the armed services were given to female nurses in 1947 and to male nurses in 1955. Military nursing played an important part in nurses' gaining recognized status.

The women's liberation movement influenced the status of nursing, as did the proposed Equal Rights Amendment. More men than in the past are now choosing nursing as a career.

The advent of new drugs and continued research have placed new responsibilities on nurses. They must have a knowledge of what the drug is, know what effects should take place, and be alert for side effects, if any. Nurses must be more aware of the technological advances taking place and their impact on nursing care as an adjunct to serving patients, families, and the community.

The economic recession, the shortage of nurses, the oversupply of physicians, and the high cost of health care have had an impact on nursing in the 1980s.

Prospective payment of hospital care provided an impetus to make changes in staffing patterns. Practical nurses and nurse aides were limited, with registered nurses returning to the bedside to do direct care. Primary care was reemphasized.

Nurses are accountable to their patients for the quality of health care they give. New roles in independent practice, rural health care, home care, free clinics, walk-in clinics, drug maintenance programs, rehabilitation, and health maintenance all broaden the nurse's opportunities and scope of responsibility.

Discussion questions

1. Do you believe the profession of nursing would have been altered if Nightingale and the monastic system had not prevailed in the nineteenth and early twentieth centuries?
2. Why has not nursing, as a profession, enjoyed an independence and an image to support what the early leaders of nursing envisioned?
3. Will the nursing profession become unified and respected as givers of primary care?
4. Who are the leaders of nursing in the 1980s and for what do they stand?
5. What impact have TEFRA and DRGs had on the delivery of health care?

REFERENCES

Briefing—one hundred years on . . . Nurs. Times **78**(19):781-782, 1982.

Brooks, J.A., and Kleine-Kracht, A.E.: Evolution of a definition of nursing, Adv. Nurs. Sci. **5**(4):51, 1983.

Bullough, V.L., and Bullough, B.: The emergence of modern nursing, ed. 2, New York, 1969, The Macmillan Co.

Dietz, L.D., and Lehorzky, A.: History and modern nursing, ed. 2, Philadelphia, 1967, F.A. Davis Co.

Dolan, J.: History of nursing, ed. 12, Philadelphia, 1968, W.B. Saunders Co.

Dooley, A.: Promises to keep, New York, 1962, Farrar, Straus & Co.

Dygert, R.E.: Tanganyika, National Geographic, pp. 321-323, Sept. 1964.

Fagin, C.M.: The economic value of nursing research, Am. J. Nurs. **82**(12):1844, 1982.

Frank, Sister C.M.: Foundations of nursing, ed. 2, Philadelphia, 1959, W.B. Saunders Co.

Giles, D.: A candle in her hand, New York, 1949, G.P. Putnam's sons.

Jamieson, E., Sewall, M.F., and Gjerston, L.: Trends in nursing history, ed. 6, Philadelphia, 1965, W.B. Saunders Co.

Kalisch, B.J., and Kalisch, P.A.: Improving the image of nursing, Am. J. Nurs. **83**:48, Jan. 1983.

Leone, L.P.: The challenge of the 80s: the pursuit of excellence in nursing, Boulder, Colo., 1962, WCHEN.

Lum, J.L.J.: Computers in nursing, J. Nurs. Adm. **8**:4-26, Feb. 1978.

Lum, J.L.J.: Labor relations, J. Nurs. Adm. **7**:4-24, July-Aug. 1977.

Lum, J.L.J.: WICHE panel of expert consultants report: implications for nursing leaders, J. Nurs. Adm. **9**:11-19, July 1979.

Mengers, G.: How's the Health Service Corps doing . . . in Appalachia, RN **35**:46-49, Sept. 1972.

Mulleris, A.C., Colavecchio, R.E., and Tescher, B.E.: Peer review: a model for professional accountability, J. Nurs. Adm. **9**:25-30, Dec. 1979.

National Commission on Nursing: Summary report and recommendations, July 1983, American Hospital Association, The Hospital Research and Educational Trust, and American Hospital Supply Corporation, Chicago.

Nightingale, F.: Notes on nursing (first republished edition), Chicago, 1974, Replica Rara Limited, P.O. Box 6626 AMF, O'Hare, Chicago, Ill. 60666.

Norby, R.B., Freund, L.E., and Wagner, B.: A nurse staffing system based upon assignment difficulty, J. Nurs. Adm. **7**:2-24, Nov. 1977.

The nurse, M.D. **8**:149, June 1964.

Nursing at the crossroads (nine articles), Nurs. Outlook **20**:1, Jan. 1972.

Palmer, I.S.: Through a glass darkly—from Nightingale to now, A.A.C.N. Publications Series 83, no. 2, p. 11, 1983.

Richards, L.: Reminiscences of America's first trained nurse, Boston, 1913, Whitcomb & Barrows.

Roberts, M.: American nursing history and interpretation, New York, 1961, The Macmillan Co.

Saint Jerome Letters, Nicene and post Nicene, father of the Christian Church, New York, 1893, The Christian literature Co.

Walsh, J.J.: The history of nursing, New York, 1929, P.J. Kennedy & Sons.

Yost, E.: American women of nursing, ed. 2, Philadelphia, 1965, J.B. Lippincott Co.

SUGGESTED READINGS

Bishop, W.J.: Florence Nightingale's message for today, Nurs. Outlook **5**:246, May 1960.

Brinton, M.W.: My cap and my cape, Philadelphia, 1950, Dorrance & Co.

Brown, E.L.: Nursing for the future, New York, 1948, Russell Sage Foundation.

Dodge, B.S.: The story of nursing (rev. ed.), Boston, 1965, Little, Brown & Co.

Edmunds, L.: Computer-assisted nursing care, Am. J. Nurs. **82**:1076, July 1982.

Fagin, C.M.: The economic value of nursing research, Am. J. Nurs. **82**:1844, Dec. 1982.

Gebbie, K., and Lavin, M.A.: Classifying nursing diagnosis, Am. J. Nurs. **74**:250-253, Feb. 1974.

Judson, H.: Edith Cavell, New York, 1941, The Macmillan Co.

Kalisch, B.J., and Kalisch, P.A.: Improving the image of nursing, Am. J. Nurs. **83:**48, Jan. 1983.

Kalisch, P.A., and Kalisch, B.J.: The image of the nurse in motion pictures, Am. J. Nurs. **82:**605, April 1982.

Kalisch, P.A., and Kalisch, B.J.: Nurses on prime-time television, Am. J. Nurs. **82:**264, Feb. 1982.

Lavin, M.A.: Cross-cultural identification and utilization of nursing approaches applicable to the delivery of health care, Int. Nurs. Rev. **20**(3):73, 1973.

Murata, J.E.: The nurse as family practitioner, Am. J. Nurs. **74:**254-257, Feb. 1974.

Palmer, I.S.: Nightingale revisited, Nurs. Outlook **31:**229, July-Aug. 1983.

Robinson, A.M.: The nurse-practitioner—expanding your limits, RN, Nov. 1973.

Styles, M.M.: On nursing: toward a new endowment, St. Louis, 1982, The C.V. Mosby Co.

CHAPTER 2
Changing patterns of nursing

". . . future (of nursing) rests with the young people who will be educated as nurses and with visionary teachers whose concepts of nursing encompass the fulfillment of the most demanding and, at the same time, most rewarding of all services—that of giving knowledgeable, humane, and comprehensive care to promote, sustain, and restore optimal health for all human beings."*

OBJECTIVE: On completion of this chapter, the student of nursing will have had the opportunity to review and consider the changes in delivery of nursing care and their implications for the future.

In the past 150 years, nursing has changed extremely slowly in respect to specific activities. However, nursing has remained constant in its nurturing of well-being to the client/patient. In this chapter the changing pattern of nursing will be discussed. It will be noted that registered professional nurses yielded many basic functions to others and now are returning to them as the practice of nursing comes more clearly into focus.

No longer do nurses scrub floors, do laundry, cook meals, or do other domestic tasks considered part of their function 100 years ago. During the past 30 years, within the hospital, the nurse has been part of a medical team, and nursing activities have been closely related to those of other health personnel. The registered professional nurse assumed responsibility for the supervision of the

practical nurse, the nurse aide, and the orderly. The registered professional nurse also assumed responsibility for the coordination of all the treatments or procedures ordered for patients by the physicians.

This left the registered professional nurse a supervisory role, giving little or no direct care to patients in a hospital setting. The registered nurse retained the administration of medication and performance of technically complex procedures. It was often said that the registered nurse "nursed the desk" rather than "nursed patients." Thus one definition of nursing evolving during the 1960s was that of care, cure, and coordination.

Two factors influenced the change in the nurse's role during the last 30 years. First, nurses saw themselves as exploited and "handservants of the doctors" and, second, as nurses became more educated in the physical and social sciences, it could be seen that nursing and medicine were two distinct entities, each a profession in its own right. Medicine was the profession of curing illness, and nurs-

*Reproduced with permission from Schlotfeldt, R.: The nursing profession: vision of the future. In Chaska, N.: The nursing profession: views through the mist, New York, 1978, McGraw-Hill Book Co., p. 404.

ing was one of restoring the patient to a state of wellness and preventing illness.

Nurses were once all things to all services. Ingeborg Mauksch once said that nursing was the dough left after cutting out cookies from an oblong cookie sheet. For example, one could clearly define the role of the physician, dietician, physical therapist, laundress, and housekeeper, but what was nursing and, most particularly, registered professional nursing?

With this background and the change occurring in health care it became important for nursing in the 1970s to define more clearly the role of the registered professional nurse and to determine the relationship to the various other disciplines in health care. As seen in Chapter 4, nursing theorists began to respond and unify what nursing is about.

Nursing was then defined as an interaction between the nurse and the individual in which a therapeutic relationship was used to assist the individual in establishing and maintaining optimal health. Nursing was a service to people that utilized the principles of physical, social, and behavioral sciences in determining which nursing measure was best for the individual, family, and/or community. Nursing was the giving of physical, spiritual, emotional, and transcultural care in a variety of settings.

It was further determined that the delivery of health care must be altered if the philosophy of restoration to optimum health was to prevail. With this philosophy, contemporary nursing took on new dimensions. Nurses were challenged to assist in altering the health care system to one that provided health care to all who live in America regardless of financial status. The challenge included (1) a change of practice settings, (2) a change from dependent to independent practice, (3) accepting the computer systems approach to the delivery of health care, (4) identifying the role of the various individuals in nursing and allied health sciences, (5) the economics of health care, (6) quality assurance care, and (7) providing a maximum number of nursing personnel in an equitable distribution throughout the country.

NURSING IN A VARIETY OF SETTINGS

Historically nursing care took place in the home, battlefield, and, later, the hospital. Community health nursing is the oldest form of providing nursing care. Women took care of their families within the home; when the mother was ill, the neighbor provided that care. Midwives were accepted health care providers. Soldiers took care of each other in the battlefield. They fought during the day and cared for the injured at night. Hospitals became the setting for care when techniques of medicine became more complex.

Home care

Nursing in the home was complex but simple. Nurses made do with what was available. Nurses did the housekeeping chores along with nurturing the ill member of the family. In nurturing, the nurse provided physical care and emotional support and sought the best-known nursing measures to ease discomfort. It was these measures which were a mixture of physicians' orders and intuition that became the nurse's domain of practice.

The provision of nursing care in the home has increased substantially in the 1980s. With shorter hospital stays, 1-day surgery, and more outpatient services in health maintenance organizations, nursing care in the home has become a necessity. Home nursing care is being provided by family members under the direction of visiting nurses.

Visiting nurses are employed by incorporated visiting nurse services, health maintenance organizations, hospitals, and professional nurse pools. Cost for the services is per visit and the amount of care given. A case load of patients provides the professional nurse the opportunity to give primary care.

The nurse in this setting brings to the home any equipment needed to provide the care required. Rental agencies for medical-nursing supplies are available to families so that patient care can be more easily provided.

Visiting Nurse services provide care by registered professional nurses, licensed practical nurses, and nurse aides. The registered nurse makes an assessment of needs. From the needs assessment, the nurse determines which of the providers of nursing will give the care. Often it becomes a step-down process, with the acuteness of the condition determining what type of nurse is needed. Home care may or may not be around the clock. It may be necessary for a nurse to be in the home only 1 or 2 hours a day or once or twice a week.

Visiting nurse services in the 1980s provide many of the same services as a hospital but at a substantially lower cost. For example, there are dieticians, physical therapist, home service aides, and social workers all available to care for specific needs that do not fall within nursing responsibility. However, it is the nurse who coordinates this care.

Nursing in the community

Public health nursing was fostered by Florence Nightingale. Although she worked diligently to foster good hospital nursing, it was she who was constantly on the alert to promote improved health practices in the community. *Notes on Nursing* shows that Nightingale, as a public health nurse, was an expert on sanitation, logistics, nutrition, and epidemiology. Nightingale said, "A District Nurse must first nurse. She must be of a yet higher class and of a yet fuller training than a hospital nurse because she has not a doctor at hand and because she has no hospital appliances at hand."

Public health or community health as a setting for the practice of nursing in the 1980s is quite different from the early days of Wald and Dock. Lillian Wald founded Henry Street Settlement on the lower east side of New York. She was from a wealthy family and well educated. She was introduced to Henry Street, center of a densely populated industrial population, while a student in nursing. She was appalled to see a family of seven and two boarders living in two small rooms. One of them was sick and lying in a bed soiled with hemorrhage of 2 days' duration. This was living proof to Wald of the acute need for home health teaching as well as changes in living conditions for the poor.

Lavinia Dock, a suffragette and activist for women's rights and nursing, spoke out for im-

proved nursing education and organized nursing to improve the welfare of the nurse and licensing laws. She fought for changes in local laws to assist the poor and to care for the ill.

Lavinia Dock and Jane Addams were close associates of Wald. Each influenced public health nursing. They demonstrated that poor health could be traced to impoverished living conditions, unhealthy working conditions, poor practices of sanitation, and impure water supplies. Nursing of the public then became more than care of the ill; it included the prevention of illness, an idea that originated from such places as Lillian Wald's Henry Street Settlement in New York and Jane Addams' Hull House in Chicago.

Today public or community health comprises a myriad of health workers all working toward the prevention of illness. The nurse functions in clinics, doing health assessments, recognizing abnormal conditions and referring patients to the appropriate source for further diagnosis and treatment, and doing health teaching to prevent illness. The nurse is vigilant for the outbreak of communicable diseases, environmental conditions that foster disease, and cultural diversities that foster poor health practices.

Community health nursing includes the school nurse, who is able to assess the health of children. The community health nursing role has changed in that the nurse is not a sanitation expert nor an epidemiologist but must have a background of environmental and biological resources with which to deal with the problems of increased drug abuse, human (spouse or child) abuse, venereal disease, the increase of once dormant tuberculosis, and polio. The vigilance of the community health nurse in case finding, screening data, and being attuned to the community and its environment has changed the pattern of community health nursing.

Community health nursing's major focus is the preventive arm of nursing practice. These nurses must be knowledgeable in all facets of nursing, including scientific principles, to make conclusions and decisions that may affect not just one individual but members of an entire family and community.

With increased emphasis on wellness, physical fitness by the public, and the unemployed not seeking illness care in the 1980s, the need for public health nursing became acute. Public health nurses are in the position to know the state of wellness within the community. They know and collect the demographics that identify the changing patterns of health care.

The economic recession provides an example of changing patterns of health care. Many affluent families became families unable to cope with the loss of money to purchase food or health care. The public health nurse became the primary care giver. With an increased demand for public health nursing, ironically, the recession hit health departments.

Health departments suffered drastically with the economic recession. Budgets were slashed, employees who resigned were not replaced, and services were diminished. Where once health departments provided cost-free service, a fee for service became a necessity.

A major concern for the late 1980s will be the state of health of all individuals. With health care benefits unavailable or changing drastically, will the United States be a healthy nation? Public health departments will have to address this situation and to make recommendations as to how to deal with millions of people who do not have food, shelter, or work in order to sustain life. Public health nurses will be seeking new avenues in meeting the challenge before them.

A vested interest in community health nursing has become a national and international affair. In the United States the U.S. Public Health Service governs health practice throughout the nation and serves with the World Health Organization to govern practices of preventive health throughout the world. Each state has a health department responsible for the specific needs of that state. There are county health and often city health departments. Nurses and nursing practice are a vital part of all agencies serving to protect the community from disease.

Hospital nursing

Hospital nursing practice in the 1980s is very different from that in the 1960s. The late 1940s saw a dramatic change in hospitals and the giving of care. Physicians played the dominant role in serving the sick. Nursing in the hospital of the 1940s was predominantly done by students with one or two registered nurses to function as supervisors and head nurses. This continued until the end of World War II, when nursing education became an issue of importance. As students became less available to staff hospitals, an acute shortage of registered nurses occurred. Many registered nurses were in private duty or military service. Thus the practical nurse or nurse aide was introduced as a substitute for the student of nursing in giving direct care.

The registered nurse did not participate in staff nursing until team nursing was introduced in the 1950s. Team nursing was introduced as a means of coordinating the efforts of registered nurses, practical nurses, and nurse aides. Since few registered nurses were available, it was believed that this approach would provide better care to the hospitalized patient. Registered nurses served as the team leaders.

Team nursing was to take the place of the functional method of giving care. In the functional method one nurse was assigned treatments, one gave medications, another administered intravenous therapy, and one did physical care. The purpose behind team nursing was to provide a combination of nursing personnel for a group of patients. The acuteness of the condition determined which of the members of the team gave the care. The team had a conference to plan for the 8 hours of care and a final conference to discuss care given and outcomes. In principle the concept was good. In reality nursing care often was fragmented and appeared to be like the functional method. This was due in part to the number and preparation of the team members in relation to the acuteness of patient care.

As medical technology advances, so did nursing

practice. As new treatments for illness were discovered, as drugs became available to treat illness, and as physicians became more involved in specialty practices, the registered professional nurse's role began to change from nurturing to highly technical tasks. The care of patients became more complex. The early days of nursing saw private duty nurses employed by the family to care for patients who were acutely ill.

Private duty care was an accepted practice of nursing until the late 1950s, when intensive care units and cardiovascular units were introduced to the hospital setting. The private duty nurse was responsible for the care of one patient for an 8- to 10-hour period. This nurse was responsible for implementing the physician's orders, maintaining the environment, and acting as confidant to the patient and family. This nurse often established a relationship with a family, caring for members of that family whenever illness occurred and nursing was needed.

Private duty nursing is all but extinct today. With intensive care units introduced in the 1950s and the technology for treating illness increasing throughout the 1960s and 1970s, the private duty approach to care has become a lost art. The "nurturing" aspect of nursing care became lost to make way for technology.

Depending on the hospital, the nurse's role in the early 1980s is different from the role in the 1960s. Hospitals vary from small local ones serving communities for simple illness, emergencies, and normal maternity needs, to larger regional medical centers that, with access to highly technical research, provide more dramatic approaches to locating major illnesses and caring for high-risk mothers and infants. The practice of nursing in each of these settings is different. In one setting the nurse will do many diverse tasks, including admission of patients, emergency care, delivery of babies, and care of the medical patient. In a medical center the nurse functions in a single unit, becoming highly skilled in one kind of nursing.

The modern hospital offers many different kinds of opportunities in nursing. The critical care unit of a hospital needs a nurse who thrives on crisis situations, can work effectively under stress, and is not rendered insensitive by caring for a continuing succession of seriously ill patients. The nurse in the critical care unit must be highly skilled in making accurate observations of the patient's condition and interpreting them correctly in terms of the needs of the patient.

The intermediate care unit of the modern hospital needs a nurse who is skilled and interested in health teaching; this nurse's daily schedule should allow plenty of time for this important function. There are fewer patients in this unit who require highly technical procedures, and crisis situations are at a minimum. Many patients in an intermediate care unit soon become ambulatory and are able to do many of the activities of daily living with little assistance from the nursing personnel.

On the self-care unit the nurse has a minimum of technical procedures to perform, but skills in human relations are used to the maximum in counseling, teaching, and providing emotional support. These nurses need a knowledge of good public health practices and of the community health resources.

The long-term care unit offers a slower pace, since it takes time to help patients help themselves. The nurse in this unit must not become discouraged by the patients' slow progress. The nurse must emphasize each patient's total needs and must know nursing in its broadest aspects.

The general hospital is a focal point for community health, and the progressive patient care concept, which has been adopted in whole or in part by almost every general hospital in the United States, envisions the general hospital of the future as a community health center—the focus for both outpatient and inpatient care. The hospital is concerned with care for long-term patients, including those with mental illness, as well as for short-term patients. It is also concerned with extending good medical and nursing care to the home by assisting in the care at home.

Nurse practitioners and physicians' assistants

In the 1960s an acute shortage of physicians occurred especially in rural and ghetto settings. Pediatricians were in extremely short supply. Dr. Henry Silver, a pediatrician, and Dr. Loretta Ford, a public health nurse of the University of Colorado, collaborated on the idea that if nurses had increased skills in assessing the difference between normal and abnormal and could improve their interviewing skills and become more acutely aware of health teaching, the care of the child in rural settings would be improved. This idea set the stage for the advent of pediatric nurse practitioners. This development became the impetus for the "practitioner" movement as a way of increasing health care to areas where physicians were in short supply.

Simultaneously at Duke University, a physician's assistant program was being developed. The physician's assistant was not a nurse but would receive a special education in health assessment and simple medical tasks. Meanwhile, in the state of Washington, a program was developed to give veterans who had been medical corpsmen added skills and to allow them to function as physician's assistants.

Physicians' assistants were educated and ultimately licensed to practice under the supervision of a physician. The American Medical Association (AMA) saw this as an answer to the shortage of physicians, as were the practical nurse and nurse aide in the delivery of nursing care.

In the early 1970s the AMA made a strong suggestion that all registered nurses be physicians' assistants. The American Nurses' Association responded quickly that nurses were giving nursing care, not medical care. The dilemma was paramount in identity of each profession.

The role of the nurse was clearly changing. The nurturing apect was being eroded with highly technical tasks to be performed. Nurses were beginning to take seriously the "role of the practitioner." Some authorities were calling the role one of expansion; others were saying it was a matter of

nurses finally fulfilling their role in a scientific manner.

Concerns in the 1980s

Defining nursing in the 1980s is not easy. Nursing combines the nurturing aspect of care with highly technical skills. The emerging definition encompasses the strong motivation for holistic care. Holism, a philosophy of man which becomes metaphysical in nature makes "man to be greater than the sum of all of his parts." To foster this philosophy, nursing then must include more than the performance of technical skills. Nursing theorists, as seen in Chapter 4, have done much to place the definition of nursing in perspective.

Nursing is the care and nurturing of the physical, social, spiritual, cultural, and emotional well-being of an individual, family, and community. The practice of nursing takes place in a variety of settings and in a number of ways. The nurse may be in an organized setting such as a hospital or functioning in a space shuttle or laboratory, as an employee or as an independent practitioner.

In the hospital, registered nurses are moving from the team-leading concept to primary care. This is described more fully in Chapter 7. The registered nurse is also in practice as an independent practitioner. The practitioner makes assessments and determines the best approach to care for the client. The practitioner is responsible for the physical setting in which the practice will take place. An office is rented or owned, and provisions are made for secretarial and bookkeeping services and supplies, or the practitioner will work in collaboration with a physician with a similar specialty.

Automation has changed the patterns of patient care. Space engineers and physicians have blended their talents and imagination in the development of all types of monitoring devices and other inventions that have affected patient care. Research on an international scale has led to many other developments. Electronic computers and ultrasonics aid the physician in making a diagnosis. Fetal and maternal cardiograms as well as fetal phonocardiography aid the obstretician.

Some devices are designed to be labor-saving tools for nurses. Electronic drug dispensers and automated infusion monitors are examples. In the future it is possible that equipment will become smaller and lighter. Recording data about patients, determining charges to patients, and processing physicians' orders are being done in many agencies. It becomes increasingly apparent that computers are destined to play a definite role in nursing service and in the care of patients.

It is necessary for nurses to understand these machines, their nature, and their function. At the present time various monitoring machines are used in surgery departments and intensive care units of some hospitals to keep a constant check on the patient's vital signs. To avoid the depersonalization effect of the automation that is a part of nursing care in hospitals, the patient needs the expressive function of psychological support, listening, understanding, and comforting care.

Jacobs and Huether (1978) believe that "today's nursing bears the burden of its heritage—diversity, fragmentation, and amorphous accompanied confusion and antiintellectualism." They further say that the "evolution of nursing science will assure the survival of nursing."*

With the evolution of a science of nursing, patterns of nursing are changing through quality assurance programs. Quality assurance measures structure, process, and outcomes of nursing either concurrently or retrospectively. Recommendations for changes in practice become the course of action required by nurses. Smeltzer defines quality assurance as "assuring the patient of a specified degree of excellence of nursing care through continuously, objectively measuring the structural process and outcome components of nursing against criteria of nursing standards."†

One approach to increase clinical nursing as a pattern of care is through the concept of the clinical ladder. Presently many nurses move from direct patient care to management of patient care by being head nurses, supervisors, directors, or administrators of service. This mode was utilized for advancement and more money. This left a dearth of well-prepared practitioners doing clinical nursing. Nurses who become experts in specific kinds of nursing care either by advanced degrees, certificate programs, or on-the-job training were limited as to advanced recognition and recommendation.

The clinical ladder concept provides an approach for nurses with clinical competence to be recognized and rewarded. It provides the opportunity for the nurse to remain at the bedside and give direct patient care. Research by the clinical nurse whose main goal is to find ways to improve the quality of care becomes a permanent part of the practice. As new standards of care are recommended, they can be tried and tested until the standard is perfected and adopted by the newest of nurses.

Family health nursing is the newest of clinical specialties. Family nurse practitioners have been on the scene for 15 years. This specialist focused on family illness. However, focus on healthy behaviors has only been introduced since 1978. Nurses such as Patterson, Zuard, and Newman began focusing on family health and identifying concepts dealing with healthy behaviors.

The faculty of The University of Akron College of Nursing in 1975 determined that family health nursing would be the focus of their graduate program. In 1980 it was accredited by the National League for Nursing. This program differs from other family practitioner programs, and thus a new specialist is being prepared. The graduate of the program is prepared with new knowledge of health, not illness. Health assessment skills along with family health theory become the cognitive skills learned. This nurse becomes skilled in assisting families and individuals within families to anticipate changes in life and to maintain healthy behaviors rather than changing from health to illness.

---

*Jacobs, M.F., and Huether, S.: Nursing science: the theory-practice linkage, Adv. Nurs. Sci. **1**(1):65, 73, Oct. 1978.
†Smeltzer, C.H.: Organizing the search of excellence, Nurs. Mgmnt. **14**:19, June 1983.

Holistic health nursing becomes more realistic with this mode of care.

The family health nurse chooses one of three leadership roles (i.e., direct care, administration, or education) with which to utilize the knowledge of family health nursing. As a primary (direct) care giver, the family health nurse evaluates the health of a family and individual through health appraisal, anticipatory dynamics, stress management, health learning, and self-care.*

The administratior or educator uses the concepts of family health nursing in studying and promoting the theories of administration or education.

THE CHALLENGE OF CHANGE

Florence Nightingale in her *Notes on Nursing* suggested the very essence of what nursing must do today—continue to progress and keep alert to the changing social structure so that nursing can meet the challenge of the twentieth century:

No system can endure that does not march. Are we walking to the future or to the past? Are we progressing or are we stereotyping? We remember that we have scarcely crossed the threshold of uncivilized civilization in nursing; there is still so much to do. Don't let us stereotype mediocrity. We are still on the threshold of nursing.

In the future, which I shall not see, for I am old, may a better way be opened! May the methods by which every infant, every human being will have the best chance of health, the methods by which every sick person will have the best chance of recovery, be learned and practiced! Hospitals are only an intermediate state of civilization never intended, at all events, to take in the whole sick population.

Miss Nightingale's challenge, written more than 100 years ago, is still as great a challenge to nurses today. Nursing care has improved, but what nurses and their nursing organizations can do in the future through education, creativity, imagination, research, and cooperation with the other health dis-

ciplines and allied professions could soar beyond our wildest imaginations.

No student could read these pages without realizing that nursing still has many unsolved problems and that the profession is changing constantly. Much of what will happen to nursing depends on nurses themselves—their courage and their fortitude. What the future of nursing service will be rests with the nurses who give that service. Nurses must meet this challenge and decide for themselves the road that is best for nursing and, most important, the method that will give the patient the best possible care.

Discussion questions

1. Discuss the major forces in the late 1980s that will affect the patterns of nursing care.
2. Discuss the difference between a primary care giver and primary nursing care.
3. Discuss the need for a two-track system for nurses to be rewarded in recognition and remuneration (i.e., clinical ladder and administration).

REFERENCES

Balint, J., et al.: Job opportunities for masters prepared nurses, Nurs. Outlook **31**(2):109, 1983.

Dirschel, K.M.: Changing a student health service to primary nursing, Nurs. Health Care **4**(5):252, 1983.

Eschback, D.: Role exchange: an exciting experiment, Nurs. Outlook **31**(3):164.

Jacobs, M.F., and Huether, S.: Nursing science: the theory-practice linkage, Adv. Nurs. Sci. **1**:65, Oct. 1978.

Prescott, P.A., and Langford, T.L.: Supplemental agency nurses and hospital staff nurses: what are the differences? Nurs. Health Care **2**(4):200, 1981.

Sultz, H.A., et al.: A decade of changes for nurse practitioners, Nurs. Outlook **31**(3):137, 1983.

Wieczorek, R.R., et al.: A clinical career pathway: the Mount Sinai experience, pt. 2, Nurs. Health Care **4**(6):318, 1983.

SUGGESTED READINGS

Abalos, D.T.: Strategies of transformation in the health delivery system, Nurs. Forum **17**(3):284, 1978.

Abdellah, F.G., and Levini, E.: Better patient care through nursing research, ed. 2, New York, 1979, The Macmillan Co.

Abu-Saad, H.: Nursing: a world view, St. Louis, 1979, The C.V. Mosby Co.

---

*University of Akron College of Nursing Family Health Nursing Program. Copyright 1981.

Alexander, E.L.: Nursing administration in the hospital health practice with a systems approach, St. Louis, 1975, The C.V. Mosby Co.

Arndt, C., and Huckabay, L.: Nursing administration theory for practice with a systems approach, St. Louis, 1975, The C.V. Mosby Co.

Barrett, E.R.: Florence Nightingale: her wit and wisdom, Mount Vernon, N.Y., 1975, Peter Pauper Press.

Blake, P.: The clinical specialist as nurse consultant, J. Nurs. Adm. 10:33, Dec. 1977.

Brownlee, A.T.: Community, culture, and care, a cross-cultural guide for health workers, St. Louis, 1978, The C.V. Mosby Co.

Elms, R.R., and Moorehead, J.M.: Will the "real" nurse please stand up: the stereotype vs. the reality, Nurs. Forum 16(2):112, 1977.

Farlee, C.: The computer as a focus of organizational change in the hospital, J. Nurs. Adm. 2:20, 1978.

Fitzsimons, V.M., and Gallagher, L.P.: Physical assessment skills: a historical perspective, Nurs. Forum 17(4):344, 1978.

Ingles, T.: The physician's view of the evolving nursing profession, 1873-1913, Nurs. Forum 15(2):123, 1976.

Kinlein, M.L.: Independent nursing practice with clients, Philadelphia, 1977, J.B. Lippincott Co.

Marram, G.D.: The group approach in nursing practice, ed. 2., St. Louis, 1978, The C.V. Mosby Co.

Richard, E.C., and Miedema, L.: The nurse practioner in the nursing home, J. Nurs. Adm. 3:11, 1977.

Riley, M., and Moses, Jr., J.A.: Coordinated care: making it a reality, J. Nurs. Adm. 4:21, 1977.

Zahourek, R., Leone, D.M., and Lange, F.J.: Creative health services: a model for group nursing practice, St. Louis, 1976, The C.V. Mosby Co.

CHAPTER 3
Evolution of nursing—education

OBJECTIVE: On completion of this chapter, the student of nursing will have an appreciation for the history of nursing education, issues in changing the system of education, and the evolution that is occurring.

NURSING EDUCATION BEFORE THE NIGHTINGALE ERA

The historical development of nursing education cannot be separated from nursing as a service, nor from the development of education as a way of life for the people of America. In the evolution of nursing as a service, it was demonstrated that as the technical advances occurred in the world, the need to know more about the body and mind created a need for formal education.

Persons giving nursing care were ill prepared; they had the motivation to serve but lacked knowledge for the reasons for their actions. The ministrations were usually simple therapeutic measures such as the use of poultices, herbs, and basic hygiene measures. The members of nursing orders were guided by definite regulations and a code of ethics, but the desire to serve was believed adequate to prepare one for the care of the ill and injured. A formal education program to prepare nurses was not needed and would not have been acceptable in the light of the standards of society of that time.

In addition, the lack of medical, technical, and scientific progress must also be considered when one is looking for the reasons for the late development of nursing education. Only as humans began to unlock the doors to the intricacies of their environment was there a need to know what caused disease and how to care for people who were ill.

Social reform led the way for the educated person. Although a larger segment of the population was educated, this education was limited to men of wealth who were philosophers, clergy, and physicians. Women were not encouraged to seek formal education. Those women who were educated had much to do with fostering preparation of nurses.

It was social reforms of the nineteenth century that led to the expressed need for preparing nurses. Technical and political developments had changed the European countries from rural to urban societies. The basic Christian philosophy fostered the concept of responsibility of the individual for the welfare of all society. Economic gains and technical progress encouraged travel and communication. Medical progress expanded. The development of the printing press made people aware of progress. Efforts toward social reform were initiated by many individuals. Evidence of these reforms is seen in the writings of Dickens and in the prison reform movement sponsored by Mrs. Elizabeth Frye. An interest in the preparation of nurses had been expressed by persons concerned with social reform. This interest was expressed in the formation of lay nursing orders of similar groups devoting their efforts to the care of the ill. The formation of the lay orders was a logical answer to the need produced by the loss of the Catholic nursing orders. Lay orders such as the Beguines in Belgium had also existed for some time. However, the need for formal preparation of the nurse practitioner had not been recognized.

The first educational program planned specifically to prepare a nurse practitioner was initiated by a Lutheran minister, Theodore Fliedner, with the assistance of his wife, Fredericke. Fliedner's interest in nursing originated from his efforts to seek solutions to the problems of the community to which he was assigned as a young minister. This community, Kaiserswerth, experienced the failure of its principal economic source shortly after Fliedner arrived to assume his duties. In the years that followed, the community evidenced many of the problems associated with economic deprivation. Reforms were needed in local government, education, and health care measures. Unable to cope with the community problems with existing resources, the young pastor traveled throughout Protestant Europe for several years seeking assistance, financial and other, for the problems of his community. These travels and his contacts with others involved in social reform enabled him to be one of the most adequately prepared persons to initiate a program for the preparation of a nurse. There is evidence of the incorporation of ideas and experiences of many in the organization of the school.

The hospital and school were established in 1836. Much of the credit for the success of this endeavor must be given to Mrs. Fliedner. She, too, had been interested in service to the poor and underprivileged before her marriage. Her ability in organization and teaching did much to make the idea of a training program for nurses a reality. She administered the hospital and school in addition to attending her family responsibilities until her death in 1842. She gave nearly all of the nursing instruction in addition to doing other tasks.

The training program had admission requirements. The applicant had to be female, at least 18 years of age, and able to certify good physical health and moral character by letters from a clergyman and a physician. A probationary period of 3 months was established. This period of probation was later replaced by required attendance to a preparatory school to enable the student to better qualify for training as a nurse.

Following the probationary period, the student began a 3-year course of instruction. Theoretical instruction was given by a physician, and Mrs. Fliedner instructed the students in the practical aspects of nursing. Classes in pharmacology were given, and the students were required to pass a state examination in this subject. The students were responsible for the care of patients during this course of study. Their assignments were rotated so that all students received similar experiences. Although many of the rotation assignments were based on tasks to be accomplished, such as laundry, housekeeping, and cooking, experience with various types of patients was also considered. Students were required to wear uniforms and received a small allowance. The services required by the patients were provided entirely by the student; therefore it can be assumed that the care of the ill was basic to the establishment of the training program. There was a strong religious service element in the training. Devotion to the care of the ill and poor was both a basic requirement for training and a guiding philosophy in practice by the deaconess. Instruction in ethics and religion was included in the course of study.

The organizational structure of the training program and practice of the deaconess of Kaiserswerth is an example of Mr. Fliedner's attempt to meld the strengths of old and new practices. This organizational structure was patterned after the deaconess structure associated with the Christian religion. Following the training period, the deaconess practiced her calling within the framework of the order. Vows were not required, and a deaconess could marry or retire; however, if active, she rendered her service through one of the established motherhouses. This practice was probably based on the fact that women still had limited social status. The women were still required to contribute within the framework of marriage or religion. Members of this order were provided with housing and maintenance but no salary. Practice in the order offered security but many restrictions. The actual practice of the deaconess was closely regulated by physicians' orders and the influence of the pastor in that community. There was still only limited evidence of the elements of professional practice as we know it today.

Many responsibilities, such as determining standards of practice, were assumed by members of the clergy or others not directly concerned with nursing practice. Later problems of the order can be traced to the lack of this element of professional nursing, but the establishment of this training initiated nursing education. From the efforts toward progress as well as the mistakes of individuals such as the Fliedners, the pattern of the present and future was shaped.

NURSING EDUCATION IN THE NIGHTINGALE ERA

The effect of the contribution of Florence Nightingale on nursing might be compared to the effects of the religious and political revolutions on the world. She questioned existing conditions and implemented changes that were revolutionary at that time. A comment from a London newspaper described the contributions:

The life and work of Florence Nightingale will remain forever a beacon of the profession of nursing. Miss Nightingale did not, as is sometimes said, create the nursing profession; that was done in large measure by the Christian Church. But she reformed it and remade it, giving it a new direction and a more lively inspiration. Her service, indeed, was personal, in that she brought her vivid and alert personality into wards and dressing stations where disorder and even despair prevailed, and by her personality—compounded of courage, discipline, and a valiant faith in and love of her fellows—exorcised the evil and established a new order of goodness and mercy. Her new order has endured because it was built on the sure foundations of knowledge and experience.*

---

*From the Florence Nightingale International Foundation, The Times (London), July 6, 1934.

In discussing the history of nursing service and nursing education separately, it is difficult to attribute the contributions of this extraordinary woman to one area of nursing more than another. Miss Nightingale expressed an interest in nursing early in her life. This interest was strongly opposed by her family, and when her background is compared with that of the individuals providing nursing care in Protestant countries, the basis for this opposition becomes evident.

Miss Nightingale was born in 1820. Her family had considerable wealth and social prestige. Her parents were well educated and able to provide the best available education for their children. Florence was an alert and intelligent girl, and with the assistance of her father, who instructed her in subjects such as mathematics, she received an even more extensive education than was common to women of her social status. She traveled extensively throughout Europe. The status of her family enabled her to make excellent social contacts that were later instrumental in the achievement of her goals in nursing.

Miss Nightingale's family continued to oppose her interest in nursing. In spite of this opposition, she was able to further her interest in many ways. She became friends with individuals concerned with the reform of social institutions such as prisons and hospitals. She also became acquainted with physicians directly involved with the exciting medical developments that were occurring at this time. These physicians were beginning ro recognize the need for a trained person in nursing and encouraged Florence in her interest. Her experience in caring for members of her family who were ill made her even more aware of the need for education in the preparation for nursing, and in 1851 she spent 3 months at the deaconess institution in Kaiserswerth. Her experience at Kaiserswerth again illustrates the benefit that can be derived from the progress and mistakes of others. When Miss Nightingale was finally able to sponsor her own school, many strengths based on her experiences at Kaiserswerth were incoprorated into the program.

In recognition of her work in Crimea, the British public established the Nightingale Fund in 1855 for the purpose of preparing better-qualified nurses. Some time elapsed before she could direct her activities toward a school of nursing. In 1860 St. Thomas Hospital in London was selected as the hospital for the training school. In this same year 15 students were admitted for training. Although Miss Nightingale did not participate directly in the instruction of the students, she determined the policies that so adequately guided the school and resulted in the establishment of an acceptable secular career for women. This school was similar to yet markedly different from the Fliedner's program of instruction. Her emphasis on the secular career rather than practice within a religious framework placed the responsibility for the preparation of nurses and the control of nursing with nurses rather than members of religious groups.

The basic requirements in Miss Nightingale's organization of the school were (1) that there should be a plan of education or training for the nurse and (2) that provisions should be made for homes that would encourage the desired personal or character development of the nurse. Miss Nightingale also believed that the school of nursing should be soundly financed to ensure adequate educational standards. Many of the problems of nursing education today are associated with inadequate financing; this clearly illustrates the wisdom of this extraordinary person.

Many ''modern'' practices were implemented in the school at St. Thomas. Remuneration was provided for lectures by members of the medical staff and for instruction given by the ward sisters (the equivalent of the head nurse of today). Records were kept of the educational experiences of the student. The basic ''work'' concept of the deaconess school was not included in the Nightingale school. Theory and clinical practice were planned to enable the student to develop the necessary skills and to know the reasons for her actions. Evaluation of the student through the efficiency report was part of the educational experience. The course of

instruction was originally 1 year but later was extended to 2 or 3 years, depending on the backgound of the student.

The provision of a residence with rigid regulations and routines had a twofold purpose. Candidates for nursing with qualifications similar to those of Miss Nightingale could be attracted to nursing if living conditions acceptable to them and their families could be provided. This alone would contribute to the acceptability of nursing as a career for women. The second purpose of the residence was to promote the standard of conduct desired in the nurse.

The organization of the school as a financially independent unit in relation to the hospital was a characteristic of Miss Nightingale's school. She believed that the student should be free from service obligations so that her education could be the principal objective of her experience in the hospital. The wisdom of this belief is evident in the examination of the problems that have existed in American nursing education in the past 75 years.

Miss Nightingale's interest in nursing and related services continued until her death in 1910. She remained in retirement but functioned as a central figure in British nursing. She opposed the central registration of nurses on the basis that an examination would not be as valid in indicating the qualifications of the nurse as would a certification by the school preparing the nurse. The examination also implied an outside element of control over nursing, and she believed this would not be sound. Perhaps if Miss Nightingale had remained in more direct contact with actual nursing practice, she might have changed her opinion. Another factor to be considered is that if the standards established through the original Nightingale school could have been implemented in other schools, the need to maintain quality nursing services through legal means such as licensure might not have been necessary. Events in the history of nursing and nursing education have proved the greatness of this nursing leader, and the future may prove that because of the needs of that time, central registration may have slowed the development of nursing as a profession.

EARLY AMERICAN NURSING EDUCATION AND LEADERSHIP

The most stable element of European nursing for several centuries was the nursing care provided through the Roman Catholic nursing orders. As settlements were established in the New World, members of these nursing orders also came and established branches in many areas of the New World. The Protestant Reformation had produced the tendency for individuals to base the selection of a residence on religious preference, so that colonial America was divided much as was Europe. The members of the nursing orders were placed in the predominantly Roman Catholic sections of countries or in predominantly Roman Catholic countries. Nursing education was not an activity of these orders in the mother countries; therefore it is logical that specific educational programs were not implemented in early American nursing endeavors. It is likely that the transfer of prepared individuals from the Old to the New World met the nursing needs of that time. Branches of the nursing orders were established in America early in the nineteenth century, further stabilizing the services provided by these groups.

The Protestant countries also contributed to nursing in America during the nineteenth century. St. Luke's Hospital in New York was staffed by members of an Anglican order in 1858. The Kaiserswerth Deaconess order was introduced into this country in 1849, and members of both Protestant groups were soon providing needed services in the Protestant areas of the United States. The initial division, based on religious conflict, of the Catholic and Protestant nursing groups did not last. Members of both groups were contributing to nursing education and service throughout the United States. Social progress within the United States soon enabled women to assume a secular career, so that the nursing orders did not assume a leadership role in nursing education as the Kaiserswerth order had in Europe.

There were other facilities for the care of the ill in early America. These were significant to the progress of nursing education primarily because they provided facilities for early training programs. Typical of these hospitals were Bellevue in New York, organized in 1736, and Blockley in Philadelphia, organized in 1731. These early hospitals usually began as a combination almshouse and infirmary to house the indigent and indigent ill in the same structure. Nursing care was actually nonexistent in these institutions. The inmates cared for each other. The individuals working in these institutions were similar in preparation and motivation to the "Sairey Gamps" of England. It was fairly common for prisoners to serve their sentences as "nurses" in these hospitals. They were voluntary hospitals organized to provide services for the ill, but the standard of nursing care was similar to that of the combined almshouse-infirmary. Various reform measures were initiated, but major changes were not effected until late in the nineteenth century. As in England, the reform measures were closely related to establishment of educational programs to prepare nurses.

America was a dynamic and progressive young country in the middle to late nineteenth century. After a stable economic and political status had been achieved, more attention was devoted to intellectual, cultural, and social endeavors. Universities were established, including some with coeducational provisions (Oberlin College, 1833). The development of social problems had created the need for reform measures, as had similar conditions in Europe. The interest and concern of the American public are evidenced by efforts of groups and individuals. Dorothea Dix had gained recognition for her work initiating reforms in mental institutions. Legislative attempts had been made to implement public health measures. Dr. Elizabeth Blackwell's graduation from medical school had encouraged other women to seek careers in fields usually restricted to men. There was a growing interest in women's rights, particularly the right of women to vote. Many of those involved in efforts toward the achievement of women's rights were instrumental in the reform of nursing practice. Considering the relationship of suffrage efforts and nursing reform, it is amusing to note that the right of women to vote did not gain the support of those at an American Nurses' Association convention shortly after the turn of the century.

Included in social reform measures were sporadic attempts at preparing individuals to give nursing care. These efforts were primarily directed toward providing basic knowledge for those individuals already giving nursing care. These attempts did not exert a lasting influence on American nursing education but did encourage the interest of influential persons. An example of this interest is a statement by Dr. Lemuel Shattuck, known for his contributions to the field of public health, in the Shattuck Report of 1950:

Institutions [should] be formed to educate and qualify females to be nurses of the sick. . . . Bad nursing often defeats the intention of the best medical advice and good nursing often supplements the defects of bad advice. Nursing often does more to cure disease than the physician himself, and, in the prevention of disease and in the promotion of health, it is of equal and even greater importance.*

Medical progress contributed to the need for more skilled nursing care, and attempts to establish programs for the preparation of nurses were encouraged and, in some instances, directly sponsored by physicians.

The first recognized program for the preparation of nurses was established through the efforts of a woman physician. Dr. Marie Zakrzewska. Her primary interest concerned the provision of facilities for women physicians, but problems in the acceptance of this endeavor and a concern for the lack of prepared nurses culminated in the establishment of a school of nursing at the New England Hospital for Women and Children in 1872. Initially a course of 6 months had been used, but this was extended to 1 year when the school was definitely estab-

lished. Dr. Zakrzewska and others assisting her had been educated in Europe, and the exposure to the school established by the Fliedners resulted in this being the guide for the program of the New England school. Some of the characteristics of the Kaiserswerth school were included in the course of instruction, but many important components were lacking. Some lectures were given by the medical staff, and Dr. Zakrzewska taught bedside nursing. The classwork was not required, and it can be concluded that the provision of care to the patients was emphasized over the preparation of the nurse. No entrance requirements were defined. The pharmacology instruction given at Kaiserwerth and much of the nursing instruction were not included.

One student, Linda Richards, graduated at the end of the first year in 1873. A description of the program from the writings of Miss Richards would indicate that it had little similarity to modern nursing education. The student's day began at 5:30 AM and ended at 9 PM. The students slept in small rooms between the wards and were "on call" for the care of their patients during the night. Time for study or recreation was not considered. Miss Richards states that only twice during the year did she have the opportunity to go to church.

A war was significant in the formation of a second school of nursing. As mentioned earlier, women were participating in social reform activities. Groups became directly involved in measures to provide care for soldiers of the U.S. Army in the Civil War. Resources for the care of the ill and injured during this war were similar to those Miss Nightingale had encountered in the Crimean War. Dorothea Dix was appointed superintendent of female nurses by the U.S. government. She was to establish a means of providing nursing services for the U.S. Army. Miss Dix found, as had Miss Nightingale, that the only prepared nurses were from religious orders and there was an extreme need for schools to prepare nurses. In response to the needs created by these conditions, one of the lay groups, made up predominantly of women, that had been providing relief measures for the soldiers expanded its organization and became the U.S. Sanitary

*Shattuck, L., et al.: Report of the Sanitary Commission of 1850 (reprint), Cambridge, Mass., 1948, Harvard University Press, p. 224.

Commission. This commission provided resources for the health of the soldiers, such as medical supplies, and assumed some functions of the Red Cross as it exists today in contributing to the welfare of those in the army. Miss Dix worked closely with this group, certainly communicating the need for programs to prepare qualified nurses. Some short-term emergency measures to prepare nurses were actually initiated during the war.

When the Civil War ended in 1865, the interest of several members of the Sanitary Commission was directed toward the solution of health problems in the New York area. The organization of Bellevue School of Nursing was a result of efforts of these individuals to improve standards of patient care at that hospital. Guidance and financial support were included in these efforts. This school of nursing was patterned after Miss Nightingale's school but was not closely similar in many respects. Consideration was given to the provision of an adequate residence, and attempts were made to recruit qualified young women and to make nursing an attractive career for women. The practice of wearing a uniform was introduced by this school. The school was under the supervision of a qualified nurse, but the training period of 1 year did not include a definite schedule of classwork or lectures. The early problems of this school were resolved, sound educational practices were implemented, and the school eventually became one of the leading schools of nursing in America. In later years a pattern of nursing education similar to that of Miss Nightingale's school was known as the Bellevue system.

Efforts of groups similar to the one responsible for the Bellevue school, social pressures, and medical progress resulted in the formation of a number of schools at about the same time that the Bellevue school was founded. These were similar in organization and sponsorship to the schools previously described. The acutal program of training would be considered deficient when compared to schools of today, but they did serve to form a strong nucleus for future nursing education endeavors. There was

no strong nursing leadership such as that of Miss Nightingale in the formation of the early schools of nursing, but the early schools eventually provided the leaders that contributed much to nursing in America. This lack of actual nursing leadership in early programs to prepare nurses was probably a primary factor in the basic differences in training programs in America and in the formation of programs different from those established in Europe. Dominant nurse leadership may have been able to prevent the exploitation of student services by establishing sound educational practices. The focus of the provision of service by the student is not surprising when it is remembered that those responsible for the establishment of early schools were primarily interested in the provision of better patient care.

It is interesting to note that the early school did not initially consider an association with an institution of higher education, even though coeducational colleges did exist. When one keeps in mind that developments in nursing, a profession primarily of women, closely parallel developments in status of women, reasons for this become evident. Education for women was not common, and education for a career even less so. Vocational preparation was not generally included in a collegiate education. The actual provision of medical education in an academic setting was not common until this century. Nursing was not yet well enough accepted as a suitable career for women that placement of it in an academic environment would be considered. Acceptance was still a problem in nursing as late as 1960.

A combination of developments led to a rapid increase in the number of schools of nursing in America during the late nineteenth and early twentieth centuries. Increases in population and the progress of medicine created the need for more and better hospitals. The need for prepared nurses increased proportionately, and more training schools were established. It was soon evident that a training school could serve as a financial asset to the hospital. The students provided an improved standard of patient care at a minimum cost. Students were used to provide the total nursing and related services in the hospital. The services of students were extended to the care of some patients in the home, with the hospital receiving the payment for these services. The very few graduate nurses in the hospital served in a supervisory or instructional capacity, and frequently this was a combined role. These graduates usually had received little or no preparation beyond that of basic nursing. These factors further served to limit the quantity and quality of the formal or structured training of the student.

This early nursing education was commonly referred to as an apprenticeship education. In reality this classification was not accurate. This method of teaching, common to the medieval period of history, implies that a person desiring to learn a skill or vocation works with a person having the desired skill or qualified in the vocation until he or she has acquired the desired skill or can assume at least the beginning responsibilities of the vocation. The preceptorship form of medical education is similar to the apprenticeship form of learning. Students in the early schools of nursing in America were taught primarily by other students. Formal lectures were given by physicians. There were some opportunities to work with practicing graduate nurses, but these were neither planned nor consistent. The lectures by the physicians were usually given at a time convenient to the schedule of patient care, and the student attended if patient care responsibilities would permit. This meant that the student attended classes in the evening after spending at least 12 hours caring for patients.

A graduate from St. Luke's Hospital in Denver (1915-1918) gave the following description of her experience. She spoke of her education as though she were a practicing nurse throughout the 3 years of her training. The hours on duty were from 7:30 AM to 7:30 PM, with 2 hours off and 1 hour for class if responsibilities permitted (patients had to be cared for first). Students had one afternoon free each week (4½ hours off on Sundays and holidays,

if possible). When on night duty, students worked from 7:30 PM to 7:30 AM for 1 month, and then they had an extra day off at the end of the month to change to day duty. Older students showed younger students the ''ropes'' and really provided the orientation on the wards in the hospital. If a student had entered training 2 hours ahead of another, she was the senior. There were no special days for entering. A beginning student was considered to be in the freshman class no matter what day of the year she entered training, and she had the same graduation day as everyone else in the class; however, she did not finish until she had 3 years of training, even if graduation day had passed. An examination in spelling, arithmetic, and letter writing climaxed the probation period.

This last comment identifies another problem area affecting nursing education. Nursing had not achieved the career desirability needed to ensure well-qualified applicants, and the status of women was not at the level that would ensure an adequate basic education of all women entering schools of nursing. Dismissals of students for illiteracy can be found on the records of schools of nursing in this period of the twentieth century.

The lack of progress in American schools are compared to the school at Kaiserswerth. Actually, little or no progress had been made, considering that approximately 75 years had passed since the beginning of the first deaconess establishment. The date of the St. Luke's Hospital graduate's training further confirms the limited progress of American nursing education, since the early schools of nursing had been in existence for approximately 40 years.

It is neither fair nor accurate to generalize and conclude that a lack of progress was common to all schools of nursing in America. Many schools were implementing sound educational practices and were preparing well-qualified practitioners. Nursing in America was gradually developing a strong leadership component. Improvement of early nursing education practices can frequently be traced directly to individual or group efforts of these early leaders. The efforts of the early leaders were also directed toward the formation of organizations that further contributed to the progress of nursing and nursing education. A description of the lives and activities of several early leaders illustrates the development toward more adequate practices in nursing education. The efforts of these early nursing leaders are also an example of the way professional progress must be made—through efforts from within nursing and by nurses.

The initiative for many changes in nursing came from Isabel Hampton Robb. Mrs. Robb had been a teacher before entering nursing. She graduated from Bellevue School of Nursing in 1883. She was made head of the Illinois Training School in Chicago in 1886 and organized the Johns Hopkins Hospital School of Nursing in 1889. She initiated many sound changes while in both of these positions. Her awareness of the problems of nursing education and of measures to solve these problems is evident in the following excerpts from a paper she presented to the International Congress of Charities, Correction, and Philanthropy at the Chicago World's Fair in 1893*:

The present history of hospitals in America shows that the hospital nursing is with few exceptions already being done by the members of regularly organized schools for nurses, and that where such schools do not exist steps are being taken for establishing them. Next, we find that the demand for trained nurses is steadily on the increase for cases of sickness in private families and what is still more important, that district nursing is being introduced into almost every large city in the country. . . .

Each school is a law unto itself. Nothing in the way of unity of ideas or of general principles to govern all exists, and no effort towards establishing and maintaining a general standard for all has ever been attempted. Some institutions consider that a two year course of instruction is essential; others place it at a year and a half; and others again at a year. In England a few schools

---

*Robb, I.H.: In papers and discussions of the International Congress of Charities, Correction, and Philanthropy, held in Chicago in 1893, New York, 1949, National League of Nursing Education.

insist upon three years. The hours of daily work also differ widely, some requiring from their pupils nine hours a day of active service; others as high as twelve and thirteen hours. The theoretical instruction is usually not included in the nine hours work, and it is difficult to speak definitely upon this subject, as the length of such a course, the subjects and the extent to which they are taught are again dependent upon the opinion upon this matter of the governing body of each particular school. We also find no general rule governing the special attainments or degree of education required from the women who present themselves as candidates. On the contrary, a woman who has been refused by or dismissed from one school for lack of education, dishonorable conduct, inefficiency, etc. frequently gains admittance into another, where the authorities have not had so high, if any, standard required from those whom they accept. But notwithstanding all these differences, each woman who graduates from any of these schools usually has a document with the high sounding name of diploma presented to her, and henceforth she is known as a trained nurse, which in nowise indicates that amount of knowledge or fitness she really does bring to her work. In fact, it is no unusual occurrence for schools to graduate nurses whom they at once, when relieved from their presence in the hospital, refuse to recommend or sustain in their work. . .

A "trained nurse" may mean then anything, everything, or next to nothing, and with this state of affairs the results are far from what they should be, and public criticism is frequently justly severe upon our shortcomings, or else is content with superficiality where like meets like. . . .

After much practical experience, I maintain that no such course of education can be thoroughly given in one year, but yet I find that very many schools limit their didactic teaching to the first year and make the second year's work of a purely practical nature and divide it between hospital work and private duty. It is absolutely necessary that class work and lectures should be carried on through the second year as well, and if this is done, then private nursing outside of the hospital is out of the question, as such interruptions would seriously interfere with any systematic teaching. I also hold that it is necessary to have the pupil under the daily observation and criticism of her teachers. This is impossible if she leaves the hospital for private duty, and one of two things must be true, viz: either she is as yet unfit to be entrusted to do her work without some supervision, or else, if she is really capable of doing this work in the second year, she should not be held by the school at all. In the latter case, why not make the term of pupilage only one year and graduate her? There is another side to this question, that of justice to the patient, but as this does not really come under the head of the standards we are just now discussing we will pass it by. . . .

There are plenty of problems to work out, and schools for nurses are capable of much finer work than has yet been done, if we to whose hands the work is now entrusted are willing to take a broad and comprehensive view of the subject. The principal of a school for nurses performs the least part of her duty, and throws away many of her privileges, if she is content to confine herself to the limitations of her own particular school. She must look into and go abroad among other schools, and teach her nurses to do the same, recognizing what is good in others and being ever ready to adopt any improvement. There is so much that we can learn from each other, and sooner or later we must also recognize the fact that we are all trained nurses, and that until something of a common standard is reached the imperfections of the few must be borne by all. Briefly, then, some of our chief aims should be to bring about a spirit of unity among the various schools, and to establish a standard of education upon which we may all be judged. . . .

In doing this, the first step should be to bring about in all our schools, as far as possible, a uniform system of instruction, so that the requirements for graduation should be about the same in each. We might well lengthen the course of instruction in training schools to three years, with eight hours a day of practical work. . . .

With this length of course it would be possible to make a better subdivision of the pupils into classes, so that every member could receive her practical teaching, her class teaching and lectures according to her grade in the school and her individual ability. There should be stated times for entrance into the school, and the teaching year should be divided according to the academic terms usually adopted in our public schools and colleges. To compel a class of students to attempt to listen to a lecture on a hot July night is barbarous. . . .

A final word as to the practical qualifications which should be required of women who present themselves as candidates to be taught nursing. A good practical English education should be insisted upon. By this is meant that the candidate should come up to the standard

required to pass the final examinations in the best high schools in the country, special stress being laid upon her ability to express herself either in writing or orally with quickness and accuracy. Her knowledge of arithmetic should be of an eminently practical nature and so that she can readily deal with problems involving fractions, percentage, bookkeeping, etc. This much is absolutely necessary. Of course more than this is desirable, as no other study develops the reasoning powers in the same practical way, and women who do not possess any education in arithmetic beyond the few simple rules, simply applied, are at once placed in a disadvantageous position upon entering upon their work in a modern hospital. Of course, if she has in addition a knowledge of languages and a broad general reading, the candidate is all the better prepared for undertaking and obtaining success in her career as a nurse.

All students, nursing and other, will appreciate Mrs. Robb's understanding of the problems of a student from her opinion of summer classes.

In addition to the initiation of sound educational practices in the schools she directed, Mrs. Robb was instrumental in the formation of the Society of Superintendents of Training Schools and the Nurses' Associated Alumnae. She actively supported state registration of nurses as a means of establishing a standard for the adequate preparation of nurses. The need for the establishment of a standard was acute. At this time there was a wide variation in basic preparation of the nurse. The course of instruction in some schools was as short as 6 weeks. Mrs. Robb believed that a basic similarity of preparation was essential if nursing was to progress. It is interesting to note that the profession is facing similar problems today, with the different programs each preparing a basic practitioner. When it became evident that state registration had not accomplished the achievement of the desired standards, Mrs. Robb worked with the Society of Superintendents toward achieving this goal. The concern of this group for the preparation of better-qualified instructors initiated an investigation of the possibility of starting some classes for nurses at Teachers College, Columbia University. A course of study, with the financial support of the Society of Superintendents, was established. The now well-known Department of Nursing and Health at Teachers College, Columbia University, resulted from these early attempts to establish sound nursing education practices.

The actual development of the nursing course at Teachers College was associated with the work of another nursing leader, Adelaide Nutting. She was a graduate of the Johns Hopkins Hospital School of Nursing and succeeded Mrs. Robb as principal of this school. Miss Nutting shared her predecessor and teacher's view on the implementation of sound standards and practice in nursing education. She contributed individually and through the Society of Superintendents (soon to be known as the National League of Nursing Education) to bring about many changes in nursing education. At the school she directed, the student's day was shortened to 8 hours, a 3-year course of study was established, and the practice of giving a monthly stipend to the student was ended. The practice of giving the student a monthly allowance was common in schools of nursing and further acted to place the student in an employee status. Since the student was considered an employee, her responsibilities to the hospital took precedence over learning activities, making the provision of a sound education difficult if not impossible.

Miss Nutting was appointed to the faculty of Teachers College, Columbia University, in 1907, becoming the first professor of nursing in the world. Under Miss Nutting's direction the school achieved international fame both through the provision of sound educational practices and through the preparation of many for leadership roles in nursing. Miss Nutting continued to work toward improved nursing education, contributing toward efforts of the nursing organization, studies, and publications.

Miss Nutting contributed to one of the early publications of the National League of Nursing Education intended to assist schools to implement sound educational practices. This book and the subsequent revisions identify both the problems and the progress of nursing education in America. It is interesting to note the title changes of each edition. The original edition was published in 1917, the first revision in 1927, and the second revision in 1937. The title of the 1917 edition was *A Standard Curriculum for Schools of Nursing*. Definite standards for the improvement of schools, outlines for courses, and even an outline for the classwork of a 3-year program were included in this first edition. The 1927 edition was entitled *A Curriculum for Schools of Nursing*. This edition was still definite in the recommended standards but indicated the expansion of nursing practice and the ability of nursing education to adapt to practice needs by the emphasis on courses in public health, disease prevention, and related subjects. The third edition, and the last, was titled *A Curriculum Guide for Schools of Nursing*. This title indicates that nursing education had progressed to the degree that a guide rather than a more rigid outline of specific courses and course content could be utilized by schools of nursing.

Many factors contributed to progress in nursing education in the middle 1920s. Minimum standards for schools of nursing had been established through more effective licensing laws. Adequate texts and nursing journals were beginning to appear. Programs had been established for the preparation of nursing educators. Nursing education was beginning to take place in colleges and universities. The initiation of projects evaluating nursing education practices was a major factor in the improvement of American nursing education. These studies provided an impetus for moving from a vocation to a profession. Sound research projects provided an evaluation of past progress as well as errors and problems. The result of these evaluations was made available to all concerned, encouraging the participation of a larger segment of nursing in activities to improve the status of the profession.

One of the earliest nursing studies was initiated to determine the requirements for health nursing. This study was later expanded to include the entire field of nursing education. This project was the responsibility of the Committee for the Study of Nursing Education, made up of physicians, nurses, and others interested in public health. It was financed by the Rockefeller Foundation. A major portion of the research was carried out by Josephine Goldmark, the secretary of the committee; thus the report of this study is frequently referred to as the Goldmark Report or Goldmark Study (1924).

The report of the Committee for the Study of Nursing Education, titled *Nursing and Nursing Education in the United States,* contained some specific recommendations for the preparation for public health nursing education practices. These included sound financing of schools, better preparation of nursing educators, and the strengthening of ties between the Association of Schools of Nursing and universities. In view of current nursing practices, it is interesting to note that this report also recommended the preparation of a worker to carry out nonnursing tasks in institutions and assist the nurse in the nursing tasks requiring less skill. This latter recommendation was not implemented in nursing until 1940, many years after the publication of the report.

In 1942 the National League for Nursing Education published *Essentials of a Good School of Nursing.* These criteria were rigid and did not allow for experimentation. A good school had an identified purpose, legal authority to exist, financial resources, prepared faculty, faculty stability, student admissions and counseling policies, student organization, student health programs, defined programs of studies, library, classrooms, and office space. Even so, in 1950 a mid-century report revealed that many schools did not meet the minimum standards. It was not until approval of schools was being done on a more systematic basis by school boards of nursing and schools were voluntarily asking for accreditation by the National League of Nursing Education that there was any noticeable change in the standards of schools.

In 1952, when there was a restructuring of all nursing organizations and the National League for Nursing (NLN) was organized, a new emphasis

was placed on the upgrading of education for nurses. Leaders in nursing continued to recognize that all schools could not be judged by the same criteria. However, it was agreed that all schools should have certain essential elements with which to build a sound educational program. These elements did not differ much from those identified by 1942, nor do they in the mid-1980s.

An earlier project of the American Medical Association stimulated a second research project affecting American nursing education. About 1910 a grading of medical schools by the organization had succeeded in eliminating many of the poorer medical schools and generally upgrading the level of medical education. In 1925 the Committee on the Grading of Nursing Schools was established, hoping to achieve similar changes in nursing education. The scope of the committee's concern was broadened to include the study of nursing duties, the need for and supply of nurses, and the status of nursing practice in general. The study extended over a 7-year period. The results of the study were published in three reports: *Nurses, Patients and Pocketbooks, An Activity Analysis of Nursing,* and *Nursing Schools Today and Tomorrow.* The actual grading of schools of nursing was not achieved, but the efforts of the committee contributed to the overall improvement of nursing and nursing education. The study of this group did eventually lead to the implementation of a program for the accreditation of schools of nursing education by the National League of Nursing Education. The first list of accredited schools was published in 1941. World War II and organizational changes slowed the actual accreditation of schools, but accreditation had been achieved in a large proportion of the schools of nursing. Today accreditation through the NLN is recognized as an important factor in ensuring an adequate standard of nursing education.

NURSING EDUCATION SINCE THE 1940s
Studies of nursing education

A study of nursing education with many implications for the contemporary nurse was published in 1948 as *Nursing for the Future* by Esther Lucile Brown. This was a report of a comprehensive study of nursing education that was directed by Dr. Brown. This study was even more significant to professional progress in that it was initiated and financed by nursing with the assistance of the Russell Sage Foundation. Brown's report approached the study of future nursing programs from the basis of health needs of society. Many of the recommendations of earlier nursing leaders such as adequate financial support of schools of nursing, increased association with institutions of higher education, and similar sound educational practices were reiterated in this report.

In 1948 Brown recommended that there be mandatory licensure and improved educational programs for practical nursing, that in-service education be expanded—with primary consideration given to interpersonal relations for all who function in the health care setting, that the term *professional* be restructured for use by schools and its graduates of institutions of higher learning, that there be a better balance of technical procedures and psychotherapeutic care, and that the hospital environment foster the nurse's professional growth and improve salaries. She further recommended the development of clinical specialists and increased research in nursing practice. Brown recommended that hospital schools be examined closely for the quality of their educational programs, be encouraged to close, experiment in shortening the period of training, and utilize the resources of junior colleges. Specialty hospitals such as children's hospitals were urged to close their schools and allow their facilities to be used as an affiliation to schools of nursing needing that kind of facililty for clinical experience. Brown strongly recommended that education for nurses be in universities with all the professional status of other disciplines.

In 1970 and 1971 Brown published two reports called *Nursing Reconsidered*. In the first she examined the changes in institutional nursing and in the second the changes in community nursing. It was evident much had occurred to change the focus of education in the intervening years since 1948.

Practical nurse education had changed. Trade and vocational schools were responsible for educating these health workers. Mandatory licensure was a reality in all states but one, Texas. Clinical specialists were being utilized, and master's degree programs were strong in their educational endeavors to prepare the practitioner. Research in nursing education and service was going forward. Brown also found that schools had examined themselves, improved the quality of their education, and were using junior and senior colleges for supportive course work. The profession of nursing had examined the term *professional* and had attempted, through the American Nurses' Association (ANA) position paper of 1965, to move in the direction suggested by Brown in 1948. In-service education and continuing education programs were evident in the health care settings. Thus it could be said that the profession had made progress in meeting the recommendations made by Brown.

Perhaps the most controversial, yet significant, research project in nursing education was the study that resulted in the development of programs in nursing in community and junior colleges. These programs were a completely new kind of nursing education. The basis for the study project was the doctoral thesis of Mildred Montag, published as *Education of Nursing Technicians* in 1951. The research project was also under the direction of Dr. Montag. Associate degree programs were generally 2 years in length, provided through a junior college, and organized to prepare a practitioner for the functions of a registered nurse. The most far-reaching effect of this project was the stimulation of other programs of nursing to examine their curriculum and teaching methods. Many changes occurred in the more traditional programs of nursing education, including experiments to shorten the 3-year diploma programs in nursing.

Federal government support of nursing education

Closely related to studies of nursing education and the increasing endeavors of nursing to adapt to the needs of society was the support of nursing education by the federal government. Federal support to nursing education was provided indirectly through the organization of the Army School of Nursing during World War I. Experience with this school indicated that a similar effort would not be adequate to meet the nursing needs associated with World War II. Some provisions for nursing education (refresher course, postgraduate education) were implemented in 1942, but the principal federally sponsored nursing education project was initiated with the passage of the Bolton Act in 1943. This act created the Cadet Nurse Program of basic education and grants for some postgraduate education. Federal support proved to be effective in increasing the number of nursing practitioners in this emergency situation. The Cadet Nurse Program was discontinued with the termination of World War II.

The stresses of World War II accentuated the problems of nursing and accelerated efforts toward the solution of these problems, as had previous wars. The need for academically prepared leaders in nursing and nursing education had been a problem and contributed to problem areas of nursing. As nurses continued to evaluate and work toward progressive patterns of practice, this need became even more evident. The efforts of nurses and the increasing concern of the government for the health of the people promoted additional legislative efforts to provide funds for the education of nurses. The Professional Nurse Traineeship Program (Public Law 911) provided funds for qualified graduate nurses to become prepared for teaching, administrative, and supervisory positions. This federal support has contributed toward further education of nurses since its implementation in 1956. Federal funds were also provided for the preparation of public health and practical nurses.

The successes of federal assistance in increasing the supply of nurses and elevating the practice of nursing with the recognition that nursing is an essential element of health care led to a series of developments that increased federal support of nursing education even further. A consultant group on nursing was appointed by the Surgeon General of the Public Health Service in 1961. The role of this group, as identified in the foreword of the study report, *Toward Quality in Nursing,* "was to advise the Surgeon General on nursing needs and to identify the appropriate role of the Federal Government in assuring adequate nursing services for our nation." The report of this committee, published in 1963, identified existing nursing resources, future needs, and recommendations to meet these needs. Included in the surgeon general's report were a number of specific recommendations for the expansion and improvement of nursing education. It was recognized by the consultants for the surgeon general that baccalaureate programs should prepare those nurses who would assume leadership positions. Until such time that education for nurses could be accomplished in institutions for higher learning, it would be necessary to "support and improve present and evolving programs of education." In the meantime the profession of nursing was to make a study of the system of education for nurses in relation to the responsibilities and skills necessary for quality care.

To follow up the 1963 report to the surgeon general, the ANA and the NLN in 1967 appointed a project director to develop a commission, independent of the two organizations, to study nursing and nursing education. Each organization contributed financially to begin the project. Other sources of income were provided to complete the study. The commission was charged to study nursing and nursing education and to make recommendations for the future. The commission director appointed people from many disciplines. Although there were nurse representatives on the commission, they did not represent either of the nurse organizations. It was believed that the commission should be given the opportunity to make recommendations without the presence of group or professional nurse pressure.

In February 1970 a preliminary report of 18 recommendations was published in the *American Journal of Nursing.* Published in September 1970, the complete report of the National Commission for the Study of Nursing and Nursing Education,

Abstract for Action, made a total of 58 recommendations that dealt with a wide range of issues in nursing. Additional money was funded to allow for implementation of the recommendations. All of organized nursing involved itself in analyzing the report and determining how the recommendations could be implemented.

The commission officially completed the task of assisting the profession in implementing some of the recommendations in 1973. A report of how the recommendations were implemented can be found in Lysaught's *Action in Nursing* published in 1974. The first year of implementation was mainly one of informing and influencing the myriad organizations and people about the findings of the commission. Not all people and organizations agreed with the findings, and they voiced this criticism openly; however, overall agreement outweighed the criticism. The commission chose to implement four priorities for nursing education, all dealing with establishing statewide master planning committees. The priorities chosen were (1) establishing nursing education within the system of higher education, (2) greater articulation between educational programs, (3) development of episodic and distributive content, and (4) advancing continued education.

How the commission's recommendations were implemented could be seen by examining individual programs such as those of the University of Nebraska College of Nursing in Omaha, Nebraska, and Brigham Young University College of Nursing in Provo, Utah. Both institutions instituted nursing programs from associate degree to the master's degree in nursing. In 1983 Brigham Young University closed their associate degree program and restructured the B.S.N. and M.S.N. degree programs. In Colorado a statewide master plan for continuing education was prepared. Hospital schools throughout the country closed and made their facilities and faculties available to junior college and senior universities. Registered nurse completion programs were developed to expressly provide an avenue for the RN to achieve the baccalaureate degree in nursing.

For the nursing needs of the nation to be supplied, expansion of associate and baccalaureate degree programs became necessary. Most schools did not have funds available; therefore one recommendation to the surgeon general was to provide federal funds for educational facilities, student loans, and payment to schools to defray the cost of instruction. The profession of nursing examined carefully the surgeon general's report and moved as rapidly as possible to right the wrongs in nursing and provide the nation with high-quality nursing services.

The recommendation of further federal support was evident in the 1963 report, and this assistance was provided through the Nurse Training Act of 1964 (Public Law 88-581). Through this act appropriations of $283 million were authorized to implement multiple approaches toward the provision of adequate nursing. Provisions of this act included the following:

1. Construction grants to collegiate, associate degree, and diploma schools of nursing for new facilities or for the rehabilitation or replacement of existing facilities
2. Teaching improvement grants to diploma, collegiate, and associate degree schools of nursing for projects that would improve, strengthen, or expand teaching programs
3. Payments to diploma schools to defray some of the costs of increased enrollments and to improve the quality of instruction
4. Traineeships for professional nurses to increase the number of graduate nurses with preparation for positions as administrators, supervisors, clinical specialists, and teachers in hospitals and related institutions, public health agencies, and schools of nursing
5. Loans to student nurses to increase the number of nurses by helping them to defray the costs of their nursing education, and to encourage them to stay in active practice by a partial cancellation clause based on their years of employment as professional nurses.

In 1967 a Program Review Committee was appointed by the Secretary of Health, Education and

Welfare to study the 1964 Nurse Training Act. It was necessary for making recommendations to Congress regarding the extension of the 1964 act beyond July 1, 1969. The committee recommended to Congress that the act be continued at least 5 years (1970 to 1974). In August 1968 Congress approved the extension of the Nurse Training Act until 1974. All provisions of the previous act were extended, with a specific change in payments to diploma schools. All schools—associate degree, diploma, and baccalaureate—were to receive $15,000 for defraying operational costs, plus an additional amount for each 2% of increased enrollment.

Although Congress approved the extension of the training act, funding was not appropriated in the amounts recommended. In January 1971 the boards of directors of the ANA and the NLN wired President Richard M. Nixon of their grave concern that curtailed funding would cause decreased enrollment at nursing schools and a more acute nurse shortage. In November 1971 funding was appropriated, but the amount was not significant. Again testimony was given by nursing organizations, and in December 1971 additional funding was appropriated.

Since 1971 organized nursing has had to struggle to secure funds appropriated by Congress from the U.S. Budget Office and Department of Health, Education and Welfare (now the Department of Health and Human Services). In 1972 the situation became so critical it threatened the viability of the majority of schools of nursing and all the graduate programs in nursing. Nursing education had become dependent on federal funding to support its educational system through capitation funds, distress grants, and program improvement grants.

In an unprecedented move, in June 1973 the NLN filed a suit against the director of the Office of Management and Budget and the secretary of the Department of Health, Education and Welfare to release the appropriated funds to schools of nursing. The complaint alleged that funds had been withheld from schools and had not been transferred to schools in time to be used for the 1973-1974 academic year. The suit further alleged that the director and secretary acted illegally in reducing the amount of funds appropriated by Congress. In December 1973, the federal court ordered the release of $21.7 million in impounded funds to schools of nursing that were members of the NLN.

In June 1974, companion health manpower bills were submitted in the Senate and House to extend the Nurse Training Act of 1971 for 5 years. One area of deep concern in the bills was the stipulation that any student accepting a federal loan or scholarship would be required to serve 2 years in a health manpower distress area in order to make a more equitable distribution of nurses. Nurse leaders spoke against this concept, not because they did not see the need for greater distribution, but because it placed undue restrictions on the student choosing nursing for a career. Late in 1974 the companion bills were approved without the restrictions on students accepting loans. Funding for the 5-year period from 1975 to 1980 would have been less than in previous years and would have created a need for innovation on the part of nursing to maintain or increase the quality of nursing education. At the last moment, President Gerald Ford vetoed the bill, saying that the measure would increase inflation and that high federal spending for nursing education would be "intolerable at a time when even high priority activities are being pressed to justify their existence." Rosamond Gabrielson, ANA president, responded by asking President Ford to "take a fresh look" at the bill vetoed. The ninety-fourth Congress submitted a new bill. Senate Bill 66 was passed by the House and Senate as one bill. President Ford vetoed the bill, again saying it was inflationary. The nursing profession, as one, spoke against the veto and apprised Congress of its displeasure. The Ninety-fourth Congress overrode the veto, making the Health Manpower Act of 1975 the first veto of President Ford to be overridden. However, again a bill was passed with funds authorized but without appropriations. Thus a separate supplemental appropriation bill had to be passed. The level of funding was substantially less than that of previous years.

Each year since 1975 has seen the profession of nursing become more politically involved in maintaining some level of federal funding for nursing education. Organized nursing (the ANA, the NLN, and the American Association of Colleges of Nursing) has worked in a united way to foster a sense of political astuteness in identifying needs of nursing education and the need for continual financial support.

President Jimmy Carter, in 1978, through his advisors, determined that a shortage of nurses no longer existed and therefore decreased the amount of federal support for the fiscal biennial 1980-82. Furthermore, President Carter pocket vetoed the appropriation bill submitted by Congress in the late 1978 congressional year. In 1979 Congress prepared another bill restoring funds that was signed by President Carter.

In 1979 Congress mandated by Public Law 96-76 that the Institute of Medicine conduct a study to ''. . . secure an objective assessment of the need for continued federal support of nursing education programs. . .'' (Institute of Medicine, 1983). The study was completed in the spring of 1983 and was presented to Congress. The recommendations dealing specifically with education were as follows:

1. No specific federal support was needed to increase the overall supply of registered nurses; therefore capitation funds would not be needed as in previous nurse training acts.
2. Funds should be made available to states to provide assistance in analyzing and planning nursing resource allocations.
3. Loans should be continued to provide students with the resources necessary to complete their nursing education.
4. Grants should be offered to nursing education and nursing services who undertake to improve collaboration.
5. Increased funding should occur in the way of fellowships, loans, and programing at the master's and doctoral levels.

6. Federal funds were necessary to develop and promote research.

The Reagan administration ''zeroed out'' financial support to nursing and nursing education because of the belief that a nursing shortage no longer existed; therefore federal financial support was not needed. However, Congress did not support that viewpoint and provided continuing resolutions for the support of nursing.

A devastating blow to nurse educators was the revelation in 1980 and 1981 that nursing students who had received government loans were the most delinquent in paying back their loans. The federal government, becoming more budget conscious, began investigating all of the student loans and found recipients of loans in health-related educational programs to be delinquent in paying back the money borrowed. In late 1983 stiff penalties were imposed on students seeking loans. Financial aid officers of educational institutions had to become more accountable in not only the giving of loans but the pay back as well.

Just what the future for federal assistance to nursing and nursing education will be is difficult to judge. However, from past history, the executive branch and Congress will be at odds as to how much assistance should be awarded nursing.

The great recession and its impact on education

The great recession of the late 1970s and early 1980s had an impact on nursing and nursing education. The amount of money from federal and state sources changed, and academic institutions could no longer afford programs that were not making money. Nursing education as a discipline received scrutiny as to cost and enrollment. Programs such as the one at Skidmore College in New York were closed because of low enrollment and being ''too costly.'' Michigan announced the closing of Michigan State University School of Nursing. An outcry of professional nurses throughout the state and the country saved that program. Other programs, such as Lutheran Medical Center Hospital School of

Nursing in Ohio, were closed without forewarning to the students or faculty. So it was across the nation. Schools of nursing were closed or threatened to be closed because of the lack of money to operate them.

It should be noted that as programs were evaluated hard decisions had to be made regarding size of program, quality programing, and duplication of programs. Not only was nursing as a discipline being evaluated, but all of academia underwent many changes. For the first time professors who were tenured were being threatened with loss of positions. New faculty positions were not available. As faculty retired or resigned, positions were not filled.

State systems such as those in Washington, Oregon, Michigan, and Ohio were in severe budget deficits. Budgets were cut 15% to 20%. Major economic problems existed. Faculty members were terminated, programs were deleted, and no new programs were approved.

In academia, strategic planning for the future became all important. The issue was, with financial resources being limited and in all likelihood continuing to be limited in the future, how should the resources be spent? Planning included evaluation of programs to determine if some should be phased out while others remained and grew. Accountability for faculty resources, programing, and outcomes of graduates were addressed. By the mid-1980s federal and state funds to all systems of education were restricted. University officials were searching for new avenues of funding to support the changes that had occurred.

Nursing education fared well in most instances. An interesting phenomenon occurred in nursing: enrollment after several years of limited increase began to climb again in 1983. With increased enrollment and limited faculty positions available, new pressures became evident. Nurse educators were faced with either accepting more students than could be adequately supervised in clinical agencies or cutting enrollment. Each institution handled this problem differently. In most instances no increase

in the number of students accepted occurred, and waiting lists began to develop. At one associate degree program in Ohio the waiting list contained over 500 names, a backlog of 2 years.

At the mid-1980s nursing education was continuing to change to meet the economic crisis.

Influence of the ANA and changes in nursing education

A discussion of nursing education and the achievement of professional progress in America would not be complete without reference to the ANA's proposed Goal 3 of 1960. Each problem and development of nursing education identified previously contributed to the formulation of this goal. Three goals were identified by the ANA Committee on Current and Long-Term Goals to serve as a guide in meeting the needs of nurses and of people for nursing service. The first two goals were concerned with the improvement of nursing practice and the recognition of the practitioner of nursing; the third goal concerned the preparation of the nurse. The committee defined the proposed Goal 3 as follows:

To insure that, within the next 20 to 30 years, the education basic to the professional practice of nursing for those who then enter the profession shall be secured in a program that provides the intellectual, technical and cultural components of both a professional and liberal education. Toward this end, the A.N.A. shall promote the baccalaureate program so that in due course it becomes the basic educational foundation for professional nursing.*

Basic to the formulation of this goal was the belief that professional practice would increasingly require a practitioner who has acquired both a liberal and a professional education. Changes in the status of women and social, educational, and medical progress were factors that support this belief. The need for this goal has been shown by other

*American Nurses' Association: Current and long-term goals for the American Nurses' Association. Committee report, New York, 1960, The Association.

professional groups, composed primarily of women who have progressed toward the achievement of educational standards implied in Goal 3. Goal 3 was presented to the membership and House of Delegates of the ANA in 1960 but was never voted on. However, in June 1964 a proposal was adopted by the House of Delegates to "continue to work toward baccalaureate education as the educational foundation for professional nursing practice."

The ANA Committee on Education presented to the Board of Directors of the organization for adoption in September 1965 a statement, "Education for Nursing." This paper became known as the "position paper" and appeared in the December 1965 issue of the *American Journal of Nursing*. The position was that education of nurses should take place in institutions of higher learning and there should be two levels of nursing practice—the technical level, obtained in associate degree programs, and the professional level of nursing practice, achieved in baccalaureate degree programs.

The practical nurse programs or vocational nurse programs now in existence would either become associate degree programs or cease to be in existence. The hospital diploma program would move in either direction, but eventually education for nurses would not occur in hospital-controlled programs.

This position had far-reaching implications for the nursing education and service of the United States. This ideal could not be realized without seriously decreasing the number of nurses needed in every community. An orderly transition had to occur as junior and senior colleges were made available to take care of the number of students enrolled in hospital diploma programs.

In 1960 there were 908 diploma programs, 57 associate degree programs, and 172 baccalaureate programs, making a total of 1137 programs in nursing in the United States. In 1972, according to *Facts About Nursing 1972-1973*, there were 1364 schools, with 524 diploma programs, 409 university or senior college programs, 408 junior college programs, and 22 independent programs. This placed 60% of nursing education in educational institutions.

In 1972 almost 95% of the junior or community colleges were publicly supported, as were 60.1% of the senior colleges, whereas only 18.7% of the hospital schools were publicly supported. Thus most financial support, as of 1972, for nursing education was provided through public funds.

The trend for change in nursing education programs continued, as shown by the statistics of 1975. In 1975 there were 428 diploma programs, 618 associate degree programs, and 329 baccalaureate programs. Some 58.1% of all education for nursing occurred in public-supported institutions, according to *Facts About Nursing 1976-1977*.

Further changes in nursing education were reported by the NLN through *Nursing Outlook*, September 1979. In 1978 there were 344 diploma programs, 677 associate degree programs, and 353 baccalaureate programs. Practical nurse programs totaled 1329, 45 less than registered nurse programs. Not only was program growth changing, enrollments were decreasing in diploma programs and increasing in baccalaureate programs. Even so, the data revealed relatively no growth in the population of any one of the programs, and zero growth in the number of graduates from all RN programs.

The ANA again confirmed its position on nursing education in 1978 by passing a resolution that by 1985 the entry to practice would be at two levels. The only level described as that of professional nursing was to be at the baccalaureate level.

The number of RN students in baccalaureate programs has consistently increased. In 1973-1974, 3003 graduated, whereas in 1977-78, 6146 completed baccalaureate programs. Baccalaureate degree education in nursing for the registered nurse had increased over 100% by the early 1980s. Many universities saw this as an avenue for increasing their own enrollments. The profession of nursing was increasingly concerned for the registered nurse who wanted a B.S.N. The concern centered around the university or college that was willing to give blanket credit for all previous nursing education and added only the general education requirements. These programs were ineligible for NLN accreditation, which in turn jeopardized the graduates in the pursuit of graduate education in nursing. At the same time a significant number of RN-B.S.N. completion programs were established and sought NLN accreditation. These programs were planned to meet the same criteria as the generic baccalaureate program in nursing.

Two noteworthy programs for RN education are the New York Board of Regents External Degree programs for A.D.N. and B.S.N. education. The programs are NLN accredited. The programs allow the student to study at home, wherever home is, and the program of studies is very rigorous. Clinical competence is tested in testing centers throughout the United States. The students have successfully passed state board examinations for licensure. Many RNs have chosen this program to secure their B.S.N. degree.

The data on the number of RNs pursuing B.S.N. education are at best a guess. RNs usually study part-time and are in the system for a number of years. It is evident, however, that the number of baccalaureate-prepared nurses has increased.

As the 1980s approached, significant changes were occurring in the preparation of the beginning registered nurse. By 1983 there were 1455 schools for the preparation of the registered nurse. According to the NLN there were 753 A.D.N. programs, 288 diploma programs, and 414 B.S.N. programs. It was further predicted that 13 diploma programs were due to close within 2 years. In 1982 there were 1319 practical nurse programs (Vaughn, 1983).

Enrollment in the schools was no longer zero based as it was in the late 1970s. Increased numbers of students were entering nursing education in institutions of higher learning. The largest number of students were being admitted to associate degree programs, then baccalaureate programs, with diploma programs third. In 1982, 116,896 students were admitted to the three basic RN programs.

These figures do not include students entering the generic M.S.N. or N.D. programs.

In 1982 there were 154 master's degree programs and 25 doctoral programs in nursing. Enrollment in each of these programs has increased; however, completion of the programs has declined, further suggesting a negative growth rate in the number of graduates.

A concern in the report of *Nursing Schools at the Mid-Century* (1950) was the number of small schools and schools with limited clinical facilities. This concern was directed at hospital schools of nursing. In the 1970s, with almost every junior college including nursing education as part of the curriculum, the same concern was expressed. Although the number of nursing programs in junior colleges has increased, there was concern about the types of controls being exercised to provide quality education. In 1974 Montag, at the Seventy-fifth Anniversary of Nursing Education Alumni of Teachers College, Columbia University, said that associate degree programs in nursing were being eroded because of the ANA position paper of 1965 and that these graduates were being used improperly by nursing services.

Thirty years have elapsed since the associate degree in nursing was introduced. Its curriculum has undergone change as nursing service agencies have utilized graduates from these programs in all capacities of nursing. Educators therefore have been forced to alter the original concept to produce the product, a marketable nurse.

There continues to be criticism of associate degree and baccalaureate graduates. Is this criticism valid? Is it impossible to use these practitioners because the profession has failed to explicate the objectives of the various nursing education programs? Is it not time to evaluate nursing education programs as was done at midcentury for the hospital-based school?

Immediately following publication of the position paper in 1965, each state developed a planning committee for nursing and nursing education. The planning committees were sponsored by the state nurses' associations either independently or jointly with allied organizations. The purposes of the state planning committees were to identify the nursing needs of the state and to determine the number and kinds of educational programs needed to meet those needs. In 1970 and in 1979 the NLN Board of Directors reaffirmed its position that all types of educational programs were needed to meet the demands of nursing. Planning for education and utilization takes time and cooperation from all persons. The board of directors made the following statements about nursing education in the 1970s:

Nursing education in the seventies must not only provide sufficient numbers of personnel prepared for the evolving functions, but it must continue to emphasize preparation for the traditional role as well.

The real challenge to nursing education is that of preparing practitioners who are flexible, creative and tolerant in their approach to assessing and solving health service problems. They must be skilled in teamwork, able to understand and cope with change, and innovative in adapting to changed circumstances. To further enhance their ability to deal constructively with change, a comprehensive coordinated continuing education system needs to be developed for practitioners, teachers, and administrators.

To prepare the numbers and kinds of qualified personnel needed for the future, the system of nursing education will need increased flexibility, additional cooperative and collaborative arrangements, broadened support, and increased emphasis on evaluation and research.*

In the spring of 1981 the Council of Baccalaureate and Higher Degree Programs of the NLN voted to send a resolution to the board of directors that sought baccalaureate education as the base for professional nursing. A position statement was prepared and was forwarded along with the resolution to the NLN board of directors. At the February 1982 board meeting the NLN board of directors accepted the resolution and prepared a position

---

*A statement by the board of directors, National League for Nursing, approved February 1972, Nurs. Outlook **20**(4):272, 1972. Copyright by the American Journal of Nursing Co.

statement on education. The position statement, which continued to support all avenues of registered nurse education, however, placed associate degree and diploma programs as fulfilling the technical role and the baccalaureate graduate as basic to the professional role. Immediately there was a great effort to have the board rescind the statement. Since that was not accomplished, the opponents of the position taken prepared four resolutions to be presented at the June 1983 NLN convention. The resolutions committee combined the four into one and recommended that the position paper not be rescinded. By a narrow margin of those members present at the convention the position statement became reaffirmed policy of the NLN. The NLN statement is given in Chapter 5.

With the NLN support, all major nursing organizations have gone on record as recognizing two levels of registered nurses. There was no timetable to the NLN position statement on education. The significance of the position statement provides new impetus in the evolving state of nursing education.

The issue of two levels had still not been resolved by 1984. The question remains as to what is technical nursing and what happens to practical nursing. From the data it appears there are three levels of nursing: (1) the vocational nurse being the practical nurse, (2) the technical nurse being the A.D.N. or diploma prepared nurse, and (3) the B.S.N. being the preprofessional, with the master's degree or doctorally prepared nurse being the professional nurse.

Higher education in nursing

For 20 years nursing has promoted the baccalaureate degree as the base for professional nursing. Simultaneously, nursing education at the master's and doctoral levels was developed and promoted as necessary for leadership positions.

In the early master's programs two leadership roles were identified as paramount, namely, education and administration. The content of the master's program was that of curriculum development, teaching, and evaluation, or adminstrative management. Then in the early 1970s it was determined that a master's degree in clinical nursing specialties was the appropriate next step from baccalaureate education. Thus formal preparation of the clinical specialist was set in motion.

To the purist in education the generalist in nursing was prepared at the baccalaureate level, the beginning specialist at the master's level, and the clinical researcher at the doctoral level. Educationally and for the benefit of clinical nursing this was sound planning. However, the clinical specialist route did not always benefit the educator or administrator who needed an additional set of theories and skills to function effectively.

By the late 1970s programs were available to the graduate student that provided a clinical specialty as core content with three leadership roles from which the student could choose: direct care (clinical specialist), educator, or administrator.

Among nurses there are some strong proponents that advanced degrees in administration should be a combination of business management and nursing and that advanced degrees in education should combine higher education and nursing.

By all standards, graduate education in nursing is young and doctoral education is in its infancy. Doctoral education is research oriented and helps to form the skills necessary to think definitively and draw conclusions, skills necessary for the clinical researcher, direct care giver, administrator, or educator.

Doctoral programs in nursing are limited in number and are not easily accessible, nor are there enough spaces for all who desire doctoral education. Therefore as nurses with master's degrees see a need for further education, doctoral degrees are secured in other fields (i.e., education, business management, philosophy, psychology, sociology, physiology, and anthropology). In 1982 there were 137 persons who graduated with doctoral education in nursing.

For further information the reader is referred to Chapter 6, Entry to Practice—Education, which treats in depth each type of educational program.

Chapter 16, Continuing Education, provides an explanation of the history and need of continuing education for the professional nurse.

NURSING EDUCATION FOR THE BLACK

Segregation in education has been a part of the American system since our country was founded. Education was originally intended for the wealthy, not the masses; for men, not women; for the professional, not the laborer. Historically, only those persons whose parents could afford to send them to school were able to receive an education. Although poor people learned to read and write, the formal educational process was denied to them. Women, it was determined, did not need to be educated, for their place was in the home. Laborers did not need formal education, since apprenticing was the appropriate way to learn a trade. The slave did not even need to know how to write, for his needs would be taken care of by the owner.

Booker T. Washington, a slave, took it on himself to learn to read and write and to secure an education. He made his own way, believing that by knowing how to read and write he and other black people could own their own land, produce their own food, and take care of their own basic needs. He was ultimately invited to be head of Tuskegee Institute, which was the first school established for the education of blacks beyond high school. At one time, there were 130 colleges for black students. Since 1964, however, many of these colleges have become integrated.

The separate-but-equal doctrine was established in 1896 when the Louisiana courts enunciated that races would be separated in railroad coaches. This separate-but-equal doctrine was enforced in 17 states and the District of Columbia on a mandatory basis and in 4 states on a local option basis. Utilizing the separate but equal doctrine, public education separated the races and thereby established a dual public education system—one for blacks and one for whites. This dual system did not end at public education but was perpetuated in private and public schools beyond secondary education. Thus nursing education, being only a part of the total, also functioned in a dual system. This dualism in education was found to be *unequal* by the U.S. Supreme Court in 1954 when it heard the *Brown vs. Topeka Board of Education* case; unequal in curricular offerings, teacher qualification, facilities, and learning resources.

As a result of the segregated system, black men and women who wanted to study nursing were denied admission to 90% of the schools of nursing. Blacks did not have primary and secondary education of the quality demanded by schools of nursing. The first college to establish a nursing program for blacks was Spelman College in Atlanta, which opened in 1881. Ten years later Dixie Hospital Training School, in cooperation with Hampton Institute of Virginia, established the second school for blacks; Providence Hospital in Chicago was also established in that same year. John A. Andrews Memorial Hospital, Tuskegee Institute, provided nursing education for blacks in 1892.

Separatism in educational institutions was only a small part of the nursing education problem for blacks; the same dual system existed in health care institutions also. There were hospitals for blacks and for whites, which made it even more difficult to secure clinical learning facilities for black students.

The pioneering black nurse Mary Mahoney gained admission to the New England Hospital of Women and Children and graduated in 1879. By 1908 there was a nucleus of black nurses who, recognizing the difficulties of the dual system of public education, which ultimately denied admission of black students into nursing education programs, formed the National Association for Colored Graduate Nurses (NACGN). There were 26 charter members, and Martha Franklin of Connecticut was its first president. Its goals were to (1) advance the standards and best interests of trained nurses, (2) break down discrimination in the nursing profession, and (3) develop leadership within the ranks of black nurses.

In 1920 the NACGN recognized that because of the separate-but-equal doctrine and the lack of equality in high schools, black people desiring to be nurses were denied admission to the better schools of nursing. Furthermore, in those schools which did educate the black nurse, minimum standards for accreditation were not being enforced by state boards of nursing. By 1936 the NACGN was urging state boards of nursing to enforce the minimum standards for accreditation even if it meant closing schools that admitted black students. This urging was taken to the ANA and the National League of Nursing Education by seeking their support to find ways of improving the schools. A curriculum committee was formed in 1936 to assist schools of nursing throughout the United States. However, improvement was slow to be accomplished.

Black students were often discouraged even from taking the required courses in the secondary schools that would qualify them for admission to the better schools. The NACGN urged the National Association for the Advancement of Colored People to work with them in improving the total educational system to wipe out the dual educational system. The NACGN then devised a plan to steer students to its better schools by counseling them to take the required courses that would qualify them for admission to schools of nursing.

Black nurses already prepared were thwarted in securing education beyond the RN diploma. They could not gain entrance into baccalaureate programs, nor were they admitted to graduate programs. Black RNs were frequently told that positions in administration and teaching were not available to them so they did not need advanced education. To compound the problem, salaries for black nurses were consistently lower than those for white nurses.

In 1935 the black nurses of Washington, D.C., faced serious educational difficulties. The nurses of Friedman Hospital wanted more education, and the only university in the area, Catholic University of America, would not admit them. If additional education was to be secured, the nurse had to move out of the District of Columbia, and even then more education was not easily obtained. Marie Brown Seymour sought help by asking a friend to determine if it was Catholic University's policy to deny admission to black nurses and, if so, what could be done to change the policy. A year later, in 1936, the way had been opened for the admission of blacks. Clara Bevely, a staff nurse at Friedman, was admitted to Catholic University of America and was graduated with a baccalaureate degree in 1944.

In 1939 the education committee of the NACGN learned that three of the schools for blacks were to be closed. The schools were John Andrews Hospital, Tuskegee Institute, Alabama; Dixie College in Virginia; and the LaMar School of the University of Georgia. These three schools supplied a great number of nurses for the area served. After obtaining the facts, the committee determined that every effort would be made to save the schools as well as to improve them. Each school was saved and improved, and in 1943 Dixie College joined with Hampton Institute to offer the first baccalaureate program in nursing for black nurses.

During this period other graduate programs were denying admission to black nurses for advanced study. The schools that were specifically singled out were Yale, Western Reserve, and the University of Maryland. Each of these schools suggested that graduates would be happier in a school closer to home. When the deans were queried, the NACGN learned that denial was primarily because the hospitals that were used for clinical experience would not allow black nurses to practice in their institutions. The problem of nursing education in universities and hospital schools of nursing was thus compounded because blacks could not be treated or work in a white hospital.

In 1945 and 1946, Western Reserve and Yale universities, respectively, admitted their first black students. Esther McCready, in 1950, instituted legal proceedings against the University of Maryland for denial of admission. On order of the Maryland Supreme Court, McCready was admitted.

Oklahoma University Medical Center admitted its first black student in 1951. Marie Fink was employed as the first black faculty member of the University of Oklahoma. By 1951 there were 330 schools admitting black students into their nursing programs, as compared to 29 in 1941.

It was not until 1954, when the U.S. Supreme Court heard the *Brown vs. Topeka Board of Education* case, that equal education became a right. Ten years later, in 1964, the Civil Rights Act made separatism of blacks and whites illegal in both education and health agencies.

The NACGN, living up to one of its stated goals, merged with the ANA in 1952, thereby paving the way for breaking down the discriminatory practices within the profession. Mabel Staupers, a black nurse, was instrumental in encouraging the NACGN to become part of the ANA. Blacks in nursing have had difficulty getting into the profession, and once in, have had little acceptance beyond the staff nurse position.

At the ANA convention of 1970, Dr. Lauranne Sams observed that of those nurses in attendance only 200 were black. She wondered about this and was encouraged to have a black nurses caucus to find out. On May 6, a caucus was held with 150 black nurses attending. From this caucus it was determined that they were concerned about and accountable to black people in a special way. There was a need for them to articulate the health needs of the black community as well as provide equal access to and mobility within the health care system.

A steering committee was formed to foster the impetus of the caucus. The committee met in December 1971 and again in March 1972 to further identify problems and map out strategies to assist the black nurse in gaining entrance into the mainstream of nursing. From these meetings, it was evident that tokenism existed rather than fulfillment of Staupers' dream of equal participation in the ANA. There had never been a black president of ANA; loss of identity had occurred, and there were only limited opportunities for black nurses to demonstrate their contributions to nursing. As the needs of black nurses were identified, it became evident that the ANA was not meeting these needs. Thus the steering committee decided to become a separate incorporated organization. In September 1972, the official National Black Nurses Association (NBNA) was incorporated.

The steering committee fostered many strategies for the ANA 1972 convention. Among them were symposia for black nurses and workshops devoted to exploring health needs of black people. The success of the steering committee was evidenced by the increase in attendance of black nurses (500 compared to 200 in 1970) and by the election of Ethelrine Shaw, a black nurse, to a vice presidency in ANA. The author had the privilege of losing this position to Shaw.

As of 1971-1972, of all those admitted to professional nursing, only 11.6% were black; a higher percentage of blacks were enrolled in practical nurse programs. As of 1972 there were approximately 20,000 black nurses.

There was still evidence in 1972 of discrimination in nursing for the black student and the prepared black nurse. The ANA House of Delegates, in the 1972 convention, voted to reaffirm its commitment of 1952 (when the NACGN merged with the ANA) to promote the welfare of black nurses. Many black nurses testified to the discriminatory practices and demanded that every effort be made to support *all* nurses and not just one segment of the profession. Among those nurses were black leaders such as Faye Wilson of the ANA Board of Directors. From the 1972 convention the ANA developed a strong affirmative action program with Ethelrine Shaw as its chairman. An ombudsman was employed in 1974 to assist black nurses in coping with the system, be it in a service or education situation.

One black nurse described her situation in an autobiography published in 1974. On applying to a professional school of nursing in 1969, she was denied admission because she lacked the necessary qualifications and was told to apply to a vocational school of nursing where she would qualify. Instead, she asked what she lacked to qualify for the professional school. She was given the qualifications and proceeded to secure the necessary educational experiences and reapplied. This time she was admitted. On discussing this with white students, she learned that they had not been made to meet the same qualifications. In other words the black student had to meet additional requirements for admission.

Since graduation, this nurse, along with 50 other black nurses, admitted to being under stress and not feeling at ease in the work situation. Ten of the 50 believed themselves qualified to be promoted and yet were passed over; 40 of these nurses felt less respected by the licensed practical nurses and nurse aides even though a large percentage of those workers were black.

In the intervening years much has been done by organized nursing to obtain equal opportunities for blacks in nursing. The National Student Nurses' Association implemented a "breakthrough" program whereby blacks would be sought and encouraged to gain admittance to nursing schools. The program was designed to assist students in succeeding in schools of nursing. Schools of nursing have made an effort to provide special preparatory course work, tutors, and preceptors for students needing assistance. Lorraine Baugh and other black nurse leaders provide consultation to faculty on the subject of retaining black students. Baugh maintains that it is one thing to admit students and another to retain them so that they become practicing nurses. Thus faculties must concentrate on how to help the student achieve the goals of the college.

The NABN is an active association and celebrated its tenth anniversary in 1981 in Cleveland. The organization's objectives are to speak out in behalf of blacks in nursing, to improve health care for blacks, and to improve the quality of education for blacks. In 1980 at the ANA convention blacks went on record as opposing the 1985 education proposal, maintaining it was discriminatory against blacks. Educational mobility was given high priority with the express belief that all persons should be able to move from a minimum level of education program and progress to a higher level, thus giving the LPN or RN access to B.S.N., M.S.N., or Ph.D. degrees in nursing.

The Western Interstate Commission in Nursing Education has not only promoted the education of the black but also developed curricular content on care of people of ethnic color. Schools of nursing were encouraged to include the content in their curricula. Since 1975 most schools have included cultural aspects in the content of the planned program of studies. All students graduating now are expected to be familiar with these. Nursing care of the black is being improved through education.

Black nurses have obtained Ph.D. degrees in nursing and other fields. They are fulfilling major leadership roles as deans of colleges of nursing and as directors of nursing in major health care facilities and in national organizations. Although black nurses have a separate organization, they are very much involved in the ANA, NLN, and other all-purpose organizations for nurses. Their leadership is evident and strong.

By the efforts of black nurses and others, Barbara Nichols became the first black president of the ANA in June 1978 and served two terms.

An interesting note in black nurse history is the lack of "documentation of the first Afro-American male nurse in the United States or even a statistical report as to its total population" (Lewis, 1981). Lewis, a black male nurse in Chicago, is a clinical specialist in ambulatory services. He writes that most black male nurses work in situations such as emergency rooms, intensive care units, and administration, where their role as a nurse is not evident. Lewis further asserts that this behavior is traced to the history of the slavery of the black male and the subservient role forced on the male. His article, "A Black Perspective: Afro-American Men in Nursing," provides a brief history on the black male nurse.

Throughout the nursing profession there are black and white leaders working to promote the black nurse, to promote the health and welfare of black people, and to end the discriminatory practices in all areas of society.

SUMMARY

Developments in nursing education during the past 160 years closely parallel the changes in the status of women in America during that period. Progress in nursing education has contributed to enabling nursing to change from a dependent, limited vocation with minimum social and legal status to an occupation on the threshold of professional freedom and opportunity for unlimited progress.

Discussion questions

1. Discuss the system of religious orders and the relationship to nursing education in the early twentieth century.
2. Discuss the impact of the need for clinical research to doctoral study in nursing.
3. Discuss what impact there might be if all registered nurse education occurred at the baccalaureate level.
4. Discuss the impact of early education of black nurses on today's nursing education.

REFERENCES

Cofer, A.: Autobiography of a black nurse, Am. J. Nurs. 75:1837, Oct. 1974.
Goldmark, J.: Nursing and nursing education in the U.S., New York, 1923, Macmillan Co.
How separate? How equal? (editorial), Change 9:11, Sept. 1974.
Institute of Medicine: Nursing and nursing education: public policies and private actions, Washington, D.C., 1983, The Institute.
Johnson, W.L.: Admission of men and ethnic minorities to schools of nursing 1971-72, Nurs. Outlook 22:48, Jan. 1974.
Lewis, M.C.: A black perspective: Afro-American men in nursing, Nurs. Leadership 4(4):31-33, 1981.
Miller, H.S.: The history of Chi Eta Phi sorority, Inc., 1932-1967, Washington, D.C., 1968, The Association for the Study of Negro Life and History, Inc.
Miller, K.: Race adjustment: the everlasting stain, New York, 1968, Arno Press and the New York Times.
Miller, M.H.: On blacks entering nursing, Nurs. Forum 12:248, 1972.
National Commission on Nursing, American Hospital Association: Summary report and recommendations, Chicago, 1983, The Association.

Pifer, A.: Viewpoint—how well has higher education served black Americans? Change **6**:9, April 1974.

Reid, I.S.: Together black women, New York, 1972, Emerson Hall Publishers, Inc.

Smith, G.I.: From invisibility to blackness: the story of the National Black Nurses' Association, Nurs. Outlook **23**:225, April 1975.

Staupers, M.K.: No time for prejudice, New York, 1961. Macmillan Co.

Vaughn, J.C.: Educational preparation for nursing, 1982, Nurs. Health Care **4**(8):460, 1983.

SUGGESTED READINGS

Anderson, B.E.: Nursing education in community junior colleges, Philadelphia, 1966, J.B. Lippincott Co.

Brower, H.T.: Potential advantages and hazards of nontraditional education for nurses, Nurs. Health Care **3**(5):268, 1982.

Brown, E.L.: Nursing reconsidered: a study of change, Philadelphia, 1970 (part I), 1971 (part II), J.B. Lippincott Co.

Bullough, V.L., and Bullough, B.: The emergence of modern nursing, ed. 2, New York, 1969, The Macmillan Co.

Dietz, L.D., and Lehorzky, A.: History and modern nursing, ed. 2, Philadelphia, 1967, F.A. Davis Co.

Fine, R.B.: The supply and demand of nursing administration, Nurs. Health Care **4**(1):10, 1983.

Galarowicz, L.: Closing a diploma school: a time for flexibility and creativity, Nurs. Health Care **4**(4):188, 1983.

Griffin, G.J., and King, J.: Jensen's history and trends of professional nursing, ed. 7, St. Louis, 1974, The C.V. Mosby Co.

Holzemer, W.L.: Quality in graduate nursing education, Nurs. Health Care **3**(10):536, 1982.

Lysaught, J., editor: Action in nursing, New York, 1974, McGraw-Hill Book Co.

Mooneyhan, E.L.: The demise of a baccalaureate program for registered nurse: lessons learned, Nurs. Health Care **4**(4):192, 1983.

National Commission for the Study of Nursing and Nursing Education (Jerome P. Lysaught, director): An abstract for action, New York, 1970, McGraw-Hill Book Co.

Nightingale, F.: Notes on nursing, what it is and what it is not, New York, 1946, Appleton-Century-Crofts, Inc. (Reprint of article originally published in 1860.)

Perry, S.E.: A doctorate—necessary but not sufficient, Nurs. Outlook **30**(2):95, 1982.

Reed, S.B., and Taira, F.: Point/counterpoint: is that doctorate necessary? Nurs. Outlook **31**(1):12, 1983.

Robb, I.H.: In papers and discussions of the International Congress of Charities, Correction, and Philanthropy held in Chicago in 1893, New York, 1949, National League of Nursing Education.

Roberts, M.M.: American nursing history and interpretation, New York, 1961, The Macmillan Co.

U.S. Department of Health, Education, and Welfare: Toward quality in nursing, needs and goals. Surgeon General's Report, Public Health Service pub. no. 992, Washington, D.C., 1963, The Department.

Vaughn, J.C., and Johnson, W.L.: Educational preparation for nursing 1978, Nurs. Outlook **27**:608, Sept. 1979.

CHAPTER 4
Evolution of theories for nursing

JOANNE MARCHIONE

OBJECTIVE: On completion of this chapter, the student of nursing will be able to utilize the various theories of nursing.

As nursing service and nursing education evolved, the need to develop a science of nursing became a goal of many nurses in leadership positions. The question "What is nursing?" has become a perennial issue. Is nursing an art, a science, or both? Is nursing an applied science, does it have its own body of knowledge? Nurse scholars of the past 2 decades have raised many questions such as these. This line of inquiry has resulted in a proliferation of articles and books on theories and theory development in nursing. Numerous conferences have also been held for the express purpose of the development and evaluation of nursing theories. This chapter will examine the current status of nursing theory from a historical-evaluative perspective.

In this chapter the student is invited to explore the following issues: (1) the nature of a theory, (2) the status of nursing theories and nursing models, (3) the evolution of nursing theory development, (4) the purposes of nursing theory, (5) evaluation of nursing theory, and (6) future directions of nursing theory development.

NATURE OF A THEORY

Theories have been viewed from many perspectives, and theory definitions have varied widely from theorist to theorist. This variability in theory definition has been attributed to the diverse philosophical approaches and value orientations of the theorists who have conceptualized and developed theories.

Theories in their most fundamental sense refer to abstract or symbolic ways of finding order in reality. They are guesses about what is being observed and experienced. All humans use this level of theorizing to label, describe, and explain their world. Kaplan suggests that theory formation may be the most important and distinctive attribute that sets human beings apart from other animals.[*]

In a more formal sense, theories are regarded as systematic accounts of the relationships among sets of variables.[†] Variables refer to objects that have the capacity to change and whose observable features can be differentiated.[‡] From this perspective a theory is defined as a set of interrelated variables,

---

[*]Kaplan, A.: The conduct of inquiry: methodology for behavioral science, San Francisco, 1964, Chandler Publishing Co., pp. 294-297.

[†]Kerlinger, F.: Behavioral research, a conceptual approach, New York, 1979, Holt, Rinehart & Winston, p. 64.

[‡]For a further discussion of four types of variables of importance to the process of theory development, see Chinn, P., and Jacobs, M.: Theory and nursing: a systematic approach, St. Louis, 1983, The C.V. Mosby Co., pp. 91-93.

definitions, and propositions that present a systematic view of phenomena by specifying relations among variables, with the purpose of explaining natural phenomena.*

Those who have defined theories for the practice disciplines have sometimes taken a more complex view. This is seen, for example, in the following theory definition: "A theory is an internally consistent body of relational statements about phenomena which is useful for prediction and prescription."†

With these two views, theories can be analyzed by examining their structure or form, their content or substance, their movement or process, and their context or surroundings.

The following example is a hypothetical situation contrived as a game‡ to assist the reader in clarifying the various ideas associated with theories and theory building.

Fig. 1 is a pictorial model of an invented object. Suppose that you, the reader, had gone out into your back yard one morning when you were home alone only to discover that a foreign object was occupying the entire land space, 8 × 8 feet. Furthermore, suppose that the height of this object was also 8 feet. Being human, you would probably try to explain the object for yourself before summoning help or assistance from another person. If you tended to think deductively, your line of questioning might proceed as follows:

1. *What is this strange object?* Inventing a name for a foreign object is the logical inclination of humans. This labeling or conceptual process is the first step in theory building.

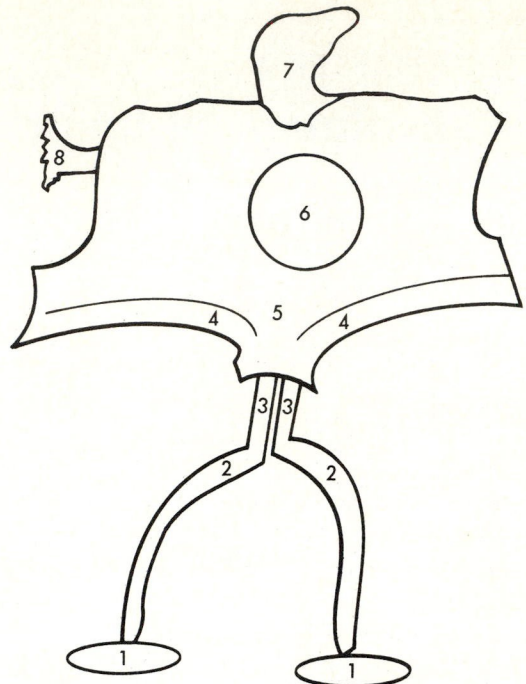

Fig. 1. Pictorial model of an invented object, metaphila.

2. *What are its component parts?* If you divided the object into numbered parts and gave each part a name, you would be able to begin to describe it to others. This division into parts and naming of the parts is called *factor isolating* and is regarded as the first level of theory building.

3. *How does each part relate to each other part, and how do these parts relate to the whole object?* When you have described each of the eight numbered parts and have discussed how each part relates to the other parts and to the object as a whole, you have completed the second level of theory building, that is, *factor-relating theorizing.*

Having answered these questions, you have now invented a symbolized structure for the foreign object. Answer the following questions. Have fun theorizing. Make up a nonsense word or familiar name for the foreign object and each of its parts.

---

*Kerlinger, F.: Behavioral research, a conceptual approach, New York, 1979, Holt, Rinehart & Winston, p. 64.
†Hempel, C.G.: Fundamentals of concept formation in empirical science, International Encyclopedia of United Science, vol. 2, no. 7, Chicago, 1952, University of Chicago Press.
‡Inspired by a similar game developed by Em Olivia Bevis and described in *Curriculum Building in Nursing: a Process*, St. Louis, 1973, The C.V. Mosby Co., pp. 130-131. It is based on the theory development work described by James Dickoff and Patricia James in the article "A Theory of Theories: a Position Paper," Nurs. Res. **17:**420, Oct. 1968.

Continue with the theory-building process. The next questions logically raised are the following: (4) What does the foreign object do? (5) How does it function? (6) Under what circumstances will it work?

Using your repertoire of previously perceived images, you would probably begin to guess its capabilities and make predictions about how it works. Invent a hypothesis about how it works and state what conditions are necessary to activate it. Describe the circumstances that would cause it to work and those which would prevent it from working according to your hypothesis. Now that you have predicted its function and identified in cause-effect statements those circumstances that would promote or prevent the object's movement, you have completed level three of theory building. You have now evolved a situation-relating level theory. This third level of theory building is concerned with predictive and promotive or inhibitive theorizing. In answering these questions, you have provided the context or subject matter for theorizing about the foreign object.

Suppose you invented a plan based on your hypothesis of how it functions, to move it or cause it to move, elsewhere. You could develop a step-by-step method for activating the object. This plan, with its step-by-step description, is sometimes called a cognitive map or paradigm. As you systematically identified each of the steps necessary to activate the object and described the sequence of movements, you creatively prescribed the movement or process of the invented object. This final level of theory building is known as *situation-producing theory*.

You are now ready to test your theory. Convinced that your paradigm will work, you begin to test its accuracy by following each step of the plan. This testing phase is the beginning of the research process. Once your hypothesis if validated or refuted, you have moved from theorizing to operationalizing the theory in the real world of practice.

You have just explained for yourself this foreign object. You have predicted and prescribed its use.

This pictorial representation of an abstract invention has now become concrete. You have given it a real meaning and you can explain it to anyone.

This exercise is easily applied to nursing and nursing phenomena. For example, suppose this object were a space person who was aware of your capabilities as a nurse. Further, suppose that this space person came to seek your assistance through a mutual communication system activated by you. Once you have discovered the answers to your theoretical questions about what the space object is and how it functions, you can begin to understand how to assist it by making predictions about what it needs. This is the essence of nursing theory. Nurse theorists have focused on theorizing about humans and their needs. The goal of nursing theorists has been the development of theories that would direct practitioners to assist humans in their attainment of health. An essential factor in assisting a human toward the goal of health is a knowledge of the environment in which the person dwells. Nurse theorists have also studied the environment. For example, time, space, gravity, relationship with others, and sensation are all necessary components for scientific inquiry into the knowledge of healthy humans. This aspect of the theoretical question is referred to as the context, surrounding, or circumstances that contribute to the totality of perceived reality about the essence and capabilities of humans.

Now that this game of theory building has been completed, a formal discussion of the elements of a theory follows.

The *structural* components of a theory, then, are the concepts or labels, constructs or variables, and propositions or designs that architecturally make up its form. *Concepts* are symbolic or abstract representations, such as the word "metaphila,"* used to describe objects of reality and their properties, events, and relationships. Concepts provide the language for communicating a theory and indicate the content or subject matter on which a theory is

---

*Name invented to describe the foreign object in Fig. 1.

based. Concepts convey general ideas about observed events and objects. Through precise and explicit definitions, theorists are able to differentiate the meaning of one concept from another.

Constructs are referred to in this chapter as more than one word that represents the manner in which one phenomenon differs from other phenomena. For example, the concept ''nurse'' takes on a totally different connotation when it is transformed into the construct ''nurse researcher.'' Likewise, the construct ''family nurse practitioner'' connotes something entirely different from the construct ''nurse researcher'' or the concept ''nurse.'' Constructs are defined on the basis of observables, and they convey more meaning than an individual concept separately.*

Concepts are defined in two ways. First, operationally, concepts are defined by assigning word meanings that link the abstract idea or symbol to the world of reality, thus making them useful or observable. Second, constitutionally, concepts are defined by assigning statements that provide meaning by linking the defined concept with other concepts in a circular fashion. Hempel† has referred to these two types of conceptual definitions as derived and primitive. Both operational and constitutive concepts are necessary to provide the structure of a theory and to link theory to research. It is only through operational definitions that a theory can be empirically validated. To illustrate the difference between operational and primitive statements consider this example: ''A nurse is a person'' versus ''A nurse is a person educated as a scientist who assists another person in the attainment of health.'' In the first, or primitive, definition the concept ''nurse'' is linked to the concept ''person'' in a circular way, leading us to ask what is a person? However, in the second definition variability has been introduced. Now the phenomenon ''nurse''

can be directly observed in action and operationalized. A theory cannot be tested empirically if none of its concepts are defined operationally, since the operationally defined concepts alone provide the researchable indexes for theory validation.

Propositions provide the design for a theory structure. Propositions are the verbal and/or mathematical statements used to connect, or link, the concepts and/or constructs of a theory. The two types of propositions most often found in a theory are axioms and postulates. Axioms are the initial statements of a theory that are regarded by the theorists as truths from which other propositions are derived. Postulates are the deductive statements of position or supposition about the types of relationships between the concepts of the theory. In relating each part of the foreign object, or ''metaphila,'' to another part and to the whole and formulating hypotheses about its action, you have formulated propositions to explain the invented phenomenon. Postulates must be proved or disproved by logical reasoning or analysis and provide the explanatory power of a theory.

Postulates that contain operationally defined concepts are labeled ''hypotheses.'' Hypotheses are the specific statements that lead to evaulation of a theory. They are predictive or prescriptive suppositions about the probable relationship and value of two or more operationally defined concepts.*

Theory content or substance refers to the subject matter chosen for study by the theorist and the assumptions held in relation to this subject matter. For example, theorist A, who has chosen an ecological model for the study of man, would be concerned with human-environment interrelationships, whereas theorist B, who has chosen a social model for the study of man, would be concerned with humans in interaction with other humans. Therefore the conclusions derived by theorist A from ecological content would be quite different from those of theorist B, whose content would be

---

*Kaplan, A.: The conduct of inquiry: methodology for behavorial science, San Francisco, 1964, Chandler Publishing Co.
†Hempel, C.G.: Fundamentals of concept formation in empirical science, International Encyclopedia of Unified Science, vol. 2, no. 7, Chicago, 1952, University of Chicago Press, pp. 206-207.

---

*Dubin, R.: Theory building, New York, 1978, The Free Press, pp. 205-207.

sociological in perspective. Nurse theorists have tended to be less interested in identifying and describing theory content than in their concern for the structural elements of theory development.*

The process of a theory has been identified as the actions or behaviors ascribed to the theorist that would move the theory forward or implement it.† King's theory of nursing process provides an illustration of the process component of theory development.‡

The process of a theory can also be found in the philosophical perspective and methodological approaches by which the theorists have chosen to move between theory building and theory testing. Two of these approaches will be examined here.

When a theorist utilizes a deductive mode for theory development, as was suggested in the metaphila game, the logical statements of a theory move from a general notion of what a phenomenon is to a particular understanding of what is happening with the phenomenon by inferential investigation. In this approach some of the proposed hypotheses may be deemed unsuitable and eliminated without investigation while the remaining hypotheses would be tested empirically and confirmed or rejected.§

In a deductive or Cartesian‖ approach to theory development the theorist identifies general state-

ments and specific antecedent conditions that serve as premises for the explanation of particular facts. This logicodeductive approach, such as that used in the metaphila game, provides the theorist with a capacity for showing logical relationships between premises and conclusions about phenomena and prevents the inference of cause-effect relationships.* The theoretical formulations of Martha Rogers in the "life process model" have been identified by Rinehart as those in which a deductive methodology has been utilized.

The inductive mode of theory development, sometimes referred to as the Socratic† approach, provides a means for the theorist to move from empirical observations or particulars to general or abstract statements about phenomena. This approach promotes data collection from reality situations such as practice arenas of nursing with the purpose of deriving inferential statements about the boundaries or parameters of the studied phenomenon, for example, humans. Inductive theories reflect an existential phenomenological philosophical perspective. That is, the theorist focuses on existing elements of study and their particular movement at a given moment in time, working in a reverse process to formulate generalizations about those phenomena. If in the metaphila game your line of questioning had begun with the situation-producing level and you had worked backward to the first level of naming and isolating the features of the foreign object, you would have utilized an inductive methodology. You may also want to try this approach to theory development. Zderad and Patterson‡ use this method in their study of humanistic nursing phenomena, while Orem§ has suggested the inductive method in theorizing on self-care.

*Phillips, J.R.: Nursing systems and nursing models, Image **9:**4-7, Feb. 1977.
†Stevens, B.J.: Nursing theory: analysis, application, evaluation, Boston, 1979, Little, Brown & Co.
‡King, I.M.: Toward a theory for nursing, New York, 1971, John Wiley & Sons, Inc.; and Daubenmire, M.J., and King, I.M.: Nursing process models: a systems approach, Nurs. Outlook **21:**512-517, 1973; and King, I.M.: A theory of nursing: systems, concepts, process, New York, 1981, John Wiley & Sons, Inc.
§Rinehart, J.: The "how" of theory development in nursing. In Theory development: what, why, how? Pub. No. 15-1708, New York, 1978, National League for Nursing.
‖The philosopher Descartes promoted the use of the logicodeductive approach to the development of theories, often referred to as Cartesian. Aristotle also fostered the deductive process as a line of reasoning.

*Kaplan, A.: The conduct of inquiry: methodology for behavioral science, San Francisco, 1964, Chandler Publishing Co.
†For the philosopher Socrates, who promoted an inductive approach to reasoning.
‡Patterson, J.: The tortuous way toward nursing theory. In Theory development: what, why, how? Pub. No. 15-1708, New York, 1978, National League for Nursing, pp. 49-66.
§Orem, D.: Nursing: concepts of practice, ed. 2, New York, 1980, McGraw-Hill Book Co.

The philosophical approach and the focus of theory development of each theory reflect the value orientation of each theorist. The selected process or methodology has provided the theorist with the freedom to move in the direction of choice and the flexibility to choose one approach in preference over another. The reader is invited to explore a similar game exercise delineated by Bevis* for an increased understanding and enjoyment of the process of theory development.

Structure, content, process, and context are interrelated elements of a theory. They are often implicit or not adequately stated explicitly. Often theorists have focused on the description or development of one or two of these elements while giving negligible attention to the others. A theory is regarded as complete or satisfactory if the structure, content, process, and context are interrelated and interwoven. Often, however, one or more of these elements has not been given sufficient attention by the theorist. One element of the theory—for example, structure—may receive sufficient description while the other components may be negligibly described or not described at all.

The nature of theories can also be understood by analysis of the heuristic devices by which they are often illustrated. For example, models, paradigms, and taxonomies are scientific, heuristic devices used to help illustrate a theory, a portion of a theory, or multiple theories. McKay has cogently differentiated these three concepts as follows: "Taxonomy is the process of classification of phenomena according to systems."† To arrange in a taxonomy is to group concepts and constructs into related properties. If all the types of foreign objects similar to the foreign object in the metaphila game were differentiated according to color, sex, capacity to function, variation in design, and so on, a taxonomy for existing metaphilae would have

begun to evolve. In nursing, theorists have built taxonomies to explain human variations.

"Paradigms are patterns or schemes which attempt to organize or describe a process," according to McKay. Paradigms can be regarded as maps or designs that move the user—a nurse practitioner, for example—to action. In the metaphila game you were able to develop a paradigm at the situation-producing level of theory building.

McKay describes models as follows: "Models are symbolic representations of perceptual phenomena . . . every model is a pattern of symbols, rules and process regarded as matching in part or in totality, an existing perceptual complex." Models are examples or analogies that are developed to provide a visual impression of something that is not directly observable. The model of the foreign object in the metaphila game gave a visual impression of a conceptual invention.

Models are differentiated according to their level of abstraction and according to the metaphor conveyed by the model. The three most common levels of abstraction used to convey a theory or theorem are iconics or pictorial models (such as that in Fig. 1 depicting the foreign object); descriptive models, also known as paradigms; and mathematical models or numerical formulations to describe a conceptual invention. The three most popular twentieth century metaphors used by scientists to convey a theory are "machine" models, "organism" models, and "field" models. Which of these did you use to characterize the foreign object? You may wish to pursue other suggested readings for a further elaboration of these heuristic devices.*

Conceptual frameworks have been defined as networks within which questions, theories, and data fit together.† These frameworks refer to the

---

*Bevis, E.O.: Curriculum building in nursing: a process, St. Louis, 1973, The C.V. Mosby Co., pp. 130-131.

†McKay, R.: Theories, models, and systems for nursing, Nurs. Res. **18:**394, Sept.-Oct. 1969.

*Meadows, P.: Models, systems and science, Am. Sociol. Rev. **22:**3-9, Feb. 1957; and Chinn, P., and Jacobs, M.: Theory and nursing: a systematic approach, St. Louis, 1983, The C.V. Mosby Co.

†Newman, M.: Theory development in nursing, Philadelphia, 1979, F.A. Davis Co.

global ideas about the individuals, groups, situations, and events of interest to a discipline. They provide the substance for theorizing and research but do not require the theorist to delineate and test the propositions that are either inherently or explicitly contained in the theory. The following lists and Fig. 2 provide both a pictorial and a descriptive model for illustrating the comparison between theories and conceptual frameworks. Newman equates conceptual frameworks with conceptual or descriptive models. A theory is a specific relationship between two or more concepts.

PURPOSE OF CONCEPTUAL FRAMEWORK

1. Provides a focus of inquiry
2. Provides a network for showing the relationship between given theories, concepts, questions, and data
3. Provides a mechanism for the identification of theory development

PURPOSE OF A THEORY

1. Provides an explanation of the phenomenon in question
2. Is testable
3. Is refutable
4. Is alterable

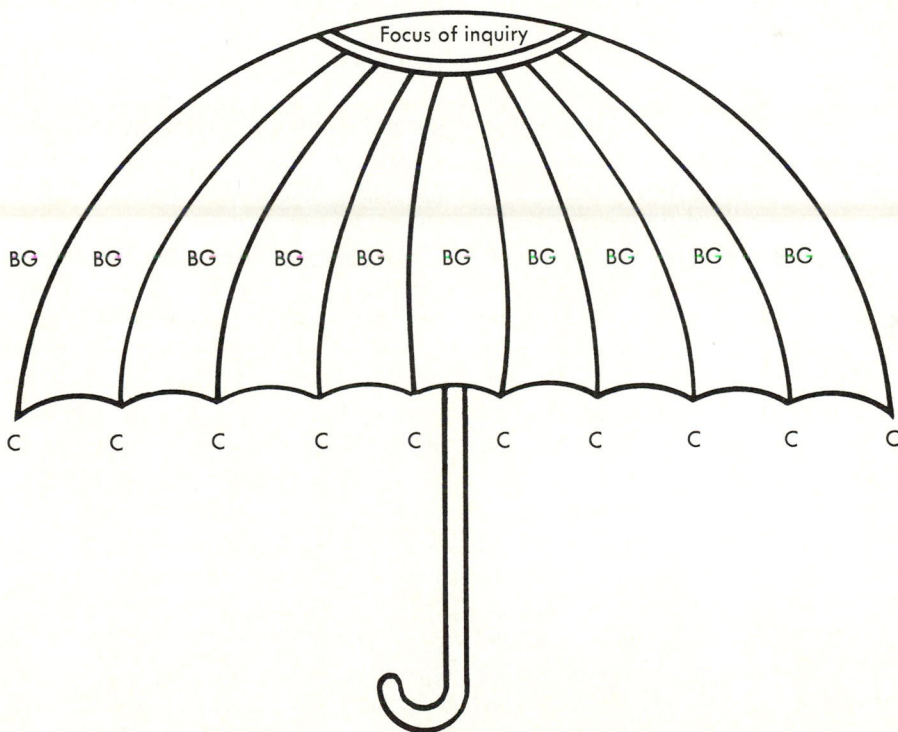

Fig. 2. A conceptual framework is a network within which questions, theories, and data fit together. It is made up of the focus of inquiry, concepts *(C)*, and broad generalizations *(BG)*. (Modified from Newman, M.: Theory development in nursing, Philadelphia, 1979, F.A. Davis Co.)

Taxonomies, paradigms, models, and conceptual frameworks alone are often insufficient to predict and control reality. Only when they are used together and when all the elements of a theory, that is, structure, content, process, and context, are made explicit and validated does a theoretical formulation reach maturity.

According to Kerlinger, theory development is the basic purpose of science.* Theory development for nursing could provide valid explanations of nursing phenomena and legitimate control of nursing practice. The challenging process of the development of nursing theory has already begun. The momentum achieved by the theorists toward the development of nursing theories in the last decade is both exciting and awesome. For a further understanding of the language of theories the reader is referred to the glossary of terms at the end of the book.

STATUS OF NURSING THEORIES AND NURSING MODELS

Newman has identified three approaches to the discovery of nursing theory that have emerged since 1962. These approaches have been identified as (1) the "borrowing" of theories from other related disciplines with the intent to integrate these theories into a science of nursing, (2) an analysis of nursing practice situations in search of conceptual relationships, and (3) the creation of conceptual systems from which theories could be derived.†

The first approach, which was encouraged by the federal funding of nurse scientist programs in 1962, often contributed "minimally" to the knowledge of nursing science. Nurse scientists prepared in other disciplines soon discovered, in attempting to test and validate relevant borrowed theories, that the data were more specifically and explicitly re-

lated to the other discipline than they were to the discipline of nursing.

Further, opponents of this first approach, while recognizing the relevance of borrowed knowledge for nursing practice, argued that nursing theory and practice would be incomplete until nurses learned to investigate questions of specific concern to nurses.*

Proponents of the second approach, that of searching for theoretical frameworks through analysis of nursing practice, asserted that change was the prime purpose or goal of practitioner-scientists (nurses) and that theoretical underpinnings could only be discovered and tested in the practice arenas.†

The third and more recent approach to nursing theory development, that of the creation of conceptual systems for theory derivation, was first described in the literature in 1970. Identifying unified man as the phenomenon of focus for nursing, Martha Rogers in an *Introduction to the Theoretical Basis of Nursing,* evolved a set of principles and postulates based on a synthesis of assumptions about man and man's environment from which theoretical questions about humans could be derived and tested.

At the same time, other nurse theorists were developing conceptual systems for the derivation of nursing theory. For example, Johnson proposed that nurses utilize an elaborate behavioral systems approach to the study of man. King promoted the use of a nursing process model that included social systems, interpersonal relationships, perceptions, and health as the variables for nursing theory development. Roy identified an adaptive model,

---

*Kerlinger, F.: Behavioral research: a conceptual approach, New York, 1979, Holt, Rinehart, & Winston, p. 64.
†Newman, M.A.: Nursing's theoretical evolution, Nurs. Outlook **20:**449-453, July 1972.

---

*Johnson, D.: Theory in nursing borrowed and unique, Nurs. Res. **17:**206-209, May-June 1968.
†Johnson, D.: One conceptual model of nursing, presented April 25, 1968, Vanderbilt University, Nashville, Tenn. (unpublished); Patterson, J.: The tortuous way toward nursing theory. In Theory development: what, why, how? Pub. No. 15-1708, New York, 1978, National League for Nursing; Rogers, M.E.: An introduction to the theoretical basis of nursing, Philadelphia, 1970, F.A. Davis Co.

whereas Orem utilized a self-care model from which theoretical questions relevant to nursing could be tested. From these seminal works, many models for nursing theory development evolved in the 1970s.*

Flaskerud and Halloran have noted that progress in developing nursing theory has slowed considerably since the proliferation of work done in the late 1960s and early 1970s. They have suggested one reason for the lag is that nurses continue to believe that theories from other disciplines are better developed than their own.†

According to Walker and Avant, a plateau seems to have been reached in nursing theory development, with nurse theorists presently focusing their attention on the differences between models and theories. This focus is seen as a deterrent to theory development. In order to promote the further development of nursing theory in the 1980s, it has been recommended that nurse theorists direct their efforts toward content analysis and testing of existing theories.‡

Some nurse theorists believe that nursing "theories" do not exist. Fawcett, for example, states that "the nursing literature yields little evidence of formulations that might be considered nursing theory" and that, although conceptual models of nursing have been demonstrated as useful for practice, "they cannot be empirically tested because of the abstract nature of their concepts."§ Menke has also suggested that nursing theory development has lacked specific direction due to lack of organization and a laissez-faire route to theory discovery.*

THE EMERGENCE OF NURSING THEORY DEVELOPMENT AND THE PIONEERS OF THEORY DEVELOPMENT

The emergence of nursing theory development can be traced to the time of Nightingale. Nightingale stressed, in her nineteenth century writings, the need for a theoretical basis on which nursing education and nursing practice must be built. Nightingale equated the laws of nursing with the laws of health and urged nurses to search for and identify these laws. She implored nurse educators and practitioners to search for principles and laws to govern practice. She encouraged nurse leaders to develop a distinct definition of nursing and developed a curriculum designed to meet the holistic needs of humans in illness and in health, which required a liberal education as its foundation.†

It was from this perspective that modern nurse leaders began their quest for nursing theory. However, the Nightingale perspective was somewhat misplaced during the turn of the century. A perspective of nursing that focused on illness and utilized a medical model to guide nursing practice was prevalent until the early 1950s.

Three nurse educators of the early 1950s who have been credited with the pioneering of nursing theory development are Peplau, Henderson, and Orlando. They utilized a conceptual framework which reflected the view that nursing had as its basic premise the interpersonal process. They attempted to formulate propositions, laws, and hypotheses based on this assumption and urged their students to test and validate these hypotheses through research. This approach was primarily developmental, and much of the knowledge base was

*Orem, D.E.: Nursing: concepts of practice, New York, 1971, McGraw-Hill Book Co.; King, I.M.: Toward a theory for nursing, New York, 1971, John Wiley & Sons, Inc.; Murphy, J.F., editor: Theoretical issues in professional nursing, New York, 1971, Appleton-Century-Crofts; and Roy, Sister C.: Adaptation: a conceptual framework for nursing, Nurs. Outlook **18:**42-45.
†Flaskerud, J., and Halloran, E.: Areas of agreement in nursing theory development, Adv. Nurs. Sci. **3**(1):1-7, 1980.
‡Walker, L., and Avant, K.: Strategies for theory construction in nursing, Norwalk, Conn., 1983, Appleton-Century-Crofts, p. 177.
§Fawcett, J.: The relationship between theory and research: a double helix, Adv. Nurs. Sci. **1:**58, Oct. 1978.

*Menke, E.M.: Theory development: a challenge for nursing. In Chaska, N.L., editor: The nursing profession: views through the mist, New York, 1978, McGraw-Hill Book Co.
†Nightingale, F.: Notes on nursing: what it is and what it is not, Philadelphia, 1860, J.B. Lippincott Co.

borrowed from the discipline of psychology. Inherent in these seminal theoretical formulations was the assumption that humans value, strive for, and have a right to independence and that nursing's goal was to foster this independence.*

Nurse leaders of the early 1960s advanced the view that the goal of nursing was to meet human needs. This conceptualization led to the publication of such texts as that of Abdellah and co-workers, which evolved conceptual frameworks that focus on the identification of "patient problems" and their need resolutions.†

A series of nursing theory conferences held at the University of Kansas beginning in 1969 resulted in a proliferation of publications related to theory development. These writings reflected a heightened search for models and theories designed to unify existing knowledge, to continue to describe and explain phenomena, and to foster the predictive and prescriptive skills needed in a practice discipline.

Courses in theory development and evaluation have been included in curricula of graduate and undergraduate schools throughout the country. Nurse theorists of the 1970s, such as Rogers, King, Orem, Johnson (see earlier citations of their work), Leininger,‡ and Roy,§ have profoundly influenced the future direction of nursing and nursing theory development.

The second annual Nurse Educator Conference held in 1978 in New York City was a historical event. It was the first time that many of the pioneer theorists were congregated to discuss the nature of nursing theory. This meeting marked another milestone in the development of nursing theories.*

THE WHY OF NURSING THEORY: NURSING THEORY FOR WHAT END?

Interest in nursing theory development emerged for two reasons: (1) nursing leaders saw theory development as a means of clearly establishing nursing as a profession, and (2) growth and enrichment of theory were important for nursing by their intrinsic value regardless of their other values.†

Nurse scientists generally agree that the basic goals of theory development in nursing are to generate knowledge that would facilitate the improvement of practice, act as a guide to research, and form the foundations of nursing education.

The primary aim of nursing theory is to add to the knowledge, understanding, and control of the world of nursing. The research activities associated with the examination of various nursing theories should result in various correlations of the phenomena of focus and the validations or refutations of the hypotheses derived from the specific theories being examined. Research has its foundation in theory, and theory is examined, validated, and/or revised through research. Therefore nursing research and nursing theory are corequisite to the generation of nursing knowledge.

King has suggested that the generation of nursing theory is not solely for the purpose of discovering new knowledge. Theories also serve as a means of (1) organizing known facts into logical systems for greater perceptual clarity, (2) finding the knowledge gaps in a specific field of study, (3) guiding

*Peplau, H.E.: Interpersonal relations in nursing, New York, 1952, G.P. Putnam's Sons; Henderson, V.: The nature of nursing, New York, 1966, The Macmillan Co.; and Orlando, I.J.: The dynamic nurse-patient relationship, New York, 1961, G.P. Putnam's Sons.
†Abdellah, F.G., et al.: Patient-centered approaches to nursing, New York, 1960, The Macmillan Co.
‡Leininger, M.: Anthropological approach to adaptation: case studies for nursing. In Murphy, J., editor: Theoretical issues in professional nursing, New York, 1971, Appleton-Century-Crofts, pp. 77-101.
§Roy, Sister C.: Adaptation: a basis for nursing practice, Nurs. Outlook **19:**254-257, April 1971.

*Gordon, M., chairperson: Nursing theory, theme of the Second National Nurse Educator Conference, New York, Dec. 1978. (Papers presented at this conference are available on tape through Teach 'em, Inc., 625 N. Michigan Ave., Chicago, Ill. 60611).
†Walker, L., and Avant, K.: Strategies for theory construction in nursing, Norwalk, Conn., 1983, Appleton-Century-Crofts, pp. 3-4.

the theorist to sources of knowledge that are relevant, (4) verifying knowledge about decision making and providing a rationale for gathering reliable and valid data that are essential for effective decision making and implementation, (5) providing a measure of effectiveness for nursing care by identifying expected outcomes and observing goal achievements, (6) developing quality assurance, (7) providing learning opportunities for nursing students to gather reliable and valid information about the health status of clients and patients, (8) developing economy of thought and an organized way of studying nursing, and (9) searching primarily for knowledge and truths that are uniquely human.*

CRITERIA FOR NURSING THEORY EVALUATION

Various formulations of criteria for the evaluation of nursing theories began to appear in the nursing literature in the late 1960s. These lists of criteria have proved useful as one means of facilitating the process of judging the merits of nursing theory and theory development. Even though there is a lack of consensus over their use, there have been some criteria for which a high degree of consensus has been reached. For example, the following criteria have generally been identified by nursing theory critics as those universal standards by which all nursing theory should be judged: (1) logical development, (2) clarity, (3) consistency, (4) significance, (5) adequacy, (6) utility, and (7) capacity for discrimination. Stevens has labeled the former three elements as criteria useful in the examination of the internal construction of a theory, and the latter four elements as criteria useful in the examination of the external evaluation of a theory.† It is also suggested that the first three criteria examine the structure and content of a theory, where-

as the latter four examine the context and the process of a theory.

Lists of criteria have often included other elements in addition to the universal elements just listed. For example, three additional criteria that have been identified by nursing theory critics, but for which little consensus has been achieved are (1) level of theory development, (2) scope of theory, and (3) degree of complexity.

Those nursing theory critics who have held the view that theory development for nursing must be predictive and prescriptive have argued that nursing theories do not exist.* They claim that most conceptual formulations in nursing merely describe or explain. However, there are those who have argued that the descriptive and explanatory levels of theory development determine the direction from which predictive and prescriptive levels emerge and thus meet the criteria of a theory.†

Several nursing leaders have argued in favor of broad-scope theories, whereas others have often taken an opposing view by citing the virtues of limited-scope theory development. For example, Ellis suggests that broadness of scope is an essential characteristic of importance to the significance of a theory. Broad-scope nursing theories would be those that would include a large quantity of generalizations or concepts about a wide variety of phenomena (e.g., a combination of cultural, biological, and behavioral observations) and contain the potential within the theory for explaining the relationships of these elements.‡ Proponents of limited-scope theory suggest that nursing theories be focused on limited aspects of nursing such as

---

*King, I.: The "why" of theory development. In Theory development: what, why, how? Pub. No. 15-1708, New York, 1978, National League for Nursing.
†Stevens, B.J.: Nursing theory: analysis, application, evaluation, Boston, 1979, Little, Brown & Co., p. 50.

*Chinn, P.L., and Jacobs, M.K.: A model for theory development in nursing, Adv. Nurs. Sci. **1:**1-11, Oct. 1978; and Fawcett, J.: The relationship between theory and research: a double helix, Adv. Nurs. Sci. **1:**1-11, Oct. 1978.
†Dickoff, J., and James, P.: A theory of theories: a position paper, Nurs. Res. **17:**197-203, May-June 1968; and Stevens, B.J.: Nursing theory: analysis, application, evaluation, Boston, 1979, Little Brown & Co.
‡Ellis, R.: Characteristics of significant theories, Nurs. Res. **17:**217-222, May-June 1968.

the alleviation of pain.* Others have called for the development of both broad- and limited-scope theories. Fawcett has noted that any model must be limited in scope because it cannot possibly deal with everything in the world of nursing.†

Degree of complexity refers to a range of variables to be included in a theory on a continuum from highly complex to relatively simplistic. Proponents in favor of highly complex theories promote nursing theories that would explain and interrelate more variables, while proponents of the relatively simplistic (frugal) approach would promote nursing theories that would explain and interrelate fewer theory variables.‡

Additional criteria have been identified by other nurse theorists. These include the following characteristics: (1) the generation of testable hypotheses, (2) usefulness as a guide for practice, (3) completeness of subject matter and perspective, (4) explicitness of underlying biases and values, (5) explicitness of relationships among propositions, (6) social congruency, (7) social significance, (8) social utility, (9) meaning and logical adequacy, (10) operational and empirical adequacy, (11) generality, (12) contribution to understanding, (13) predictability, (14) pragmatic adequacy, (15) testability, (16) usefulness, (17) identification of implicit values, (18) generation of information, and (19) use of meaningful terminology.§

Most recently Fitzpatrick and Whall‖ and Fawcett,* using two distinctively different approaches, have delineated sets of guidelines for the systematic analysis of conceptual models. They address the usefulness of the model rather than the testability of the theory.

The criteria chosen by evaluators or critics of nursing theory have often reflected the value orientation and personal biases of the evaluator. These various lists of criteria provide a wide spectrum of options for judging theory. The reader is encouraged to explore the various evaluative perspectives for critiquing nursing theories and models.

ISSUES AND FUTURE DIRECTIONS OF NURSING THEORY DEVELOPMENT

Much has been written related to nursing theory and theory development since the time of Nightingale. Issues continue to emerge in an effort to discover and define the laws of nursing. Controversy persists over such issues as the following:

1. What is the central concern of nursing?
2. Is nursing the science of health?
3. Is nursing a basic or an applied science?
4. What is the relative importance of the nursing process as a basic concept?
5. What are the commonalities and differences among nursing models?
6. Should the goal of nurse theorists be the development of a unified theory of nursing or should it be a pluralistic approach to nursing theory development?
7. Should current efforts be directed toward theory building or theory testing?

Nightingale conceptualized nursing as the science of health. The four basic concepts introduced in her model were person, nursing, environment, and health. These four concepts are identifiable in the nursing theories and models of contemporary theorists, although noticeable shifts in emphasis have occurred since Nightingale's time.

For example, Nightingale's model placed its em-

*Jacox, A.K.: Assessing pain, Am. J. Nurs. **79**(5):895-900, 1979.

†Fawcett, J.: Analysis and evaluation of conceptual models of nursing, Philadelphia, 1984, F.A. Davis Co., p. 42.

‡Stevens, B.J.: Nursing theory: analysis, application, evaluation, Boston, 1979, Little, Brown & Co., p. 66.

§Duffey, M., and Muhlenkamp, A.F.: A framework for theory analysis, Nurs. Outlook **22**:571, Sept. 1974; Johnson, D.: Development of theory: a requisite for nursing as a primary health profession, Nurs. Res. **23**:372-377, Sept.-Oct. 1974; and Hardy, M.: Theories: components, development, evaluation, Nurs. Res. **23**:100-107, March-April 1974.

‖Fitzpatrick, J., and Whall, A.: Conceptual models of nursing: analysis and application, Bowie, Md., 1983, Robert J. Brady Co.

*Fawcett, J.: Analysis and evaluation of conceptual models of nursing, Philadelphia, 1984, F.A. Davis Co.

phasis on the environment and health, whereas the models of Peplau and Orlando focused on the concept of nursing or more specifically the nurse-person relationship.*

Ellis† has commented on the limitations of conceptual models that continue to focus on the interpersonal process. She suggests that this way of focusing preserves a traditional view of nursing as a human-to-human helping relationship without adequately formulating the specific goals or the contextual space that explains nursing as a distinctive type of helping relationship.

A more recent shift in emphasis is evident in the focus on person as the central phenomenon of interest to nursing. This person focus is most dominant in the works of Rogers,‡ Newman,§ Parse,‖ and Fitzpatrick.¶ Models with person focus have also been criticized for their lack of clarity in the definition of humans. For example, Ellis# noted the inadequacy of defining humans in terms of energy fields or behavioral systems and recommended that conceptualizations of humans be defined in terms of human striving, human resilience, and human bonding.

The centrality of the concept of health has also received considerable scholarly discourse among contemporary nurse theorists. Current emphasis on health is understood by some theorists to suggest

a developmental stage toward integration and synthesis of the other basic concepts. An innovative conceptualization of health has been developed by Newman.*

Contemporary nurse theorists have also begun to include family as one of the important concepts for consideration in nursing theory development.†

Gudmundsen has argued cogently in favor of pluralism in nursing theory development. She has stated:

The idea of one theory of nursing, or one theory of nursing practice is not compatible with the concept and the purposes of scientific theory or scientific explanation, just as there is no validity to the idea of a theory of medicine or a theory of physics . . . nursing is not an entity into itself. . . . Nursing is a concept and as such possesses certain features. For a concept to be useful it must be specific.‡

Dickoff and James, speaking in support of a pluralistic approach to theory development, suggested that nurse theorists use a matrix to examine the repertoire of theories available for nursing. In this matrix the vertical items would include all of the available theories and the horizontal axis would identify notable factors germane to current nursing. The outcomes from this approach would encourage both intensification and extension of the theoretical formulations in nursing.§

Although the matrix approach has not specifically been used, nurse theorists and practitioners have employed a similar methodology in their recent collaborative work to classify nursing diagnoses. Significantly, the third National Conference

*Peplau, H.E.: Interpersonal relations in nursing, New York, 1952, G.P. Putnam's Sons; and Orlando, I.J.: The dynamic nurse-patient relationship, New York, 1961, G.P. Putnam's Sons.
†Ellis, R.: Conceptual issues in nursing, Nurs. Outlook 30(7):406-410, 1982.
‡Rogers, M.: An introduction to the theoretical basis of nursing, Philadelphia, 1970, F.A. Davis Co.
§Newman, M.: Theory development in nursing, Philadelphia, 1979, F.A. Davis Co.
‖Parse, R.: Man-living-health: a theory of nursing, New York, 1981, John Wiley & Sons, Inc.
¶Fitzpatrick, J.: A life perspective rhythm model. In Fitzpatrick, J., and Whall, A.: Conceptual models of nursing: analysis and application, Bowie, Md., 1983, Robert J. Brady Co.
#Ellis, R.: Conceptual issues in nursing, Nurs. Outlook 30(7):406-410, 1982.

*Newman, M.: Theory development in nursing, Philadelphia, 1979, F.A. Davis Co.
†Clements, I., and Roberts, F., editors: Family health: theoretical approach to nursing care, New York, 1983, John Wiley & Sons, Inc.
‡Gudmundsen, A.M.: The conduct of inquiry into nursing, Nurs. Forum 18:52-59, 1979.
§Dickoff, J., and James, P.: New views of traditional roles. Presented at the Second National Nurse Educator Conference, New York, 1978. (Available on tape through Teach 'em Inc., 625 N. Michigan Avenue, Chicago, IL 60611.)

on Classification of Nursing Diagnoses, held in 1978, marked the first time in the history of nursing that 14 nurse theorists representing multiple and disparate views met together for the common purpose of reaching a consensus on one conceptual framework for the classification of nursing diagnoses.*

Nursing models are currently being used to develop new theories and to guide research and practice. And today there exists a community of nursing scholars and theorists who have collaborated and inspired one another in the activities of nursing theory development. Several of these scholars now view theory testing as the vital next phase to follow this initial development of nursing theory.†

SUMMARY

For more than 2 decades now, nurse theorists have developed a number of theories for nursing. Because of this effort, nursing knowledge has increased and nursing science has expanded toward greater understanding of humans and their health potential.

In the course of nursing theory development many issues have been raised relative to the nature of nursing. As pioneers and neophytes in nursing have responded to these issues, a refinement of the original ideas and the creative development of new nursing theories have evolved. Nursing and nursing theory development have been profoundly influenced by such theorists as Roger, King, Orem, Johnson, and Roy.

Discussion questions

1. Discuss the nature of a theory.
2. Discuss the purpose of a conceptual framework.
3. Discuss one of the nurse theorists' work as it relates to nursing practice.

4. Discuss why nursing theories have become a part of nursing practice.
5. Discuss how a theory is evaluated and if it is useful to nursing practice.

SUGGESTED READINGS
General theory references

Burr, W.R.: Theory construction and the sociology of the family, New York, 1973, John Wiley & Sons, Inc.

Dewey, J.: Logic: the theory of inquiry, New York, 1938, Henry Holt & Co.

Dubin, R.: Theory building, revised ed., New York, 1978, The Free Press.

Gibson, Q.: The logic of social enquiry, New York, 1960, The Humanities Press.

Glaser, B.G., and Strauss, A.L.: The discovery of grounded theory: strategies for qualitative research, Chicago, 1967, Aldine Publishing Co.

Hanson, N.R.: Patterns of discovery, New York, 1958, Cambridge University Press.

Hempel, C.G.: Fundamentals of concept formation in empirical science, Chicago, 1952, University of Chicago Press.

Kerlinger, F.N.: Foundations of behavioral research, ed. 2, New York, 1973, Holt, Rinehart & Winston.

Merton, R.K.: Social theory and social structure, revised ed., New York, 1957, The Free Press.

Popper, K.P.: The logic of scientific discovery, New York, 1961, Science Editions, Inc.

Popper, K.R.: Conjectures and refutations: the growth of scientific knowledge, New York, 1965, Harper & Row, Publishers.

Skidmore, W.: Theoretical thinking in sociology, New York, 1975, Cambridge University Press.

Stinchcombe, A.L.: Constructing social theories, New York, 1968, Harcourt, Brace & World, Inc.

Wiener, P.P., editor: Readings in philosophy of science, New York, 1953, Charles Scribner's Sons.

Nursing theory texts

Abdellah, F.G., et al.: Patient centered approaches to nursing, New York, 1960, The Macmillan Co.

Chaska, N.L., editor: The nursing profession: views through the mist, New York, 1978, McGraw-Hill Book Co.

Chinn, P.L., and Jacobs, M.: Theory and nursing: a systematic approach, St. Louis, 1983, The C.V. Mosby Co.

Clements, I.W., and Roberts, F.B., editors: Family health: a theoretical approach to nursing care, New York, 1983, John Wiley & Sons, Inc.

Fawcett, J.: Analysis and evaluation of conceptual models of nursing, Philadelphia, 1984, F.A. Davis Co.

Fitzpatrick, J., and Whall, A.: Conceptual models of nursing: analysis and application, Bowie, Md., 1983, Robert J. Brady Co.

---

*Kim, M.J., and Moritz, D.A.: Classification of nursing diagnoses: proceedings of the third and fourth national conferences, New York, 1982, McGraw-Hill Book Co.

†Walker, L.O., and Avant, K.C.: Strategies for theory construction in nursing, Norwalk, Conn., 1983, Appleton-Century-Crofts.

Hardy, M.E., editor: Theoretical foundations for nursing, New York, 1973, MSS Information Corp.

Harmer, B., and Henderson, V.: Textbook of the principles and practices of nursing, New York, 1922, The Macmillan Co.

Kim, M.J., and Moritz, D.A.: Classification of nursing diagnoses: proceedings of the third and fourth national conferences, New York, 1982, McGraw-Hill Book Co.

King, I.M.: Toward a theory for nursing, New York, 1971, John Wiley & Sons, Inc.

King, I.M.: A theory for nursing: systems, concepts, process, New York, 1981, A Wiley Medical Publication.

Murphy, J.F.: Theoretical issues in professional nursing, Des Moines, 1971, Meredith Corp.

Newman, M.: Theory development in nursing, Philadelphia, 1979, F.A. Davis Co.

Nightingale, F.: Notes on nursing: what it is and what it is not, Philadelphia, 1860, J.B. Lippincott Co.

Orem, D.: Nursing: concepts of practice, ed. 2, New York, 1980, McGraw-Hill Book Co.

Orlando, I.J.: The dynamic nurse-patient relationship, New York, 1961, G.P. Putnam's Sons.

Parse, R.R.: Man-living-health: a theory of nursing, New York, 1981, John Wiley & Sons, Inc.

Patterson, J.G., and Zderad, L.T.: Humanistic nursing, New York, 1976, John Wiley & Sons, Inc.

Peplau, H.E.: Interpersonal relations in nursing, New York, 1952, G.P. Putnam's Sons.

Riehl, J.P., and Roy, C., editors: Conceptual models for nursing practice, ed. 2, New York, 1980, Appleton-Century-Crofts.

Rogers, M.E.: An introduction to the theoretical basis of nursing, Philadelphia, 1970, F.A. Davis Co.

Stevens, B.J.: Nursing theory: analysis, application, evaluation, Boston, 1979, Little, Brown & Co.

Vaillot, M.C.: Commitment to nursing, Philadelphia, 1962, J.B. Lippincott Co.

Verhonick, P.J., editor: Nursing research I, Boston, 1975, Little, Brown & Co.

Walker, L.O., and Avant, K.C.: Strategies for theory construction in nursing, Norwalk, Conn., 1983, Appleton-Century-Crofts.

Wiedenbach, E.: Clinical nursing: a helping art, New York, 1964, Springer Publishing Co.

Wooldridge, P., et al.: Behavioral science and nursing theory, St. Louis, 1983, The C.V. Mosby Co.

Zderad, L.T., and Belcher, H.C.: Developing behavioral concepts in nursing, Atlanta, 1968, Southern Regional Education Board.

Selected journal references

Abdellah, F.G.: The nature of nursing science, Nurs. Res. **18:**390-393, Sept.-Oct. 1969.

Ahad, M.A.: Evolution of nursing science: implications for nursing worldwide, Image **13:**56-59, June 1981.

Andreoli, K.G., and Thompson, C.E.: The nature of science in nursing, Image **9:**32-37, June 1977.

Beckstrand, J.: A critique of several conceptions of practice theory in nursing, Res. Nurs. Health **3:**69-79, June 1980.

Brodish, M.S.: Nursing practice conceptualized: an interaction model, Image **14:**5-7, Feb-March 1982.

Bush, H.A.: Models for nursing, Adv. Nurs. Sci. **1**(2):13-20, 1979.

Chinn, P.L., and Jacobs, M.K.: A model for theory development in nursing, Adv. Nurs. Sci. **1:**1-12, Oct. 1978.

Clark, J.: Development of models and theories on the concept of nursing, J. Adv. Nurs. **7:**129-134, March 1982.

Collins, R., and Fielder, J.: Beckstrand's concept of practice theory: a critique, Res. Nurs. Health **4:**317-321, Sept. 1981.

Crawford, G., Dufault, Sister K., and Rudy, E.: Evolving issues in theory development, Nurs. Outlook **27:**346-351, May 1979.

Daubenmire, M.J., and King, I.: Nursing processes models: a systems approach, Nurs. Outlook **21:**512-515, Aug. 1973.

Dickoff, J., and James, P.: Theory in a practice discipline. I. Practice oriented theory, Nurs. Res. **17:**420, Sept.-Oct. 1968.

Dickoff, J., and James, P.: A theory of theories: a position paper, Nurs. Res. **17:**197-203, May-June 1968.

Donaldson, S.K., and Crawley, D.M.: The discipline of nursing, Nurs. Outlook **26:**118-120, Feb. 1978.

Duffy, M., and Muhlenkamp, A.F.: A framework for theory analysis, Nurs. Outlook **22:**571, Sept. 1974.

Ellis, R.: Characteristics of significant theories, Nurs. Res. **17:**217-222, May-June 1968.

Ellis, R.: Conceptual issues in nursing, Nurs. Outlook **30**(7):406-410, 1982.

Fawcett, J.: The 'what' of theory development. In Theory development: what, why, how? New York, 1978, National League for Nursing.

Fawcett, J.: A declaration of nursing independence: the relation of theory and research to nursing practice, J. Nurs. Admin. **6:**36-39, June, 1980.

Fawcett, J.: A framework for analysis and evaluation of conceptual models of nursing, Nurse Educator **6:**10-14, Nov.-Dec. 1980.

Flaskerud, J.H., and Halloran, E.: Areas of agreement in nursing theory development, Adv. Nurs. Sci. **3**(1):1-7, 1980.

Hadley, B.: Evolution of a conception of nursing, Nurs. Res. **18:**400-403, Sept.-Oct. 1969.

Hardy, M.: Theories: components, development, evaluation, Nurs. Res. **23:**101-106, March-April 1974.

Hardy, M.: Evaluating nursing theory. In Theory development: what, why, how? New York, 1978, National League for Nursing.

Jacox, A.: Theory construction in nursing—an overview, Nurs. Res. **23:**4-13, Jan.-Feb. 1974.

Johnson, D.: Development of theory: a requisite for nursing as a primary health profession, Nurs. Res. **23:**372-377, Sept.-Oct. 1974.

Johnson, D.: State of the art of theory development in nursing. In Theory development: what, why, how? New York, 1978, National League for Nursing.

King, I.M.: Nursing theory—problems and prospects, Nurs. Sci. **2:**394-403, Oct. 1964.

King, I.M.: A conceptual frame of reference for nursing, Nurs. Res. **17:**27-31, Jan.-Feb. 1968.

King, I.M.: The why of theory development. In Theory development: what, why, how? New York, 1978, National League for Nursing.

Levine, M.E.: The four conservation principles of nursing, Nurs. Forum **6:**47-49, 1967.

Levine, M.E.: Holistic nursing. In Germain, L.D., and Alfano, G.J., editors: The nursing clinics of North America, vol. 6, pp. 253-264, Philadelphia, 1971, W.B. Saunders Co.

Mathwig, J.: Nursing science, Image **3:**9-14, Feb. 1969.

McKay, R.: Theories, models, and systems for nursing. Nurs. Res. **18:**293-400, Sept.-Oct. 1969.

Patterson, J.G.: The tortuous way toward nursing theory. In Theory development: what, why, how? New York, 1978, National League for Nursing.

Patterson, J.G., and Zderad, L.T.: All together complementary synthesis, Image **4:**13-16, Oct. 1971.

Peplau, H.E.: Operational definitions and nursing practice. In Zderad, L.T., and Belcher, H.C., editors: Developing behavioral concepts in nursing, Atlanta, 1968, Southern Regional Educational Board.

Phillips, J.R.: Nursing systems and nursing models, Image **9:**4-7, Feb. 1977.

Putnam, P.A.: A conceptual approach to nursing theory, Nurs. Sci. **3:**430-442, Dec. 1965.

Quint, J.C.: The care for theories generated from empirical data, Nurs. Res. **16:**109-114, Spring 1967.

Reilly, D.: Why a conceptual framework? Nurs. Outlook **23:**566-569, Sept. 1975.

Rinehart, J.: The 'how' of theory development in nursing. In Theory development: what, why, how? New York, 1978, National League for Nursing.

Rogers, M.: Euphemisims in nursing's future, Image **7:**3-9, June 1975.

Roy, Sister C.: Adaptation—a basis for nursing practice, Nurs. Outlook **19:**254-257, April 1971.

Rubin, R.: A theory of clinical nursing, Nurs. Res. **17:**210-212, May-June 1968.

Schlotfeldt, R.M.: Reflections on nursing research, Am. J. Nurs. **60:**492-494, April 1960.

Schlotfeldt, R.: This I believe—nursing is health care, Nurs. Outlook **20:**245-246, April 1972.

Siegel, H.: Misconceptions about conceptual frameworks: a point of view, Nurs. Health Care **4**(1):16-17, 1983.

Smoyak, S.A.: Toward understanding nursing situations: a transaction paradigm, Nurs. Res. **18:**405-411, Sept.-Oct. 1969.

Vaillot, M.C.: Nursing theory, levels of nursing and curriculum development, Nurs. Forum **9:**234-249, 1970.

Walker, L.O.: Toward a clearer understanding of the concept of nursing theory, Nurs. Res. **25:**428-435, Sept.-Oct. 1971.

Wiedenbach, E.: Comments on beliefs and values: basis for curriculum design, Nurs. Res. **19:**427, Sept.-Oct. 1970.

PART TWO
CONTEMPORARY PERSPECTIVES

Florence Nightingale   Nursing is a progressive calling: year by year nurses have to learn new and improved methods, as medicine and surgery and hygiene improve; year by year nurses are called upon to do more and better than they have done. In our nursing, if we are not making progress every year, every month, every week, take my word for it, we are going back.

To a student of nursing the contemporary scene is of utmost importance. An elliptical view of the history of nursing has been presented, and now attention will be turned to the nursing world of the 1980s. It will be seen that nurses are gaining more autonomy of practice, that entry to practice requires more knowledge in a variety of sciences and arts, and that without research, nursing cannot become a profession in its own right. It will be further seen that ethical issues, collective bargaining, and politics in nursing have invaded the individual nurse's domain and are not just for nursing as a collective body.

Throughout Contemporary Perspectives, the student will see evidence of the evolution of nursing growing from infancy to young adulthood. The continuum of professionalization is moving past the middle with significant progress. The student will also become aware of the problems that confront nursing in becoming an autonomous profession. A question that can rightfully be asked is "Will nursing become a profession for a few, or will it be an occupation for the masses who perform nursing tasks and who exhibit professional behaviors?"

CHAPTER 5
Issues in nursing—an overview

OBJECTIVE: On completion of this chapter, the student of nursing will have an elliptical view of the issues confronting nurses and nursing.

In the preceding chapters the history of nursing service and nursing education was provided as a base to examine the issues in nursing today. As the history is examined and the issues identified, one begins to wonder if the concerns of today are the same or different from those of the past. From the late 1890s to the present, leaders of nursing have been concerned with standards of nursing practice, the education process for the professional nurse, and the welfare of the individual nurse. These issues are the same today—only more complex.

Definining nursing has plagued the profession for the past 30 years and continues to be an issue to resolve. The role of the professional nurse continues to change as nursing theories evolve and become a part of nurses' practice. Leaders and practitioners of nursing have continuously worked to redefine nursing as the practice of nursing becomes secure with a scientific base. Nurse practice acts throughout the United States have been updated to bring them into line with the changing role of the nurse. The medical profession and others have not accepted the changes in nursing easily. Although the medical profession has continuously relinquished technical skills to nurses, it has not accepted the fact that nurses have their own body of knowledge and can practice independently. The impact of these changes has created conflict and confusion within and outside the profession of nursing.

In the late 1980s the prevailing issues are cre-dentialing of nurses with specific skills and knowledge, autonomy of nursing practice, functional redundancy, and reimbursement for nursing services. In the 1970s the issues were human rights, nurses' rights, and the delivery of health care services. The issues of the 1970s were not resolved and bear consideration in this chapter as a historical perspective. Futurists such as Alvin Tofler and Daniel Bell tell us that to plan for the future the past must be examined.

As future leaders, students of nursing need to have the historical perspective of the past and knowledge of the dilemmas of the present to plan for change and deal with the issues of tomorrow systematically and scientifically. Part One of this book, Evolution of and Trends in Nursing, set the stage for this chapter and all others in Contemporary Perspectives.

ISSUES OF THE 1970s
Human rights

The human rights issue began in the early 1800s with such movements as women's suffrage, emancipation of blacks, and the upgrading of medical and nursing care. Each of these movements has had moments of quiescence and eruption. With eruption some change took place only to be followed by a period of acceptance and satisfaction with the status quo. In 1954, when Brown of Topeka, Kansas, challenged the educational system, a whole series of movements was started in the areas of education, work systems, equal rights of men and women, human rights in the areas of research, and the patient's rights for medical and nursing care. Miss Brown, via her parents, challenged the Topeka Board of Education for equal education, maintaining that as a black she was not receiving an education equal to that of the white student and that, through the doctrine of separate but equal education, she was denied good teachers, facilities, and learning resources. The U.S. Supreme Court heard the case and decreed that all children, regardless of race, must be given an equal education and that separate was inherently unequal. Thus the movement to integrate school systems throughout the country began. Through this case, also, discriminatory practices with regard to sex, race, color, and creed were examined, and the Civil Rights Act of 1964 was enacted. Through this act, the black people of our country, as well as other minority group members, were legally given equal rights to work, education, and housing.

In the Civil Rights Act other human rights were identified, such as equal pay for equal work whether done by men, women, blacks, or white. From this legislation, the women's liberation movement gained new impetus. Women found many discriminatory practices in existence, such as the difficulty of establishing credit or purchasing a home in their own right. In an effort to rectify these inequities, the Equal Rights Amendment (ERA) was proposed and passed in the U.S. Congress. Ratification by 38 states was required by 1978 in order for it to become an amendment to the constitution. Ratification did not occur, and Congress elected to extend the period to June 30, 1982. In 1979, 35 states had ratified the ERA, with some states discussing the possibility of rescinding previous action.

The ERA was not ratified in 1982. There continues to be activity on the part of the proponents of ERA to reintroduce the amendment. Under the Reagan administration equal rights for women in the executive branch erupted in the summer of 1983. Although Reagan has appointed many women to positions of importance, it is well known that the president did not support the ERA amendment. However, nursing did achieve something in having a nurse appointed as administrator of health care financing in the U.S. Department of Health and Human Services. Carolyn K. Davis, R.N., Ph.D., is a nurse, nurse educator, and administrator in higher education. She has become well known in setting the stage for changes necessary to meet the government's participation in financing health care. Dr. Davis continually admonishes those who are administering health care that costs need to be controlled. New rules and regulations have been put into effect. These rules (i.e., Tax Equity and Fiscal Responsibility Act [TEFRA] of 1982 and Diagnostic Related Groups [DRG]) will have far-reaching effects on medicine, nursing, and health care agencies in the delivery of health care.

The ERA movement is not dead. Activists will continue to promote the worth of women. In turn, this will provide nursing, a predominantly female profession, support in its effort to be recognized. In fact, at the July 1982 ANA convention, the delegates interrupted their convention in Washington, D.C., to demonstrate their support of the ERA amendment.

The issue of equal rights has specific meaning to nursing, which is predominantly a woman's profession. Female nurses in positions such as administration do not receive pay equal to that of male administrators in similar positions; however, male nurses found that when they moved into nursing administrative positions, their salaries were consistent with those of other male administrators. Black nurses were denied career mobility as well as being products of inferior educational programs. Thus the Civil Rights Act of 1964 had specific meaning to the profession of nursing and demanded that nurses look internally to discriminating practices for the individual nurse and the delivery of nursing care.

Minority groups formed coalitions within nursing and identified a lack of health care to various culture groups within the United States. They found the educational system, economic rewards, and career mobility to be major issues in nursing. The profession of nursing had to eliminate discriminatory practices and provide equal rights in the delivery of nursing care and career satisfaction to the individual nurse.

Ethical issues created the most concern for nurses. The issues of abortion, euthanasia, death and dying, use of human transplants, and research on human beings caused deep emotional and intellectual dichotomy for the individual nurse as well as for the professions of nursing and medicine.

The ethical issues demanded examination of the right of each individual to receive adequate health care; the right of individuals to have a say in their care; the right of the individual to choose, with sufficient knowledge, whether to participate as a subject in a research project; and the right of the individual nurse to choose how he or she could meet the needs of each patient.

Euthanasia continues to be a moral issue facing society. It can also be viewed as the right to die with dignity, the right to be spared unending pain, or the right to choose a quality life or no life. The use of heroic medical measures such as cardiac or respiratory resuscitation to prolong life beyond a quality existence must be examined. Does the patient or family have the right to determine if heroic measures should be performed or continued? A question that needs to be pursued with regard to human rights is, ''What is 'quality of life,' and what does each individual have a right to expect in the way of care that sustains, restores, or maintains optimum health for that individual?''

The use of human transplants presented another ethical issue for the nurse. Society appears to have accepted human organ transplants as morally justifiable. However, the ethical issue centered around the questions of who decides when, for whom, and under what conditions these operations are performed. Moreover, in this issue is encompassed the question of when to seek permission to obtain donor organs.

What did all of this mean to nursing? One had only to review nursing literature, letters to editors, journal articles, and newspapers to know that nurses, individually and collectively, had mixed attitudes toward these various issues. Students and practicing nurses had to confront these issues and make decisions regarding their own beliefs, incorporating them into the practice of nursing. The technical skills of nursing care, and knowledge of how, why, and when various procedures are done can be taught. But educators needed to provide students with the skills and knowledge necessary to develop a valuing system to use in determining how they would approach the ethical issues involved. See Chapter 9 for elaboration of the issue.

Nurses' rights

Nurses' rights centered around the issue of the nurse being able to practice as a primary giver of care. Because of the maldistribution of health workers, the shortage of physicians and nurses, and the movement for national health insurance, nursing was forced in the mid 1960s to examine the role of the nurse. Nurse practitioner programs that emphasized the nurse's ability to provide physical assessment, make nursing diagnoses, and implement nursing care without the assistance of a physician were developed, which provided a changing role for the nurse.

Along with the nurse practitioner programs, physician assistant and pediatric associate programs were organized to provide extended physician care in areas where shortages of medical personnel existed. As physician assistant and nurse practitioner programs proliferated, a change occurred in the roles of the physician and nurse. As the role of the health assistants or associates developed, new dilemmas for the physician and nurse were created.

The leaders of nursing in 1970 began developing a role for nurses that would allow people to seek out the nurse's assistance in a primary situation rather than through the traditional visit to the physician. Thus the primary role, or independent nurse practitioner role, began to evolve. The idea was that the nurse was a health care worker with a broad background in all dimensions of human beings who knew how to make physical assessments with regard to the health care required and whose educational background was forward moving. The question was, "Why not let the nurse be the first one to see the patient, assess the needs, and determine whether medical or nursing care was necessary?"

The issue of the independent practitioner in 1970 opened up a whole new avenue of concerns. One problem was to determine whether the education of the practitioner should be at the undergraduate or graduate level. Ultimately, it was decided that as faculty were prepared to teach physical and emotional assessment, this should be included in the baccalaureate curriculum. Because both faculty and practicing nurses needed training in assessment, continuing education courses had to be planned and financed before this new aspect of nursing practice could be offered to the nursing population.

Simultaneously, it was evident that nurse practice acts were self-limiting, necessitating revision of definitions of nursing. New York and California, in 1972, were first to prepare new definitions and successfully secure passage through the legislative process. Other states followed, adopting either the New York or California model to meet the needs of their own nurse practice acts.

Defining the roles of the nurse, physician, and those of the 300 other types of health workers created a real dilemma as to who was responsible for what, for whom, and under what circumstances. And yet, realistically, breaking from traditional roles and adding new ones was a means of securing some kind of health worker for all geographical areas, as well as making health care available to all who needed it.

Other issues in the area of nurses' rights dealt with (1) the misuse of the variously prepared nurses, (2) determining the necessity for providing continuing education programs for all nurses whether actively practicing or not, and (3) the inclusion of graduates from associate degree and diploma programs into baccalaureate nursing programs. The hostility among nurses from these various programs dissipated the unity needed to accomplish the goals of nursing. Career mobility, which holds out some hope of drawing these nursing factions closer together, is being made an issue, and certainly the pressure is on to make this a right rather than a restriction. As Shirley Chater said in her keynote address of the 1975 NLN convention, much of nursing time has been consumed with naming, gaming, and blaming, rather than taking what is and moving forward. See Chapters 3 and 6 for further clarification of this issue.

The welfare of the individual nurse has been of concern to the profession of nursing and became an issue in 1946 when the ANA first adopted the Economic and General Welfare Program. Since that time the issue has broadened to encompass the constraints on nurses with regard to the medical profession and the antiquated delivery of health care. The ANA has maintained that nurses themselves should obtain high standards of practice and should be in control of their own practice. The ANA Economic and General Welfare Program gained new impetus in 1974 and began paving the way for nurses to be in command of their destiny while moving the role of the nurse into a health care system that provides health care to all. See Chapter 10 for an expanded discussion of collective bargaining.

Leaders of nursing in the 1970s were not any better supported in these problems than were Florence Nightingale, Linda Richards, Adelaide Nutting, and others throughout the past 175 years. But for professional status to be reached and maintained, nursing must have the following: (1) a strong scientific, theoretical base of knowledge; (2) a strong service orientation; (3) the recognized authority by the professional group with community sanction; (4) a code of ethics that is enforced; (5) a professional organization that is supported by the group it serves; and (6) ongoing research.

The issue in nurses' rights was whether nurses were willing to expend the effort necessary to become a full-fledged profession by meeting the six criteria or be satisfied to allow the profession to continue with the constraints placed on nursing by the existing system of health care. Nursing research had just begun to gather a scientific body of knowledge that was unique to nursing. Although nursing had a strong service orientation, it was not an independent service; nursing and nurses were still taking direction from the physician and administrator of health care agencies. Nursing was recognized as a profession in title only. Unless nurses become primary givers of care, nursing will not gain full sanction as a profession. The ANA Code of Ethics has been in existence since 1950; however, it had not been enforced, and most nurses were not familiar with its contents. Although nursing has had a professional organization from which the officers speak out for nursing, it was not supported by even a majority of practicing nurses. Thus professional status could not be reached, and nursing cannot reach this status until nurses become united by enforcing a code of ethics, having a unique body of knowledge, and gaining independence as practitioners.

The issues for nurses' rights were basic to the need for service, education, and welfare. Again, the nursing literature was reviewed, and it was found that nurses were concerned with continuing education, the need for certification, developing clinical expertise, and promoting standards of excellence through the Academy of Nursing and/or the certification program of the ANA. They were concerned with changing the delivery of health care to provide the professional nurse with the right to say where nurses were assigned and to determine the kind of nursing care a patient needs. Nurses were involved with promoting health legislation that made health care a right and with legislation that provided nurses with legal rights to have a say in their own welfare. See Chapter 11 for a discussion of politics in nursing.

Delivery of health care

The delivery of health care was of major concern in the 1970s. There was a collage of differing, independent agencies, hospitals, clinics, and public health agencies, each with its own unique system. These systems did not provide a unified approach to health care that would give an individual, family, or extended family the opportunity to receive a continuum of care, from prevention to restoration of optimal health.

National health insurance was frequently discussed as one means of altering the system. Health systems organizations were implemented to foster community planning.

Physicians consistently rejected the idea of federal health insurance plans. Organized nursing, the ANA, and the NLN consistently supported the principle of federal health insurance. Almost all plans before Congress were rejected because they were inadequate or because the cost to implement them was prohibitive. There was one concept that everyone agreed with and that was the right for all citizens to have access to health care.

Nursing supported the need for change in the delivery of health care and provided impetus in new approaches to the delivery of care by nurses. Nursing also supported the concept that focusing on the prevention of illness was a means of providing a healthy nation.

The answers to an evolving health care system are not easily reached. Lucille Petry Leone, in 1962, suggested that in the 1980s hospitals would be family health centers. There is evidence that perhaps her prediction will materialize. Medical centers are changing their names to health care centers, signifying a unified approach to dealing with the issue of a "system" of health care. Family practitioners are being prepared as medical specialists and family health nurses as nurse specialists, which, in turn, has stimulated the development of family practice clinics.

ISSUES IN THE 1980s AND INTO THE 1990s

In the early 1980s there was a resurgence of two issues addressed in the 1970s: entry to practice and credentialing of nurses. By the mid 1980s the cost of health care and functional redundancy were the issues. The credentialing of nurses with specific skills and knowledge remains to be addressed as does the issue of new graduates' entry into nursing.

Entry to practice

The entry to professional nursing became an issue in 1965 and returned to the scene in 1978 when the ANA resolved to have the minimum preparation for professional nursing a baccalaureate degree, which was to be implemented by 1985. The New York State Nurses Association has supported legislation for this change since 1975, and each time it has been voted down by the state legislators. Opposition comes from nurses who believe that the present system of registered nurse (RN) education is good and from physicians and hospital administrators who support hospital-based programs and see no need to change.

The Ohio State Nurses Association House of Delegates voted in 1976 to accept 37 Concepts of Change that would be translated into a new nurse practice act that would legislate change of the educational system for nursing education by 1985. In 1983 no legislation had been introduced dealing with the education issue.

In opposition to this issue new nurse organizations appeared whose main purpose was to maintain the inclusion of diploma nurse education as a way to become a registered professional. However, specialty organizations such as the American Association of Operating Room Nurses and the American Association of Nurse Anesthetists voted to support baccalaureate education as the entry to professional nursing. Even the National Student Nurse Association, composed of students from all types of programs, voted to support baccalaureate education as a base for professional practice.

Early in 1979 the NLN appointed a task force to identify differences in competencies and practice roles in each of the programs. The task force reported in July of 1979 that differences did exist in the knowledge base as well as practice bases. Further differences were found in the accountability of the graduate. "As the amount and type of education and experience increase the degree of re-

sponsibility and liability likewise increases."*

Until 1983 the two major organizations, ANA and NLN, were polarized as to the entry to practice issue. In June 1983 the NLN membership ratified the position statement accepted by the NLN board of directors in February 1982. The following is the position taken:

The quality of nursing and health care has been a concern of the National League for Nursing since its inception in 1952. In view of this concern, NLN has constantly striven to improve the quality of the nursing education programs that provide the manpower necessary to meet society's needs for nursing care.

Democratic society being always in flux, a number of changes in the demographic, economic, social, cultural, and political environments are affecting the delivery of nursing and health care. Consumers' awareness about and expectations of health care continue to grow as knowledge about health is more and more widely disseminated through popular channels. The League has constantly sought not only to identify these changes, but also to incorporate appropriate responses to them within its goals and programs.

A striking and continuing shift has occurred in the responsibility for health care provision. Activities once exclusively medical are now considered to lie within the province of nursing as well; nursing, in turn, has relinquished certain of its responsibilities to other health care providers.

The social forces impinging upon nursing place demands for greater responsibility and accountability on both the profession and the individual practitioner. Increased sharing by nurses of accountability for the quality and cost of health care compels greater concern not only for the education of graduates of nursing programs—that they be adequately prepared to make independent decisions based on sound knowledge and experience—but also for their appropriate utilization within the health care system.

In light of these changes, the NLN reaffirms its goal of improving the standards for quality nursing education, nursing service, and health care delivery.

Nursing as an occupation, in the broadest sense, covers a wide range of activities that may be viewed as a continuum beginning with simple nurturing tasks, pro-

---

*NLN task force cites differences in competencies and practice roles, NLN News **72:**3, July-Aug. 1979.

gressing through increasingly complex responsibilities, and culminating in critical decision-making activities. To meet the reality of this wide range of responsibilities and activities, a corresponding range of nursing practice roles is required; these have come to be referred to as vocational, technical, and professional nursing practice.

For each nursing role, adequate pre-service preparation must be required. Since professional nurses are expected to provide the leadership for all nursing personnel, they need a broad background of knowledge and of clinical skills that will equip them to make the independent judgments and critical decisions necessary in a complex health care delivery system.

Given the need for such a broad background in the arts and sciences, as well as in nursing, professional nursing practice requires the minimum of a baccalaureate degree with a major in nursing. Preparation for technical nursing practice requires an associate degree or a diploma in nursing. Preparation for vocational nursing requires a certificate or diploma in vocational/practical nursing.

Therefore, to meet the varied needs of the public, the National League for Nursing supports the education of nurses in programs that differ in purposes and lengths and that prepare for varying kinds of practice entailing different degrees of responsibility.

Moreover, to meet society's needs and the changing personal career goals of nurses, opportunities should be provided for individuals to progress within the nursing field. A clear definition of the purposes and a general agreement on the content of each nursing program will facilitate educational mobility for graduates.

More nurses with graduate preparation (i.e., master's and doctoral degrees) are required to provide leadership in nursing service, nursing education, and nursing research. In turn, greater numbers of baccalaureate graduates are required—not only by the increased complexity and scope of care, but also as a base for progression into graduate programs for the eventual assumption of leadership positions.

Community involvement in planning the development of nursing programs is essential to assure the approximate mix of nursing personnel to meet the needs of each community.*

The educational issue continues to be an emotional one. It affects the lives of many, and a "divide and conquer" situation has been created. Nursing is divided by the vested interests of each group in so many ways that the enemy (whoever that may be) will conquer. The unity needed to provide direction for the future of nursing is dissipated. For some the concern is not that eventually nursing education will occur in the institutions of higher learning, but they object to the target date of 1985 and do not wish it to be legislated. Others see no reason to change, believing that hospital-based programs are producing a professionally prepared nurse. Those in associate degree education are concerned because they do not want to prepare less than registered nurses, albeit that the original intent of these programs was to prepare technical nurses.

According to the ANA cabinet on nursing education, by 1985 "five percent of the states will have implemented the baccalaureate degree qualification, rising to 15% by 1988 and to 50% by 1992."* The cabinet called a meeting of nurse representatives in July of 1983 to plan strategies for achieving the goals of the association.

As of 1983 no state has been successful in legislating the entry to practice issue. It is my opinion that legislating the entry issue now would not be in the best interest of the profession. In 1976 I predicted that by 1992 the last diploma program would close, only 4 years after the maximum number of years suggested by goal 3 of the ANA.† This prediction was based on the number of diploma programs in 1972 and the number of diploma programs closing. Evaluating the number of diploma programs in 1983 and the projected number to close by 1985, the prediction made in 1976 is on target. The change is occurring through evolution.

It is my posit that the profession will be pronouncing the Ph.D.-prepared nurse as the only nurse eligible to meet the profession's standards.

---

*NLN position statement on nursing roles—scope and preparation, Feb. 1982, 10 Columbus Circle, New York, N.Y.

*Selby T.L.: ANA reps meet to develop education plan, Am. Nurse **5**(8):1, 1983.
†DeYoung, L.: Foundations of nursing, ed. 3, St. Louis, 1976, The C.V. Mosby Co., p. 137.

The language of the past has consistently been that baccalaureate education is the *base* for professional nursing. To legislate the educational issue would box the profession into law. The issue in the 1990s will be the utilization of the baccalaureate-prepared nurse as the preprofessional, and the master's-prepared nurse seeking full status with a Ph.D in nursing.

Credentialing study

In 1974 the ANA House of Delegates directed the association to study the feasibility of accrediting basic and graduate education. Accreditation of nursing education has been the responsibility of the NLN since its formation in 1952. The ANA invited conferees, including the NLN, to two meetings. In 1976 the ANA appointed an independent study committee to assess the existing system of accreditation, certification, and licensure in nursing. The contract was awarded the School of Nursing at The University of Wisconsin at Milwaukee, and Dr. Marguerita Styles was named to chair the committee.

The findings of the committee were made public in 1979. The following Principles of credentialing in addition to the principle that credentialing exists primarily to benefit and protect the public, guided the study committee*:

1. In addition to benefiting and protecting the public, credentialing also benefits those who are credentialed.
2. The *legitimate interests* of the involved occupation or institution and of the general public should be reflected in each credentialing mechanism.
3. *Accountability* should be an essential component of any credentialing process.
4. A *system of checks and balances* within the credentialing system should assure equitable treatment for all parties involved.

5. *Periodic assessments* with the potential for *sanction* are essential components of an effective credentialing mechanism.
6. *Objective standards and criteria* and *persons competent* in their use are essential to the credentialing process.
7. Representation in credentialing systems of the *community of interests* directly affected by credentialing mechanisms should assure consideration of the legitimate concerns of each group.
8. *Professional identity and responsibility* should evolve from the credentialing process.
9. An *effective system of role delineation* is fundamental to any credentialing mechanism for individuals.
10. An *effective system of program identification* is fundamental to any credentialing mechanism for institutions.
11. *Coordination* of credentialing mechanisms should lead to efficiency and cost effectiveness and avoid duplication.
12. *Geographic,* including interstate, *mobility* should be improved by the credentialing of the individual.
13. Widely *accepted definitions and terminology* are basic to an effective credentialing system.
14. *Communications and understanding* between health care providers and society should be facilitated through the credentialing process.

The committee further set forth credentialing definitions and their requirements for licensure, registration, certification, educational degrees, accreditation, charter, recognition, and approval. The most far reaching of the committee's recommendations had to do with a credentialing center. The purpose of the center "would be to study, develop, coordinate, provide services for, and conduct credentialing in nursing."*

The ANA received the report and accepted the recommendation of the committee to form a task force to further study the report and promote im-

---

*Credentialing in nursing: a new approach, report of the Committee for Study of Credentialing in Nursing, Am. J. Nurs. **79:**674, April 1979. (Reprinted with permission of the American Nurses' Association.)

*Credentialing in nursing: a new approach, report of the Committee for the Study of Credentialing in Nursing, Am. J. Nurs. **79:**680, April 1979. (Reprinted with permission of the American Nurses' Association.)

plementation of the recommendations. In so doing, the ANA invited NLN to participate The NLN board of directors at their preconvention meeting in 1979 declined the invitation; however, the membership brought the issue to the floor for vote and the majority voted for the NLN to particpate in the next phase of the credentialing study.

During the first 2 years (i.e., 1980 to 1982) all the major nursing organizations met to consider a credentialing center as envisioned. Consensus was not reached. Each organization had vested interests in what would become a part of the center; for example, NLN has for 35 years been the body to accredit schools and they were not willing to relinquish that responsibility.

In 1982 the ANA delegates at their convention voted to "ensure a system of credentialing in nursing."* This became a bylaw change of the organization. Just what or how the bylaw will be implemented continues to be unclear; however, should a center be formed as envisioned, significant changes in all major nursing organizations would occur in the 1990s.

Cost effectiveness and employment needs

A major issue in the health industry is the cost of illness care. As medical technology has developed more sophisticated treatment, and as inflation has spiraled, the cost of illness care has also risen. In the early 1980s it is a major issue, particularly in hospitals. Health care in the United States has, up until the 1980s meant hospitalization and treatment of illness. The average patient cannot afford the cost of care for simple illnesses.

The committee developed broad position statements on which decisions could be made. They took the following positions on entry to practice†:

*The A.N.A. bylaws as revised by the 1982 house of delegates, Am. Nurse **14**(10):15, 1982.
†The statements of the committee quoted in this discussion are from Credentialing in nursing: a new approach, report of the Committee for the Study of Credentialing in Nursing, Am. J. Nurs. **79**:680, April 1979. (Reprinted with permission of the American Nurses' Assocation.)

1. Education for entry into practice should be defined by the professional society.
2. Therefore the positions taken by the ANA in 1965 and 1978 should be used as a guide for the definition.
3. The professional society, with broad consultation, should continue periodically to assess society's needs for nursing to redefine practice and educational preparation accordingly.

They made the following statement on educational mobility: "mechanisms for the credentialing of individuals and educational programs should encourage the achievement of the highest aspirations of individuals insofar as they are consonant with their abilities, and should remove artificial barriers to this attainment."

On control of credentialing, they made the following statements:

1. It is an appropriate role for state government agencies regulating nursing (nursing boards) and with responsibility for protecting the public to license individuals for practice.
2. It is an appropriate role for the profession, with broad consultation, to credential and/or set standards for the credentialing of:
   a. Individuals:
      i. For entry into professional practice.
      ii. For entry into specialty practice.
   b. Institutions and agencies offering educational programs which prepare:
      i. For entry into professional practice.
      ii. For entry into specialty practice.
   c. Institutions/agencies providing organized nursing services.
3. It is an appropriate role for the federal government to determine that agencies, institutions, programs, and individuals eligible for funding and reimbursement are appropriately credentialed according to the roles defined above.

On cost of credentialing, the committee stated:

Although the cost of credentialing mechanisms and processes may be subsidized in part by government, philanthrophy, and professional societies, the costs of credentialing are ultimately reflected in the costs of health care; therefore:

1. Credentialing should be limited to that required to serve the public welfare.

2. A coherent, articulated, comprehensive system, considering all persons involved in nursing practice, should result in minimal credentialing and related costs.

3. Individuals are responsible for maintaining their own competence and for the learning required to maintain that competence and for the costs of associated credentialing.

4. Agencies and institutions providing nursing education and nursing service are responsible for maintaining the quality of those programs and services and for the costs of associated institutional and program credentialing.

5. Cost studies of credentialing and public oversight of relationships between credentialing (and other regulatory mechanisms) and health outcomes should continue to be done.

On accountability, they enumerated the following points:

1. Accountability, within the framework of the standards set by the professions, is an essential dimension of credentialing.

2. Accountability includes aspects of shared governance, as well as reporting, explaining, and justifying.

3. The structural components of credentialing bodies and credentialing processes should provide for both intraprofessional and extraprofessional accountability.

4. The involvement of public members on credentialing bodies should fulfill the purpose of challenging the assumptions upon which the credentialing processes rest, with the view toward having them serve the public interest in contrast to that of the profession.

5. Accountability as it relates to credentialing must encompass the notion of having appropriate mechanisms for redress for the public and individual practitioners or agencies, in cases wherein either is ill-served.

On competence, they stated:

1. A comprehensive credentialing system should assure initial and continued competence of the nursing practitioner.

2. Research on existing and emerging methods of assessing competence should be ongoing.

3. The employing agency or institution is responsible for providing an environment in which continued competence and improved practice are encouraged.

4. The delineation of practice privileges and continued periodic review of such privileges in agencies and institutions has a role in assuring practitioner competence in his/her particular nursing responsibility.

Our society is illness oriented. Former Secretary of Health, Education and Welfare Joseph Califano, on taking his cabinet post, made it his platform to change society from an illness orientation to a health orientation. The belief was that if illness could be prevented, national health insurance could be afforded.

Hospitals have examined their practices and found physicians ordering many more diagnostic studies than necessary. Measures were introduced to discourage this practice. Patient stay days were examined. It was found that patients were being kept in the hospital longer than necessary; so patient stay days were decreased. All this has affected nursing. As the patient stay decreased, the level of acuteness of illness increased, which demanded a higher concentration of RN care. The need for RNs has increased, and there has been a decrease in the need for nurse assistants and licensed practical nurses. See Chapter 2 for a discussion on the cost of health care.

Issues surrounding cost control of health care

In 1980 the ANA adopted a social policy statement that addressed social concerns of nursing, nature and scope of nursing practice, and specialization in nursing practice.

The social policy statement examined the issues and identified some specific areas of concern. Among the issues were authority for nursing practice, working relationships, health as it becomes the center of nursing attention, and rules that will govern the cost of health care.

An outcome of the statement provides a definition of nursing that encompasses four characteristics of nursing. The statement defines nursing as "diagnosis and treatment of human responses to actual or potential health problems," and the four characteristics of nursing are identified as

"... phenomena, theory application, nursing action, and evaluation of effects of action in relation to phenomena."*

The social policy statement further identifies two types of practitioners: the generalist and the specialist. The generalist provides the bulk of nursing care while the specialist focuses on "specific clusters of phenomena." The specialist is educated at the master's and doctoral level.

Cost control of health care affects who gives care and whether such care is economical. Chapter 2 discussed "downtime" for the individual who is not an RN; Levi calls this phenomenon "functional redundancy."† Levi, in studying the process of professionalization, has concluded that so long as anyone can do nursing tasks there is functional redundancy. RNs may be educated to do all nursing care; however, the LPN and nurse assistant are also doing many of the same tasks. Thus the RN is in competition with others and has no monopoly over "any set of socially significant or even insignificant roles."

Levi postulates that for the status of nursing to be elevated to a profession the first thing to do is "try to remove the possibility of functional redundancy." It was seen in Chapter 2 that an all-RN staff was more cost-effective than a mixed staff of RNs and other nurse workers. If this be the case, then reimbursement for nursing service in dealing with cost control and delivery of quality care would make sense for the profession to move forward in 1990.

An issue surrounding functional redundancy is the one of technical and professional nursing. Coupled with the social policy statement on generalist and specialist, maybe the issue of technical and professional would be resolved if functional redundancy was eliminated. Just as there are no technical and professional physicians, why does the profession of nursing need a technically prepared

nurse who is different from the professional nurse? The credentialing issue would also take on new meaning. Only those nurses could practice nursing as a specialist if additional education and certification had been secured.

The social policy statement raises an issue on the new graduate as a generalist. The question to be examined is "Is the new graduate ready to function as a generalist on graduation?" There are many nursing service administrators and staff who say they are not prepared and support the extern-internship for the new graduate. The proponents of internships maintain that the new graduate would have controlled settings in which to practice.

If professionalization occurs with arduous theoretical study and application, and if autonomy of a profession occurs because the generalist and specialist have knowledge and skills no one else has, then perhaps there is a real case for internships for all new nurses. As a means of quality control and cost effectiveness, internship should be explored in the late 1980s.

SOME AREAS FOR CONSIDERATION

The future of health care, which includes care given by nurses, is in the hands of legislative leaders. The system provided will be implemented by health workers. Nurses will need to take the issues of human rights, nurses' rights, and the delivery of health care into perspective so that the future of professional nursing can survive.

The following statements need to be considered as the future is being planned:
1. Quality health care is considered a right for everyone rather than a privilege of those who can afford it.
2. Manpower must be provided to meet the needs of consumers of health care services.
3. Each nurse must resolve the ethical issues in order to provide health care.
4. Society has changed its attitudes and values relative to health and medicine.
5. The advances in medical care need to be evaluated in relation to the role nursing will take.

*Nursing—a social policy statement, Kansas City, Mo., American Nurses' Association, p. 9.
†Levi, M.: Functional redundancy and the process of professionalization, J. Health Politics Policy Law **5:**2, Summer 1980.

In November 1983 the ANA determined the need to advance a national health policy agenda. To this end the ANA desires to foster "political savvy" among nurses. The agenda identified is as follows: access to care, financing health care, funding basic needs, funding nursing education and nursing research, human rights, economic and general welfare of nurses, and health hazards.*

The professional nurse should be cognizant not only of the technical aspects of nursing but also the theoretical and philosophical aspects of the profession. By examining the past and the present, the future can be planned and made to function as desired by the profession.

The health industry has become the major industry of the United States as well as the largest employing industry. It supports in excess of 300 different types of health workers. As this growth has occurred, the roles of the physician, the nurse, and other health workers have blurred; federal control has increased through legislation regarding regulation of agencies, utilization of facilities, and medical peer review; technology has affected delivery of health care by increasing the cost of health care and the complexity of care; and preventive medicine is evolving as the focus of health care.

A unified approach to health care that offers a continuum from prevention of illness to the restoration of optimum health can be accomplished by not accepting the status quo and by rigorous research of the problem and implementing the findings.

SUMMARY

The issues in nursing today are not necessarily different from those in the past, but they are far more complex. The issues of human rights, nurses' rights, and an effective health care system need everyone's attention. Although the status quo maintains equilibrium, a consistent pattern of change is necessary to move the delivery of health care in

such a way that all citizens will receive adequate care. Professional nurses need to be aware of all issues facing the profession and society and to contribute to the solutions through planned change.

Discussion questions

1. Discuss the value of a credentialing center and the impact such a center would have on licensure, accreditation of educational programs, and certification.
2. Discuss the human rights issue as it presently influences nursing as a predominantly female profession.
3. Discuss what "autonomy of nursing practice" means.
4. Discuss the ANA Code of Ethics and its internalization by a practicing nurse.
5. Discuss functional redundancy in relation to achieving the goal of nursing as a profession.

SUGGESTED READINGS

Aydelotte, M.K.: Nursing education and practice: putting it all together. J. Nurs. Educ. **2**:21-27, Nov. 1972.

Aydelotte, M.K.: The future delivery system and the utilization of nurses prepared in formal educational programs. In Chaska, N.: The nursing profession, New York, 1978, McGraw-Hill Book Co.

Bell, D., et al.: Toward the year 2000: work in progress, Boston, 1968, Beacon Press.

Christy, T.E.: New privileges . . . new challenges . . . new responsibilities, Nurs. '73 **4**:8-11, Feb. 1974.

Credentialing in nursing: a new approach, Am. J. Nurs. **79**:674, April 1979.

Fagothey, A.: Right and reason: ethics in theory and practice, ed. 7, St. Louis, 1981, The C.V. Mosby Co.

Fletcher, J.: Ethics and euthanasia, Am. J. Nurs. **73**:670, April 1973.

Fry, S.T.: The social responsibilities of nursing, Nurs. Economics **1**(1):61, 1983.

Jacox, A.: Address to the next generation, Nurs. Outlook **26**:38, Jan 1978.

Levi, M.: Functional redundancy and the process of professionalization, J. Health Politics, Policy and Law **5**:2, Summer 1980.

Lewis, E.P.: A role by any name (editorial), Nurs. Outlook **22**:89, Feb. 1974.

Lewis, E.P.: The issue that won't go away, Nurs. Outlook **27**:107, Feb. 1979.

Lysaught, J.P., editor: Action in nursing, New York, 1974, McGraw-Hill Book Co.

---

*Am. Nurse **15**(10):1, 5, 1983.

McCarty, P.: The 80's: What lies ahead for nursing? Am. Nurse **12:**1, Jan 1980.

Moore, W.W.: The professions: roles and rules, New York, 1970, Russell Sage Foundation.

Nichols, B.: Open letter to the nurses of America, Am. J. Nurs. **80:**61, Jan. 1980.

Orem, J.Y., and Lindbeck, R.S.: Nurse participation in medical peer review, Nurs. Outlook, **22:**27-30, Jan. 1974.

Popiel, E.S.: Nurse practitioners: a new program in continuing education, J. Nurs. Ed. **12:**29-36, Jan. 1973.

Roe, A., and Sherwood, M.: Nursing in the seventies, New York, 1973, John Wiley & Sons, Inc.

Sheahan, Sister D.: Scanning the seventies, Nurs. Outlook **26:**33, Jan. 1978.

Styles, M.M.: Dialogue across the decades, Nurs. Outlook **26:**28, Jan. 1978.

Styles, M.M.: On nursing: toward a new endowment, St. Louis, 1982, The C.V. Mosby Co.

Toffler, A.: Future shock, New York, 1970, Random House, Inc.

CHAPTER 6
Entry to practice—education

OBJECTIVE: On completion of this chapter, the student of nursing will have an understanding and appreciation for the present-day system of nursing education, that is, postsecondary and higher education.

The educational issue of entry to practice has been with the profession for 20 years. Chapter 3 familiarized the reader with the evolution of nursing education, and this chapter will discuss what presently constitutes the educational routes to practice.

To enter the practice of nursing an individual can choose practical (vocational) nursing or registered nursing education. Practical nurse education can be achieved in senior high schools, junior colleges, and vocational education schools. Registered nurse education can be achieved through junior or community colleges, hospitals, and 4-year colleges or universities.

POSTSECONDARY AND HIGHER EDUCATION

Nursing education follows the system of education in the United States, namely, postsecondary education and higher education. Postsecondary education is any educational endeavor following high school. This level of education can be found in corporations to train specific kinds of workers, for example, MacDonald's and IBM each have highly sophisticated programs to train their personnel. The purpose of postsecondary education is to provide an individual with a trade or vocation with which to earn a living. Practical nursing and two of the registered nurse programs fall in this category. Associate degree nursing programs and hospital-based

programs can be classified as postsecondary education.

Higher education is usually found in the 4-year colleges and universities. There are some who classify higher education only in universities where graduate education takes place. With this classification, nursing programs found in 4-year colleges and universities are considered in the system of higher education.

EXTERNAL CONTROLS

The system of nursing education is governed by a variety of state, regional, and national controls. State governing bodies such as state boards of nursing, boards of regents, and departments of education govern whether a program can function. In most states, all nursing programs must have approval from the state board of nursing. Practical nurse programs will additionally have approval from either a department of education or a department of vocational education or both, depending on the system within the state. Registered nurse education will additionally have approval from a board of regents, department of education, or both, again depending on the state system.

Regional accreditation of nursing education occurs when the educational institution in which it is housed receives its approval.

Nationally, programs may choose to be accredited through the National League for Nursing. This is voluntary; however, approximately 90% of all programs elect to meet the criteria for their respective programs.

The impact of external controls on nursing education is a forceful one. Standards of excellence are expected to be met. Thus graduates of approved and accredited programs can expect a sound education.

In 20 years nursing has essentially achieved its goal of having nursing education in the mainstream of the education system (i.e., postsecondary and higher education). However, the profession has not achieved the goal of all education in the mainstream of higher education.

LEVELS OF EDUCATION

What remains for nursing is to determine if the goal for two types of nurses (or levels) is appropriate. Presently there are three levels of nurses identified in the nursing literature: vocational, technical, and professional. In examining the general system of education the vocational level is fairly clear and concise. Vocational education (i.e., postsecondary) is the providing of skills with knowledge for practice in an occupation such as nursing.

Technical education is not so clear. Technical education can be found in high technology with the most profound theoretical background. For example, an engineer is well disciplined in high technology or a surgeon becomes a highly skilled technician.

Professional education becomes more clear than technical. Professional education builds on a base of liberal education in the social-physical sciences and the arts and humanities.

With an understanding of the general system of education, nursing needs to address what is technical education for nurses and what is professional education for nurses?

If baccalaureate education is the base for professional nursing, then what is the base for technical education? Another question that could be posed is, "At what point is there a difference in what a technical nurse does and what the professional

nurse does?" A final question might be, "Are all of the beginning entry points to practice nursing technical education? And if so, what is professional nursing?"

The system of higher education includes the academically prepared nurse at the doctoral level, the only professionally prepared nurse. In order to achieve the doctoral level, one must have a baccalaureate degree and a master's degree, both in nursing. Perhaps in the late 1980s and 1990s the profession needs to address the ramifications of one level only for nursing.

Legitimizing nursing as a profession can only be done when functional redundancy is reduced or removed altogether. Chapter 5 discusses functional redundancy. The questions posed help the student to examine with an inquiring mind the issue that has consumed more energy and time than any issue in nursing.

PRESENT SYSTEM OF NURSING EDUCATION

The present system of nursing education includes practical nurse education, registered nurse education, and graduate education.

Practical nurse education has two entry approaches, the senior high school and postsecondary schools. Registered nurse education may occur through one of five types of programs: associate degree, diploma, baccalaureate, nurse doctorate, and master's degrees. Each of these programs will be described in the following pages. Graduate education in nursing includes master's and doctoral programs.

Practical nurse program*

Practical nursing as it is known today is a young vocation; however, its evolution has spanned centuries, and its cultural heritage is rich in tradition and service to humankind. Beginning in response to a need to meet basic human needs, early practical

*Contributed by Gay Lindsay, Director, Practical Nurse Program, Akron, Ohio.

nursing programs varied widely in length, course content, and basic organization. Their objective was to train attendant nurses to provide care in the home.

During the 1940s, a decade that saw the world involved in war, a turning point in the recognition of the practical nurse as a contributor in nursing service occurred. The shortage of professional nurses clearly indicated the need for another level of nursing. Nursing leaders agreed to assume responsibility for formulating principles and policies for the control and use of the practical nurse.

In the beginning, schools were under the sponship of private agencies, but the availability of federal funds (Smith-Hughes Act of 1917) soon placed the education of practical nurses with the public schools. In 1947 a job analysis for the practical nurse occupation was published by the U.S. Office of Education. Soon, a curriculum guide followed and programs to educate instructors were developed.

By the end of the 1940s many states had passed laws providing for licensure of the practical nurse. Practical nursing organizations were established, and the National League of Nursing Education prepared achievement and licensure tests that enabled evaluation of learning experiences and attested to the practical nurse graduates' abilities.

The rate of educating practical nurses increased rapidly during the 1950s, 1960s, and 1970s. Currently there are 1319 state-approved programs, and the total enrollment as of Oct. 15, 1982 was 61,517 students.*

Today's over 500,000 employed LPNs are prepared to assist professional nurses and to work under supervision in giving patient care to people of all ages and cultures in various stages of dependency.

A statement of the competencies of graduates of educational programs in practical nursing was developed by the National League for Nursing Council of Practical Nursing Programs in 1979. This document describes the minimum expectations of new graduates in accomplishing the nursing process and includes the following:

Practical nursing students are prepared in educational programs that stress clinical experiences primarily in structured care settings such as hospitals and nursing homes. Clinical practice is correlated with basic therapeutic knowledge and introductory content from the biological and behavioral sciences. Planned and supervised experiences are directed toward teaching students to perform nursing measures with precision, safety, and efficiency consistent with current nursing concepts and practices. Communication skills and mental health concepts are integrated into the total curriculum. Qualified nurse educators guide students in the nursing process and care planning.*

Legally, practical nurses are limited to performing those acts for which they have received educational preparation.

Qualifications for the practical nurse are maturity, an ability to use sound judgment, and a high school diploma. Often, schools use standard preentrance tests to determine a potential student's aptitude for practical nursing.

At present, practical nurse education in the majority of states is a minimum of 1 year in length, usually a calendar year. Most programs include courses in body structure and function, general psychology, microbiology, basic nursing, medical-surgical nursing of adults and children, maternity nursing, personal and vocational relationships, nutrition, pharmacology, mental health nursing, and geriatrics. The supervised experience includes patient care in medical-surgical, pediatric, and maternity nursing and may include specialties such as labor and delivery, nursery, and operating and recovery rooms.

The cost of education for the student varies, but in general it is less than that of other nursing education programs. Such financial assistance as Basic Education Opportunity Grants, Supplemental

*Vaughn, J.C.: Educational preparation for nursing, Nurs. Health Care **4**(8):461, 1983.

*Competencies of graduates of educational programs in practical nursing, Pub. No. 38-1686, New York, 1979, National League for Nursing.

Educational Opportunity Grants, Guaranteed Student Loans, Veteran's Education Benefits, and scholarships is available.

The opportunities for practical nurses are many. They can work in private duty nursing; in general hospitals or in specific fields such as obstetrics, pediatrics, surgery, general medicine, and psychiatry; in nursing homes and physicians' and dentists' offices; in the Peace Corps and armed forces; in community health agencies; in industry; and in many other areas.

Liscensure for practical nurses exists in all states, the District of Columbia, Guam, Puerto Rico, and the Virgin Islands. Pennsylvania in 1919 was the first state to pass such legislation, and the District of Columbia in 1960 was the last. In some states these laws are permissive and protect the title of practical nurse only. An increasing number of states have mandatory licensure. Twelve jurisdictions have separate laws governing the practice of practical nursing. In all others the laws are not separate from the Registered Nurse Practice Act.

The National Federation of Licensed Practical Nurses is the membership organization for the LPN and vocational nurse. In 1970 the federation adopted revised, expanded functions of the LPN. These functions include increased responsibility, such as being a team leader.

Approval for schools of practical nursing occurs first through a state board of nursing. All schools must be approved by the appropriate state board. National accreditation may occur through the National Association for Practical Nurse Education or the NLN Council of Practical Nursing Programs, which added that service in 1964.

Although practical nurse programs do not prepare the practitioner to go on to professional nursing, there are some practical nurses who, after completing this part of their education, have continued on to become registered professional nurses. Because the practical nurse program is a program within itself, it is not considered a stepping-off program for professional nursing.

In 1968 the NLN Council of Diploma Programs passed a resolution to make every effort to admit the LPN to diploma programs and to allow previously learned material to be challenged by examination. This was an attempt to assist the practical nurse to move from one level of nursing to another without undue hardship.

Since 1970 a greater effort has been made on the part of all registered nurse programs to admit the LPN and allow this individual to challenge course work through competency-based modules. Articulation is becoming easier without jeopardizing standards.

Registered nurse education

The entry to practice nursing with a registered nurse license can be accomplished in five different and distinct types of programs. The newest approach is by way of a nurse doctorate to be found only at Case Western Reserve, Frances Payne Bolton School of Nursing, Cleveland, Ohio.

A second approach designed specifically for the nonnurse college graduate is the master's degree in nursing, which provides basic nursing education. In May 1982 there were six such programs throughout the country.* Yale and Case Western Reserve University programs date back to 1923 with a resurgence of interest in 1960 when Pace University at New York Medical College admitted its first class under Frances Reiter. Throughout the years of 1923 to 1970 Yale and Case Western Reserve Universities have altered their programs; for example, Case Western Reserve University first had a master's basic degree in nursing, then a bachelor's degree, and now the nurse doctorate.

Taken in most recent historical context the next approach is associate degree nursing education. Associate degree education was founded in 1952 and 1953 with eight schools and now provides the largest number of RNs.

The fourth approach is that of a generic baccalaureate nursing education. These programs date back to 1909 with their greatest growth and emphasis since the 1950s.

---

*Slavinsky, A.T., and Diers, D.: Nursing education for college graduates, Nurs. Outlook **30**(5):293, 1982.

The oldest form of registered nurse education is that of diploma nurse education. Although the number of these programs has significantly decreased, the number of graduates each year remains significant.

The following pages provide an account of each of these programs in order of historical development. There are many similarities and yet subtle differences. The one truism for all graduates of these programs is that they are prepared to care for people with the same basic technical skills of nursing and take the same state board examination with which a license to practice nursing is secured.

Diploma programs.* Diploma education for nursing occupies a significant position in preparing RNs to meet the current and future needs of society.

The oldest form of education for nursing, this type of education can be traced back to Florence Nightingale, who consistently indicated that nurses needed preparation and that they should not be people just coming from the street or the home with little or no background in the care of the sick. Hospitals established schools of nursing leading to a diploma when the needs of nursing demanded that practitioners caring for patients have some form of education. Although at the outset, diploma programs controlled by hospitals reflected an apprentice type of training and had as a primary objective the meeting of the service needs of the controlling hospital, today's diploma programs assume a rightful position of offering education that fits into the mainstream of postsecondary education.

Today's diploma programs in nursing are usually controlled by a hospital. However, there are some schools that are independently incorporated with an identifiable board of control and a financial base that is separate from the hospital. It is therefore more appropriate to acknowledge this type of education as a school, controlled by a hospital or independently controlled, that offers an education program leading to a diploma rather than by a hospital diploma school of nursing.

---

*Contributed by Marilyn Burkart, Assistant Director, Division of Diploma Programs, National League for Nursing.

Today's diploma program in nursing is hardly recognizable from its counterpart of 25 to 30 years ago. Although close proximity to the clinical setting continues to be given major emphasis, today's programs are not unlike those of any other educational institution with regard to students, faculty, resources, and sources. However, there are features that characterize and give credence to this form of nursing education. The following statement, entitled *Characteristics of Diploma Education in Nursing,* revised and adopted by the Council of Diploma Programs of the NLN in 1978, serves the important purpose of informing the prospective student and the consumer about the unique characteristics of diploma education for nursing*:

The diploma program in nursing serves the interests and goals of qualified students who desire an education that is centered in an acute-care setting dedicated to the care of patients. The characteristics of the diploma program in nursing are:

The school is in the unique position of offering a readily accessible clinical laboratory that promotes the students' understanding of the hospital climate and resources and the interrelation of other health disciplines.

The primary purpose of the school is to develop the potential of students as individuals and as competent beginning practitioners of nursing in acute care facilities and in a variety of health care settings.

The school may enter into cooperative relations with colleges or universities for educational courses and/or services. The school may also enter into cooperative relationships with health care institutions and agencies in order to provide learning experiences for students.

The school provides the necessary educational resources, facilities, and services to students and faculty.

The philosophy and objectives of the school give consideration to the personal and professional development of the students and serve as the basis for the development of the curriculum.

The faculty, including nurse and non-nurse members, are cognizant of concepts and trends in nursing, nursing education, and general education. They have academic preparation and experience in nursing, nursing education, and/or other special fields of interest that ensure a quality educational program.

---

*National League for Nursing, 1978.

The faculty are committed to the improvement of nursing education as it relates to nursing practice and the delivery of health care and have a unique opportunity to promote changes in nursing practice in hospitals and other health care agencies.

Admission requirements include graduation from high school or its equivalent, with successful completion of certain prerequisite courses, satisfactory achievement on pre-entrance examinations, and satisfactory assessment of personal qualities and health status.

Students are selected by the faculty and are admitted directly to the program in nursing.

Students are given the opportunity to demonstrate the knowledge and skills acquired in previous educational experiences for course exemption or advanced placement in the educational program.

The faculty, utilizing trends and changes in education and health care, plan, organize, implement, and evaluate the curriculum within the framework of the philosophy, objectives, and policies of the school of nursing.

The curriculum is designed to develop the knowledge and skills essential for beginning practice as a registered nurse in acute, intermediate, long-term, and ambulatory health care facilities.

The curriculum includes courses in the theory and practice of nursing and courses in the natural and social sciences. Learning is reinforced through the application of scientific and nursing principles for implementing the nursing process in the care of individuals and groups with nursing and health needs.

Early and substantial patient care experiences are provided in the hospital and in a variety of community agencies which serve to foster within the student a strong identification wih nursing.

The graduates of diploma programs (1) are eligible to take the examination leading to licensure as a registered nurse; (2) utilize the nursing process which includes assessment, planning, implementation, and evaluation of nursing care for individuals and groups of patients; (3) have an understanding of the hospital climate and the community health resources necessary for extended care of patients; (4) understand the role of other health disciplines and are contributing members of the health team; and (5) adjust with minimal difficulty to the role of beginning registered nurse practitioners in acute, intermediate, long-term, and ambulatory health care facilities.

Competency to practice is the expectation of the graduate of the diploma program in nursing, the employer of the graduate, and the patient or consumer of the service. To guide faculties in diploma programs in nursing, as well as students, employers, and the public, in their understanding of the knowledge, skill, and competencies of graduates of diploma programs, the NLN Council of Diploma Programs in 1978 adopted the following outline, *Role and Competencies of Graduates of Diploma Programs in Nursing:*

The graduate of the diploma program in nursing is eligible to seek licensure as a registered nurse and to function as a beginning practitioner in acute, intermediate, long-term and ambulatory health care facilities. In order to fulfill such roles, graduates should demonstrate the following competencies*†:

Assessment
Establishes a data base through a nursing history including a psychosocial and physical assessment.
Utilizes knowledge of the etiology, pathophysiology, usual course, and prognosis for the prevalent illnesses and health problems.
Establishes priorities when providing nursing care for one or more patients.
Recognizes the significance of non-verbal communication.

Planning
Formulates a written plan of nursing care based on the assessment of patient needs.
Includes in the nursing care plan the effects of the family or significant other, life experiences, and social-cultural background.
Involves the patient, family and significant others in the development of the nursing plan of care.
Incorporates the learning needs of the patient and family into an individualized plan of care.
Applies principles of organization and management in utilizing the knowledge and skills of other nursing personnel.

*National League for Nursing, 1979.
†Competency, as used in this document, is the ability to apply in practice situations the essential principles and techniques of nursing and to apply those concepts, skills, and attitudes required of all nurses to fulfill their role, regardless of their specific position or responsibility.

Implementation

Meets the health needs of individuals and families.

Utilizes concepts, scientific facts, and principles when providing nursing care.

Performs technical nursing procedures.

Initiates appropriate intervention when environmental and safety hazards exist.

Initiates preventive, habilitative, and rehabilitative nursing measures according to the needs demonstrated by patients and families.

Performs independent nursing measures and/or seeks assistance from other members of the health team in response to the changing needs of patients.

Collaborates with physicians and members of other disciplines to provide health care.

Documents nursing interventions and patient responses.

Utilizes effective verbal and written communication.

Communicates pertinent information related to the patient through established channels.

Assists the physician in implementing the medical plan of care.

Applies knowledge of individual and group behavior in establishing interpersonal relationships.

Teaches individuals and groups to achieve and maintain an optimum level of wellness.

Utilizes the services of community agencies for continuity of patient care.

Protects the rights of patients and families.

Evaluation

Evaluates the effectiveness of nursing care and takes appropriate action.

Initiates and cooperates in efforts to improve nursing practice.

Professionalism

Recognizes the legal limits of nursing practice.

Demonstrates ethical behavior in the performance of nursing.

Practices nursing in a nondiscriminatory and nonjudgmental manner.

Respects the rights of other to have their own value systems.

Accepts responsibility and accountability for professional practice.

Pursues independent study and continuing education.

Demonstrates flexibility in functioning in a changing society.

Adjusts with minimal difficulty to the role of employee.

What are schools with diploma programs like today? They are no different from any other schools and share the same problems and challenges as other educational institutions. Diploma programs are no longer 3 calendar years in length; they may vary from 1 year (a specialized program for licensed practical nurses) to 2 academic years, to 2 calendar years, to 3 academic years. All schools stipulate graduation from high school or equivalency as a requirement for admission. Regardless of the length, all schools offering diploma programs in nursing include courses in nursing and courses in the biological, physical, and social sciences planned so that the new graduate can function in the position and setting designated in the objectives of the school. Some schools have a prerequisite of 1 year of college or requirements of college courses in the areas of general education and physical, biological, and behavioral sciences before admission to the nursing major. Other schools contract for college courses within the confines of the curriculum, while still others teach their own courses.

Thus students graduating from a diploma program in nursing can earn a number of legitimate college credits in the above areas or are prepared to challenge for exemption from these courses if they continue their education beyond the diploma program. With regard to admission, schools do not discriminate because of age, sex, religion, national origin, race, marital status, or handicap, and the heterogeneity of the student body reflects this. Efforts are made to allow students to transfer from one program to another without a great loss of time, and more and more emphasis has been placed on providing opportunities for students to be admitted with advanced standing. Students in diploma programs represent diverse backgrounds and a variety of educational experiences before admission. These may range from licensure as a practical nurse to a master's degree in mathematics.

The school offering the diploma program in nursing, similar to other kinds of educational insitutions, offers a variety of services to students, including housing, health guidance, and counseling as well as access to libraries and learning resource centers. Even though housing facilities are available, it may not be a requirement for students to be in residence. In fact, many schools encourage students to commute, which is in keeping with the needs of the variety of students who choose this type of education. Older and married students often find that this type of educational program allows them to reach their goal without radically changing their way of life.

Students are encouraged to participate in organizations aimed at promoting leadership at the local, state, and national level. Opportunities are provided for them to be active in community affairs and to carry out functions related to their interests and needs. Faculty in diploma programs are creative, energetic, and committed to this type of nursing education. They are active in their efforts to improve their abilities as teachers, and they plan to carry out ongoing faculty development programs especially designed to attain these purposes.

The curriculum or planned program of studies is the most vital part of the diploma program in nursing and demands the greatest attention of the faculty. Based on a specific set of objectives, evolving from the philosophy and objectives of the school, the curriculum includes courses arranged in sequence to take into consideration the needs of the learner. Thus courses progress from simple to complex, known to unknown, normal to abnormal.

The nursing courses, planned within a framework developed and accepted by the faculty, include content related to nursing foundation, nursing history, ethics, fundamentals of nursing, and medical, surgical, obstetric, pediatric, and psychiatric nursing. Leadership in nursing or the management

of nursing care for groups of patients is especially important to the curriculum, since this content and experience is essential to the kind of position the graduate of the diploma program in nursing is being prepared to assume.

The courses in general education and the biological, physical, social, and behavioral sciences are basic to the nursing courses and provide the foundation of knowledge necessary to understand al facets of the patient and family.

Learning experiences in the clinical setting are the most important part of the nursing courses, since it is in this laboratory setting that the student, directly supervised and evaluated by the instructor, has the opportunity to apply the content learned in the theory portion of the course. The clinical laboratory is vital to the diploma program in nursing, and the close proximity to the hospital provides opportunity for the student to have early exposure to this setting as well as quality experience in sufficient quantity throughout the program. Learning experiences are also planned in a variety of other settings such as the community, extended care facilities, physicians' offices, and other similar agencies and institutions.

The hours spent in the clinical laboratory are carefully arranged in a specified ratio to the theory hours to attain the objectives of the courses and the curriculum and to meet the learning needs of the students. Competency to practice is essential to the attainment of objectives.

Faculty are responsible for supervising a designated number of students assigned to the clinical portion of each nursing course. The number of students, usually fewer in the first nursing courses in the curriculum, provides for careful selection of the most meaningful learning experience in the clinical setting for the student and allows the instructor and student to share in developing and implementing the nursing care plan for the assigned patients. Ample opportunity is provided for the student to use the nursing process in implementing and evaluating the care plan for each patient.

Thus the school offering the diploma program

in nursing is making a contribution in preparing nurses to meet the current and future needs of society.

Baccalaureate degree programs. In the early years of collegiate education there were two types of programs in nursing that led to the baccalaureate degree. The first, a preservice program, was called the basic degree program and was designed for individuals who had had no previous education in nursing. The second was usually called a general nursing program and was designed for graduates of approved diploma and associate degree programs who wished to extend their general education and professional background and prepare for first-level positions in nursing, including public health. Both of these programs provided the necessary foundation for graduate study in nursing.

By the latter part of the 1960s, faculties in collegiate schools of nursing had begun to make changes that presaged the events of the 1970s. The first major change was the emphasis on a single curriculum pattern applicable to both preservice students and graduate professional nurses who wanted to continue their education. The graduate of an approved diploma or associate degree program was allowed to apply for admission, have any previous work evaluated, and, if admitted, had the option of earning credit in required courses by successfully passing either standardized or teacher-prepared examinations. It was believed that this was an effective method of utilizing previously learned knowledge and skill, since the student would then move on to the next course of study and gain new learning experiences that were designed to meet the objectives of the baccalaureate degree program.

The baccalaureate programs in nursing during the 1960s were designed to prepare nurses to be professionally and technically competent members of a health team while providing students with the liberal education necessary to function effectively as individuals and as members of society. The philosophy of most baccalaureate educators of that period was cogently summarized by Tschudin when she indicated that the graduate of a baccalaureate program in nursing could be expected to do the following*:

1. Perform common, important nursing procedures
2. Carry out nursing procedures not previously encountered and devise new ones to meet varying circumstances or technological advances
3. Function effectively in the absence of established policies, set routines, and written procedures
4. Be oriented primarily to patients rather than tasks or routines and establish priorities in the care of a group of patients
5. Function effectively in widely varying, complex nursing situations and give guidance and directions to those with lesser preparation
6. Identify and study the technical problems of nursing, drawing on research findings and scientific methodology
7. Plan, evaluate, and make decisions for the improvement of nursing care
8. Assume initiative and accept personal responsibility for making nursing decisions when changing circumstances in the care of patients indicate the inadequacy of established routines
9. Assume responsibility for the quality of nursing care provided by themselves, or others, for the patients for whom they care
10. Collaborate with the physician in achieving his therapeutic goals and in developing nursing care plans for his patients

By 1970 there were indications that programs in nursing, while emphasizing the sound foundation in the biological and social sciences, were also examining critically the reason for which the program existed. As stated by Aydelotte,

one must examine the basic goals, the *purpose* for which professionals are prepared, for which their roles exist, and for which society has tendered its support. The purpose is certainly not the enhancement of the professional elite and the profession itself. Rather, the purpose evolves from the needs in our society for specific human

*Reprinted, with permission, from Tschudin, M.S.: Educational preparation needed by the nurse in the future, Nurs. Outlook **12**:32, April 1964.

services. Society has assigned to nursing the primary tasks of assessing patient wants and needs; designing and executing care practices to meet these; and the further function of instructing patients and others in the maintenance of health, the avoidance of malady, and the extension of care. While patient wants and needs will vary in kind and amount and are dependent upon a number of social and economic factors as well as cultural forces which are operating, there is an obligation impinging upon the profession to meet these assigned ends.*

An early indicator of this changing from emphasis on facts and techniques to a process whereby client needs were assessed and analyzed before the planning of nursing interventions was the statement regarding baccalaureate education issued by the NLN Council of Baccalaureate and Higher Degree Programs in 1968†:

General assumptions regarding baccalaureate education in nursing

The significant characteristics of baccalaureate education in nursing derive from a base in general education that "must consciously aim at these abilities: effective thinking, communication, the making of relative judgments, and the discrimination of values."‡ The professional major in nursing builds upon, incorporates, and extends these abilities and introduces content essential for the practice of professional nursing.

The baccalaureate program provides students with the opportunity to acquire: (1) knowledge of basic theories, skills, and techniques of the nursing profession; (2) knowledge of the broad function the profession is expected to perform in society; (3) competency to select and to apply relevant information from various disciplines; (4) competency in communicating with members of other disciplines and the general public; (5) ability to

assess and to provide for nursing care needs; (6) ability and motivation to evaluate current practices and to try new approaches; and (7) an adequate foundation for graduate study in nursing.

Characteristics of baccalaureate programs in nursing

A baccalaureate program in nursing corresponds to the general pattern of other baccalaureate programs that are offered by the institution. In addition, such a program is characterized by the usual features of undergraduate education in a professional discipline. These include:

1. Admission based on the policies of the educational institution.
2. Instruction throughout the program by persons qualified for college teaching in their respective disciplines and employed as faculty by the institution of higher education.
3. Learning experiences, resources, and facilities for general and specialized education in an environment where a community of scholars share interests, purposes, and opportunities.
4. Courses in the humanities, the natural sciences, and the social sciences, some of which serve as a base for the development of the major, some of which are included as electives at various levels in the program, and none of which is restricted to students in the nursing major.
6. Development of students' potential as individuals, citizens, and professional practitioners.
6. Continous evaluation of the purposes of the program and its effectiveness in meeting those purposes.
7. A total curriculum and a sequence of courses developed according to a rationale that can be supported by the faculty.
8. Adequate foundations for graduate study in the major field of concentration.

The faculty is responsible for developing a curriculum that exhibits these characteristics of general education. In addition, the faculty in a baccalaureate program in nursing is responsible for developing a curriculum in which the courses comprising the major apply previous and concurrent learning to the study of nursing and assist the student to progressively synthesize and apply this learning in nursing practice.

---

*Aydelotte, M.K.: Nursing education and practice: putting it all together, J. Nurs. Educ. **11**(4):21-27, 1972.
†Characteristics of baccalaureate and graduate education in nursing. Reprinted, with permission, from Nursing Outlook, July 1968.
‡General education in a free society. Report of the Harvard Committee, Cambridge, Mass., 1945, Harvard University Press, p. 73.

In 1978 the statement of characteristics of baccalaureate nursing education was revised and described as follows*:

The baccalaureate program in nursing, which is offered by a senior college or university, provides students with an opportunity to acquire: (1) knowledge of the theory† and practice of nursing; (2) competency in selecting, snythesizing, and applying relevant information from various disciplines; (3) ability to assess client needs and provide nursing intervention; (4) ability to provide care for groups of clients; (5) ability to work with and through others; (6) ability to evaluate current practices and try new approaches; (7) competency in collaborating with members of other health disciplines and with consumers; (8) an understanding of the research process and of its contribution to nursing practice; (9) knowledge of the broad function the nurse profession is expected to perform in society; (10) a foundation for graduate study in nursing.

Nurses are prepared as generalists at the baccalaureate level. They provide within the health care system‡ a comprehensive service that assesses, promotes, and maintains the health of individuals and groups. These nurses are prepared to: (1) be accountable for their own nursing practice; (2) accept responsibility for the provision of nursing care through others; (3) accept the advocacy role in relation to clients; and (4) develop methods of working collaboratively with other health professionals. They practice in a variety of health care settings—hospital, home, and community—and emphasize comprehensive health care, including prevention, health promotion, and rehabilitation services, health counseling and education, and care in acute and long-term illness.

---

*National League for Nursing, 1978.
†Throughout this statement, theory is used in the universal sense.
‡The health care system involves social, cultural, economic, and political components of society. It can be conceptualized from a local individual perspective of nurse and client/family along a continuum to the broad, national health care scene. For the most part, the graduates of baccalaureate programs in nursing work within the local health care system although fully aware of the regional and national health care scenes. The master's graduates in nursing are proficient working within the local health care system and have learned to extend their influence and effectiveness to and through the regional and national levels.

Baccalaureate nursing programs are organized according to conceptual schema consistent with the stated philosophy and objectives of the parent institution and the unit in nursing. These programs provide the general and professional education essential for understanding and respecting people, various cultures, and environments; for acquiring and utilizing nursing theory upon which nursing practice is based; and for promoting self-understanding, personal fulfillment, and motivation for continued learning. The structure of the baccalaureate degree program in nursing follows the same pattern as that of baccalaureate education in general. It is characterized by a liberal education base at the lower division level on which is built the upper division major. In baccalaureate nursing education, the lower division consists of foundational courses drawn primarily from the scientific and humanistic disciplines inherent in liberal learning. The major in nursing is built upon this lower division general education base and is concentrated at the upper division level. Upper division studies also include courses that complement the nursing component or increase the depth of general education.

Consistent with the foregoing characteristics and directly related to criteria as outlined in the *Criteria for the Appraisal of Baccalaureate and Higher Degree Programs in Nursing*, the graduate of the baccalaureate program in nursing is able to do the following*:

1. Utilize nursing theory as the basis for making nursing practice decisions
2. Use nursing practice as a means of gathering data for refining and extending that practice.
3. Synthesize theoretical and empirical knowledge from the physical and behavioral sciences and humanities with nursing theory and practice.
4. Assess health status and health potential; plan, implement, and evaluate nursing care with clients—individuals, families, and communities.
5. Improve service to the client by continually evaluating the effectiveness of nursing intervention and revising accordingly.
6. Accept individual responsibility and accountability for nursing intervention and outcome.

---

*National League for Nursing: Characteristics of baccalaureate and graduate education in nursing, New York, 1978, The League.

7. Evaluate research for applicability of its findings to nursing actions.
8. Utilize leadership skills through the involvement of others in meeting health needs and nursing goals.
9. Collaborate with citizens and colleagues on the interdisciplinary health team to promote the health and welfare of people.
10. Participate in identifying and effecting needed change to improve delivery within specific health care systems.
11. Participate in identifying community and societal health needs and in designing nursing roles to meet these needs.

The baccalaureate program in nursing is a comparatively new development. Although there were many nursing programs associated with colleges earlier, it is generally agreed that the first baccalaureate program in nursing was established at the University of Minnesota in 1909. That this was not followed by a noticeable increase in the number of baccalaureate programs in the United States was probably due to the fact that, at that time, hospital programs were a well-established tradition and nursing educators found it difficult to convince the public that nursing education, like legal or medical education, was a public responsibility and therefore should be accomplished in educational institutions supported by the public. Historically, many of the early so-called collegiate programs were developed solely to furnish the nursing service for the medical center of the university rather than to provide primarily for the education of the nursing student. Many of these early programs were little more than hospital programs, either preceded by or followed with a circumscribed series of courses within the college or university. World War I provided the initial impetus and World War II proved the need for the professionally educated nurse and forced the federal government to help finance the preparation of nurses. The National Defense Education Act of 1956 served to reiterate the interest of the government in nursing, and in 1963 the report of the Surgeon General's Consultant Group on Nurs-

ing served to firmly establish the need for baccalaureate education in nursing and appeared to indicate the continuing interest of the federal government in this type of nursing program. However, in the final document, *Toward Quality in Nursing,* the consultant group recommended that a national study of nursing education, with emphasis on the responsibilities and skills required to provide high quality care, be undertaken. The initial result of this recommendation was the formation of a joint committee of the ANA and the NLN to investigate the ways and means by which such a study could be undertaken. Coincidentally, in 1965 the ANA went on record with the position that all nursing education should be placed within the mainstream of the American educational system. Perhaps as a result of the impact of this position, or as a result of the recognition that the problems of nursing and nursing education were indeed wide-ranging, the ANA voted in 1966 to provide the monies to launch the study. The story of the funding of the National Commission for the Study of Nursing and Nursing Education is discussed elsewhere, but the report of this commission published in 1970 vis-à-vis baccalaureate education effectively laid to rest any doubts about the validity of nursing education within the college or university setting.

Baccalaureate programs in nursing are offered by a department, school, college, or division of a senior college or university. A retrospective look at those programs offered up to and including the 1950s indicates that a majority of the programs were conducted under an apprentice plan. Today, the educationally centered, college-controlled program is an accepted pattern. As a result of the acceptance of nursing as a respectable academic discipline, and perhaps also of the demands of students in all disciplines during the 1960s, the program in nursing is conducted in a manner congruent with any other baccalaureate program within an institution. Students of nursing attend general education courses with other students in other disciplines; tuition and fees are assessed in the same manner, and nursing students abide by the same rules and regulations in regard to living arrangements that apply to all other students. Scholarships and loans previously available to other students are now available to the nursing student with the same criteria for availability applied.

The professional nursing courses are taught by the faculty of the school, college, or division of nursing and may be conducted in either a classroom, hospital, community, or community agency. The laboratory for clinical learning experiences may be a hospital but more often is a community agency. Learning experiences, as in other college laboratories, are designed to meet the educational needs of the student.

In the late 1960s and early 1970s a trend appeared in baccalaureate education toward nontraditional approaches to education that, on the whole, made education more flexible, open, and accessible to more students. In most programs the applicant needed to meet admission requirements established by the college or university. Although it might be said that, in general, these requirements included high school graduation with academic units in specified areas, increased numbers of students were being admitted on the basis of successful completion of the GED (high school equivalency test). The Scholastic Aptitude Test of the College Entrance Examination Board remained the most frequently used preentrance examination for high school students, but it appeared to be used less often as a criterion for entrance and more frequently as a tool for effective counseling of the students. CLEP (college-level examination program) programs also provided the prospective college student with an opportunity to complete the initial general education requirements before entrance. In some programs a preentrance interview was being used to determine a prospective student's depth of interest in nursing and willingness to accept the responsibility of self-direction and initiative in the nursing program.

More flexible programing and admissions continue to be an issue in the 1980s. In the 1960s the impetus for change was to provide more equal opportunities in education, to allow more student participation, and to utilize newer approaches to teaching. The issues in the 1980s are flexible programming and variety in admission requirements to accommodate the adult learner. Thus the tradition of baccalaureate education exists with nontraditional programming.

Basic degree programs in nursing vary greatly in terms of the length of the program, the organization of the curriculum, the theoretical framework on which the curriculum is based, and the manner in which general education and professional nursing courses are presented throughout the program. Most programs are 4 academic years in length; about one third of these require an additional summer session. Only a few programs are longer than 4 academic years and two summer sessions.

The movement toward increased flexibility is evidenced by the increased numbers of programs that accept graduates of diploma and associate degree programs and the numbers that now permit study on a part-time basis. Most programs still attempt to maintain a 1:1 ratio of professional and general education courses. In programs that espouse an integrated or nursing modeled curriculum, students have general education and professional education courses throughout the 4-year program. In others the emphasis may be on general education courses in the first 1 or 2 years of college and professional nursing courses in the remaining 2 or 3 years. In almost all programs it is possible for the prospective student of nursing to accomplish the first year in a junior or community college and then transfer to the program in nursing without loss of time or credit. Increasingly, students are electing programs in which the first 2 years of the required work can be accomplished in either a junior college or another senior college of their choice. There appears to be a trend developing toward articulated programs. In these programs all students enter the associate degree program initially. At the completion of this phase, the student is eligible to take the state board examination for licensure as an RN. The opportunity then is presented for the student to continue in the program, and, on completion, be awarded the baccalaureate degree. Additional indicators of the increased flexibility and a desire to plan programs that will meet individual as well as societal needs are (1) the inclusion of basic research methodology in the baccalaureate curriculum, (2) the opportunities being presented in some programs to develop a degree of specialization within a clinical area, and (3) the development of courses at the baccalaureate level that will prepare the graduate in primary care skills.

Collegiate programs in nursing will still vary in regard to admittance policy. In some the beginning student will be admitted directly to the program in nursing; in others the student will be admitted initially to another college (general education, university college, etc.) and on completing general university requirements will be transferred to the program in nursing.

The emphasis today, as previously, is on broad comprehensive preparation in nursing. Perhaps even more today than previously, the graduate is being prepared to function at a beginning level in all areas of the health delivery system. This graduate should function effectively in positions of beginning leadership and should be able, after having had some experience in nursing, to assume beginning administrative positions without additional formal preparation. Since the emphasis in all basic degree programs is on clinical nursing, it should be emphasized that baccalaureate education does not prepare the nurse to function as a teacher, supervisor, or administrator of nursing services. Students are introduced to concepts of teaching and administration as these concepts relate to the nursing process. Although nursing program graduates may advance to beginning administrative positions, such as head nursing, with additional preparation, they are primarily prepared to function with the patient.

On completion of the program, the student is awarded the baccalaureate degree in nursing and, like students in other programs, is required to pass the state board of nursing examination for licensure in the state in which he or she plans to work.

Associate degree programs.* Associate degree nursing education made a profound impact on the entire health professions field in the United States from a modest beginning of eight schools participating in a research project during 1952 and 1953.

The idea for this type of nursing education was described first by Mildred Montag in *The Education of Nursing Technicians*. This idea was given a chance to be tested in a research project. A research grant was given to Teachers College, Columbia University, in 1952 to determine if it might be possible to prepare people for nursing practice within the framework of existing junior community colleges. Junior colleges had been preparing students for years to meet both student and community needs.

This kind of educational program broke all the traditional patterns of nursing education. It placed the entire responsibility of the educational process on the educational institution and the future practitioner rather than on the service institution. The ideas for this kind of program were original and young—as were the schools in which the programs were located. The junior college is the United States' unique contribution to higher education, and the movement is a vigorous one dating back only to the early part of the twentieth century. Any description of the junior college movement includes an analysis of the need for diverse types of educational opportunities at the post–high school level. The junior college was a natural setting for this type of program, with its prime responsibility being to meet community needs. What better way to attempt to meet the nursing needs of a community than to introduce a nursing curriculum into a school already accustomed to incorporating new programs and using existing courses?

To launch a research project to test the feasibility of this type of preparation for nursing took courage,

---

*Contributed by Ruth Swenson, formerly Director, Associate Degree Program, Webster State College, Ogden, Utah.

for over the years nursing had built up a heritage of many traditions. In the face of opposition but with much enthusiasm, eight schools undertook the task of building and testing a new type of curriculum in nursing, under the guidance of the research project staff at Teachers College. The purpose, according to Montag, was ''the developing and testing of a new type of program preparing young men and women for those functions commonly associated with the registered nurse.''

Each school established its own curriculum within the framework and requirements of its own college. The designing process was an exciting one, for the entire college faculty participated. Here was the beginning of the merger of specialized and general education. The general pattern has been to divide the required credits into approximately 50% nursing courses and 50% general educational courses.

In most of the programs there is concurrence of general education and nursing courses, with the philosophy that each enhances the other and that students grow and mature as they associate with students and instructors from other disciplines. The nursing courses are fewer and broader, with emphasis on principles. No time is wasted on needless repetition, since every experience needs to be a meaningful one for the student. Experience with patients is considered laboratory time, and the hours and credits are calculated as for a physics or chemistry laboratory. This clinical experience is well planned, increasing in complexity as the students demonstrate readiness for greater challenge.

The instructors must be excellent teachers and skilled practitioners in the care of patients and in interpersonal relationships. Their co-workers include both college and hospital colleagues, other health agency workers, and the entire community.

The students meet the college's graduation requirements and are granted an associate degree at the completion of the program. Programs vary in length; some schools require 2 academic years and others add one or both summers.

The eight original schools varied in many ways. Some were state controlled; others were privately controlled. Most were coeducational; one was for women only. There were large schools and small schools, and they were located in various parts of the country. This was considered a good cross section for the sample to be tested. Those who participated in the research project undertook it with open minds. If the graduates had not measured up to established criteria, the programs would have been discontinued. But they did measure up well in comparison with graduates of other programs with similar experience. The complete report of the project from inception to completion is described in Montag's book *Community College Education for Nursing*.

These programs are shorter than either baccalaureate or diploma programs, and they are a complete entity. The graduate is prepared to sit for the licensing examination and accept a position in nursing. It is important to remember that the 2 years do not represent the first 2 years of a baccalaureate degree program. There is a growing movement, however, to help students build on previous educational experiences. The LPN, in many schools, is given advanced placement in an associate degree program. Many schools are currently involved in new research to test innovative but sound approaches to open curriculum patterns. Another trend is the use of challenging examinations both in general education and in nursing courses. Successful achievement on examinations may make it possible for students to have specified courses waived and receive advanced placement. The external degree is still another new approach to help students complete specified course work outside the campus.

Another change has been the location of the programs. It is estimated that about 75% of the programs continue to be in junior or community colleges, whereas 25% are now located in senior colleges or universities. Regardless of the location, the admission requirements, standards, curriculum development, and graduation requirements are all consistent with school patterns. One of the prime requisites is the total responsibility, including financial, of the college for the program. This means that the students majoring in nursing pay the same tuition, carry the same credit load, and meet the same responsibilities as other students. It means, too, that students are entitled to the same high level of education with qualified instructors as students majoring in any other field.

There is no fixed pattern in the development of the curriculum. Most of the schools have been able to achieve an approximately even distribution of credits between general education and nursing courses. The general education courses include the humanities and the life, physical, and social sciences.

With the growth of other health occupations curricula on the campuses, there has been another movement—core classes. Since students majoring in related fields have certain related educational needs, courses have been developed in the life and physical sciences to meet these needs more directly.

Organizational patterns are beginning to change, also, with the advent of divisions or schools of allied health programs. A department of nursing may now be located in a school or division of allied health programs, rather than a science division. Nursing students are learning to work with students in other allied health fields, which, one hopes, will carry over into their future professional practice.

The graduates of these programs are prepared to function in hospitals, outpatient departments, physicians' offices, and clinics in the positions commonly called general duty or staff. These graduates are classified as technical nurses. They serve as members of nursing teams. A major leadership role is not one for which the schools claim preparation. The fact that some of the graduates function well in leadership roles does not change the preparation role. At graduation, as with all other new workers, there is a transition period from student to worker that needs to be met with sound orientation programs. More agencies are now recognizing this essential link and are offering this needed orientation for new workers.

The associate degree program is a well-established type of educational program in nursing. Support and direction have been offered by the NLN with consultation help and with joint committees with the American Association for Junior Colleges. Various foundations also assisted certain universities in preparing faculty to teach in the junior college programs. The movement seems to have established itself. It has moved into the community college and the university and become an integral part as easily as a chameleon picks up the color of its surroundings.

In 1978 the Council on Associate Degree Programs approved a statement on the competencies of the associate degree nurse on entry to practice. The council defined five interrelated roles: provider of care, communicator, client teacher, manager of client care, and member with*in* the profession of nursing. In addition, several assumptions basic to the scope of practice were enumerated*:

> The practice of graduates of associate degree nursing programs:
> —Is directed toward clients who need information or support to maintain health.
> —Is directed toward clients who are in need of medical diagnostic evaluation and/or are experiencing acute or chronic illness.
> —Is directed toward clients' responses to common, well-defined health problems.
> —Includes the formulation of a nursing diagnosis.
> —Consists of nursing interventions selected from established nursing protocols where probable outcomes are predictable.
> —Is concerned with individual clients and is given with consideration of the person's relationship within a family, group, and community.
> —Includes the safe performance of nursing skills that require cognitive, psychomotor, and affective capabilities.

---

*National League for Nursing: Competencies of the Associate Degree nurse on entry into practice, New York, 1978, The League.

—May be in any structured care setting but primarily occurs within acute- and extended care facilities.

—Is guided directly or indirectly by a more experienced registered nurse.

—Includes the direction of peers or other workers in nursing in selected aspects of care within the scope of practice of associate degree nursing.

—Involves an understanding of the roles and responsibilities of self and other workers within the employment setting.

In the years since associate degree nursing education has existed, proponents have refined the functions to coincide with the times as well as to be prepared for the future.

Other entry points to the practice of nursing

There are two other entry points to the practice of nursing often forgotten in the preparation of the RN. Students who already have a baccalaureate degree in another discipline do have the option of seeking a university program that offers the master's degree in nursing or the nurse doctorate as the initial entry to nursing.

These programs prepare the generalist at graduate level. Basic skills of nursing are included; however, theoretical expectations in application of knowledge, and independence in learning are at the graduate level. Students take the same state boards as all other entry students. First positions are often at the same level as other prepared graduates.

The nurse doctorate can only be achieved at Case Western Reserve University, Frances Payne Bolton School of Nursing, Cleveland, Ohio. It is the belief of this faculty that the only educationally professionally prepared nurse is at this level. Their program is fashioned on the concept of medical, dental, and law education. Professional education occurs only when a baccalaureate degree in other disciplines has been achieved. This program was initiated in the late 1970s and graduated its first class in 1982.

Registered nurse programs. As the number of programs admitting the RN has increased in the last few years, so have the options available to this student. A new development has been a baccalaureate program designed specifically for the graduate nurse: the RN completion program. The programs started as a part of the NLN open curriculum project, which was aimed at helping students achieve career mobility. Another approach has been the program developed by Michigan State University in which RNs in a tricounty area of that state can earn a bachelor's degree in nursing without going to the main campus or leaving their jobs. The program is designed to provide a way for nurses to take general education and other courses either through local colleges or the Michigan State University continuing education service. The curriculum is identical to that offered on the main campus, and the program is fully accredited by the NLN.

A vexing question, as yet unanswered, is that of college credit for work accomplished in a hospital diploma program. Most colleges and universities do not award college credit for work accomplished in nonacademic settings; however, there are increasing numbers of programs that permit the graduate nurse to earn credit by examination. Each program establishes the criteria by which this credit is awarded. Most colleges and universities now allow the student to test for credit in general education as well as in professional nursing courses up to the senior year. Although the credit by examination or credit by competency programs may differ, usually the student applies to take an examination in the course before registering for that course. The student who passes the examination successfully is awarded credit in that course. The examination may be a written one or one that tests clinical competency. If the examination is not passed successfully, the student is required to take the course. Although to some this may appear to be an arduous task, currently it is the fairest if not the most efficient way to evaluate the graduate nurse's ability and standing. Students who are graduates from associate degree programs in nursing that are not articulated with a baccalaureate program should expect to have their programs evaluated individually and advanced standing credit or deficiency assigned accordingly.

RN completion programs are intended as articulated programs for the associate degree and hospital-prepared nurse. In each program the content for nursing is considered lower division academic work. Therefore nursing content offered for the baccalaureate degree builds on previous knowledge, adding either new concepts or in-depth knowledge. The student will continue to meet university general education requirements as well as prerequisites and corequisites for nursing courses.

To summarize, the RN has four options in achieving the baccalaureate degree: (1) the generic program, (2) a satellite program offering the generic program off the main campus, (3) completion programs designed especially for the RN, and (4) external degree programs such as offered in New York State.

In an effort to address the issue of RNs who wanted academic degrees without repetitive learning and state legislators becoming more involved with the issue of education, some universities began addressing articulation of the RN bypassing the baccalaureate degree and securing the master's degree in nursing.

The University of California, San Francisco School of Nursing initiated such a program. It was the first school to create a program whereby the previous foundation was recognized "to support educational mobility and to strengthen the leadership abilities of nurses."*

A second such program began in the fall of 1983 at Case Western Reserve University, Frances Payne Bolton School of Nursing, Cleveland, Ohio.

This movement characterizes the need for educational mobility and recognizes the diversity that exists in nursing education today. To this end the

---

*Articulated bachelor/masters of science in nursing (for registered nurses), University of California, San Francisco School of Nursing promotional material, 1983.

NLN board of directors approved the following statement in 1982:

> Educational mobility, a characteristic of today's society, has strong implications for nursing, whose scope of practice currently encompasses vocational, technical, and professional nursing. Preparation for practice of each type can best be provided through appropriately designed, high-quality programs that are specific to their purpose and complete in themselves.
>
> Individuals who wish to change career goals should have educational opportunities to advance from one type of nursing practice to another. These opportunities will benefit individuals by allowing them to expand their scope of practice and thus move into areas of great responsibility. Society will be assured that nursing care needs will be met by knowledgeable and competent practitioners.
>
> In addressing these needs, educational institutions are responsible for setting policies on admission, graduation, and transfer and earning of credits. The faculty in each institution is responsible for applying these policies to their individual programs and developing curricular patterns and content in keeping with their beliefs and the purposes of the program. In a plan for educational mobility, opportunity should be provided for students to validate previously acquired educational and clinical competencies to facilitate advanced placement.
>
> The NLN supports the concept of educational mobility and encourages the preservation of this right of individuals to self-fulfillment.*

Graduate education. Considering the fact that graduate education in America in any discipline is not more than 100 years old, the development of graduate programs in nursing has been remarkable. The early recognition of the need for prepared teachers and supervisors precipitated the founding of the Department of Nursing and Health at Teachers College, Columbia University, in 1903. Although this program in no way could be considered graduate education, other postgraduate courses in teaching and administration modeled on those at Teachers College began to be organized in other

---

*Position statement on educational mobility. Approval by the National League for Nursing Board of Directors, Feb. 1982.

universities. Since the courses were highly specialized and the prerequisites for admission were extremely rigid, these programs did not meet the educational needs of graduate nurses nor did they meet the need of the profession for leadership preparation. Although attempts were made during the 1930s to define the levels of educational preparation needed, the occurrence of World War II focused a great deal of attention on the development of all levels of nursing education. During the war years (1941-1945) much attention was given to advanced nursing curricula in the universities. It was recognized that nursing was attempting to define its status in society as a profession and that advanced educational preparation was one of the means by which prepared leadership could be provided.

As stated previously, before 1950 almost all baccalaureate degree programs were specialized in nature. At that time the baccalaureate programs provided for beginning practice in the public health nursing field or for administration, teaching, and supervision in hospitals and schools of nursing. About this time, leaders in nursing education began to recognize the need for broad, comprehensive education at the baccalaureate level, which then placed specialization at the graduate level. There was much confusion and disagreement as to the level on which clinical and functional preparation should be placed, and the situation was one in which programs at the same academic level prepared for positions at various levels of nursing, and programs at different academic levels had the same objectives. At this time there were both baccalaureate and master's degree programs that prepared for administrative, supervisory, and teaching positions. In 1952 the Work Conference on Graduate Nurse Education, sponsored by the NLN, attempted to remedy the situation and define levels of preparation. The report stated ''that the baccalaureate program should prepare the nurse for general professional nursing, the master's programs for specialization.'' The report also defined specialization in programs leading to the master's or higher degree as ''building upon previously developed

competencies for successful functioning in a specific field of concentration.''* The decision of the board of directors of the NLN in 1959 to no longer accredit programs on the baccalaureate level that provided for both clinical and functional specialization enforced the stand for uniformity in specialization.

In concert with these developments, increased attention was given to the development of master's and doctoral degree programs of a truly graduate caliber. In 1959 the NLN established the following:

At the Master's level each program provides an experience in carrying through a systematic study centered around a problem of interest to nursing. This study provides experience in research methodology as a basis for being an intelligent participant in a research project and an intelligent consumer of research findings. Programs of advanced study in nursing leading to a doctoral degree provide for intensification and depth of knowledge in the area of specialization and in related areas as well as training in research methodology.†

In a document prepared by the Graduate Seminar of the Western Council on Higher Education for Nursing in May 1958, the following was stated:

Nursing leaders must maintain the quality and efficiency of nursing care. Therefore, their preparation in nursing and their specialities is of the utmost importance. In nursing, as in other education fields, the teacher must have a more expert grasp of the subject matter than her students. Similarly, the supervisor and nursing consultant must be prepared with a clinical competence beyond the experience of those whom they guide. Graduate nursing education must be based on an understanding of the natural and behavioral sciences that are included in the baccalaureate programs in nursing.‡

*National League for Nursing, Division of Nursing Education: Report of Work Conference on Graduate Nurse Education, New York, 1952, The League, pp. 17 and 18.
†National League for Nursing Council of Baccalaureate and Higher Degree Programs: Characteristics of graduate education, New York, 1959, The League.
‡Western Council on Higher Education for Nursing, Graduate Seminar: Guidelines for developing master's degree programs in nursing in the west, Boulder, Colo., 1958, Western Interstate Commission for Higher Education.

The graduate nurse of today whose career goals include teaching or supervision or who wishes to function as a clinical specialist has for some time been aware of the need for graduate preparation.

The entrance of the federal government into nursing by virtue of making scholarships and grants available to nurses who wished to continue their education during the 1950s and 1960s greatly increased the number of nurses with graduate preparation. Although the need still exists, and in spite of vigorous promotion by nursing leaders and explicit recommendations made by the National Commission on Nursing and Nursing Education, monies available to students from federal sources decreased during the latter part of the 1960s and the early 1970s. In spite of this, graduate programs proliferated during this period.

Graduate departments of nursing schools offer a variety of programs in clinical specialty areas, teaching, and supervision. Recently there has been a resurgence of interest in graduate programs that prepare nurses for administrative positions in nursing service. In all programs increasing emphasis is being given to clinical preparation as well as clinical research. Although it is recognized that the nurse researcher is prepared only at the doctoral level, the need for the prepared nurse research consumer or facilitator is reflected in the curricula in master's programs today. In the majority of master's programs in nursing there are three components: clinical content, functional specialization, and research. Along with an increase in the clinical content has come an increase in the degree of specialization with a clinical specialty. Whereas 10 years ago a student might elect a clinical specialty area such as medical-surgical nursing, the student today is more likely to be specializing in cardiovascular nursing, geriatric nursing, or another subspecialty. Changes discussed previously as related to baccalaureate programs are being reflected in the graduate programs. There is evidence of a great deal of experimentation, and the changes in education (open curricula, external degrees, nonguided study, articulated curricula, etc.) are influencing the direction of graduate education in nursing. As in the baccalaureate programs, the concept of part-time, self-paced education at the master's level is being noted with increasing frequency.

In 1978, the Council of Baccalaureate and Higher Degree Programs went on record as supporting the following characteristics of graduate education leading to a master's degree in nursing*:

The master's program in nursing is offered by an institution of higher education and is built upon a baccalaureate curriculum that has included an upper division major in nursing. It provides students with an opportunity to: (1) acquire advanced knowledge from the sciences and the humanities to support advanced nursing practice and role development; (2) expand their knowledge of nursing theory† as a basis for advanced nursing practice; (3) develop expertise in a specialized area of clinical nursing practice; (4) acquire the knowledge and skills related to a specific functional role in nursing; (5) acquire initial competence in conducting research; (6) plan and initiate change in the health care system‡ and in the practice and delivery of health care; (7) further develop and implement leadership strategies for the betterment of health care; (9) actively engage in collaborative relationships with others for the purpose of improving health care, and (9) acquire a foundation for doctoral study.

Individuals prepared at the master's level in nursing improve nursing and health care through their expert practice and through the advancement of theory in nursing. The concurrent study of appropriate graduate-level cognate courses serves to broaden the students' understanding of relevant knowledge from other disciplines.

---

*National League for Nursing: Characteristics of graduate education in nursing leading to a master's degree, New York, 1978, The League.
†Throughout this statement, *theory* is used in the universal sense as it applies to all disciplines.
‡The health care system includes social, cultural, economic, and political components. It can be conceptualized from an individual perspective of nurse and client/family to the broad national health care scene. For the most part, the graduates of baccalaureate programs in nursing work within the local health care system although fully aware of the regional and national health care scenes. The master's graduates in nursing are proficient in working within the local health care system and have learned to extend their influence and effectiveness to and through the regional and national levels.

These courses, combined with the expansion of nursing theory that was acquired at the baccalaureate level, permit students to focus their graduate study on aspects of nursing practice and on a functional role that meets their interest and objectives. This combination of relevant graduate cognate courses and advanced nursing theory provides knowledge for the development of expert nursing practice in specialty areas of the students' choice.

Provision for acquiring specialized knowledge and skills in an area of nursing practice may vary in extent and depth depending upon the student's goals of specialization. Those preparing for specialized practice roles may concentrate in a single area and have greater opportunities for practice than students advancing their nursing knowledge and expertise as a necessary element of the functional roles of teaching or administration. Research and consultation skills are integral to the functional roles of specialist, teacher, or administrator, although preparation in these areas is characteristic of postmaster's study in nursing. Areas of clinical study should reflect societal needs for nursing services and be sufficiently broad in scope to enable persons so prepared to serve in a variety of settings and locales. It is recognized that some specialty areas in nursing will require depth of knowledge in a delineated area of practice, while others, such as those concerned with services to diverse populations, families and groups, call for an advanced level of generalized knowledge and practice.

The relationship between clinical and functional preparation is of criticial importance. Although advanced clinical preparation is at the base of master's preparation in nursing, it alone is not enough. Functional preparation at the master's level may focus on such areas as the role of specialist, teacher, or administrator. Such preparation is most effective when it provides opportunity for the student to practice functioning within the role. Such role preparation offers knowledge of: (1) the theory of the role; (2) the usual role expectations; (3) the functional dimensions of the role; (4) role ambiguities and conflicts; and (5) strategies for effective role implementation.

In the master's program, opportunity is provided for the student to build upon previously acquired knowledge of the research process, both in conducting research and in helping others to utilize research findings. It is expected that the master's student in nursing is capable of identifying researchable nursing problems. The student may conduct replication or pilot studies, or may synthesize a conceptual framework from a review of the literature to design a circumscribed, original study. Knowledge of data anlysis is essential both for the implementation of a study and for the intelligent comprehension of research. Opportunities need to be provided to acquire research skills, which can be accomplished in a variety of ways depending upon individual students' needs and goals.

The graduates of master's programs in nursing apply the concepts of change in contributing to the enhancement of nursing and health services. They are actively involved in initiating change and constructively handling the conflict generated when such change is undertaken.

The leadership strategies developed and implemented for the betterment of health care encompass the range of activities needed to influence both nursing education and nursing practice constructively. Furthermore, these strategies are designed to promote the personal and professional investment of self and to employ professional standards and ethical conduct. The leadership strategies emanate from a broad theoretical base and enable the leader to prescribe, decide, influence, and facilitate changes for nursing and health. The direction and scope of leadership are directly related to one's field of operation and to the publics served. The roles of change agent and consumer advocate are also effected through the selection and implementation of a broad range of appropriate strategies.

The interdisciplinary collaborative role of the graduate of a master's program is characterized by initiation and interpretation. Master's-prepared nurses utilize newly acquired functional role skills to design, initiate, and assume a leadership role as well as a collaborative role. They take an active part in delineating the goals and standards of the group and in designing the mode and terms of operation. One of the major responsibilities of a master's graduate in nursing is to interpret the role and function of nurses to others.

The learning climate for study at the master's level enables students to experience a collegial relationship with peers in their own and other disciplines. Opportunities to relate with faculty facilitate a partnership in learning that promotes intellectual curiosity and creative inquiry and aids in meeting individualized learning goals.

The master's program in nursing is conceptually organized to flow from the philosophy and objectives of the total program and to guide curricular decision making and selection of learning experiences. Such a conceptual scheme also protects the integrity and consistency of the master's program irrespective of the number and variety of specializations, provides a basis for program evaluation, and insures some common learning experience for all students. Because of the diversity of clinical and functional specialties in master's programs, the behaviors expected of graduates should consist of both the behaviors expected of all master's graduates and the specialized behaviors expected of graduates from particular specialties.

These characteristics were developed by the professional nurse membership of the Council of Baccalaureate and Higher Degree Programs and are an expression of professional accountability to the consumer, both student and client.

In addition to the nurses being prepared at the master's level, increasing numbers are being prepared at the doctoral (Ph.D.) level. Since nurses are seeking doctoral preparation in many areas other than nursing (administration of higher education, sociology, law, etc.), it has been impossible to compile accurate figures on the number completing degrees within any given year. It is known, however, that the number of nurses earning a doctoral (Ph.D.) degree in nursing is increasing, as is the number of institutions offering doctoral (Ph.D.) programs in nursing. In 1982, 25 institutions offered a doctoral program in nursing. Of those, two schools offered the nurse scientist program. In 1982, 34 universities were considering the opening of doctoral (Ph.D.) programs with six to be operational by 1984. Thus a total of 31 universities were offering Ph.D. or nurse scientist programs by 1984.

Doctoral programs in nursing are gaining in maturity as theories of nursing are developed and tested. Research in nursing had to occur before doctoral education could be developed and thus supported in the academic world. Content and approach vary in each of the programs offered. One may focus on usual clinical areas such as medical-surgical nursing while others emphasize such nontraditional areas as transcultural nursing. All emphasize research; some also emphasize theory de-velopment. Master's education supports specialization in a given area, but doctoral education narrows the area of specialization even further, making it possible for the doctorally prepared individual to become an expert in a given area through research.

Doctoral programs are not accredited in the same manner as other nursing programs. Neither state boards of nursing nor the NLN has jurisdiction over this level of education. First, the university and the state higher education commission must give approval to begin the program. When the university is visited for its continued accreditation through the regional academic accrediting body, the program in nursing is reviewed and given recognition as a program in an accredited institution.

Academic degrees need to be distinguished from professional degrees. Academic degrees are the bachelor of arts/science, master of arts/science, and doctor of philosophy. Professional degrees are the master of nursing and nurse doctorate. In nursing, professional degrees are offered at the baccalaureate and master's level. Until the fall of 1979, nursing did not have a professional degree at the doctorate level. Schlotfeldt, of Case Western Reserve University, Cleveland, Ohio, supported the thesis that the "time is right for the development . . . of pre-service nursing which merits the award of a professional doctorate . . . the nurse doctorate, or N.D. degree."* With that pronouncement the professional doctorate was launched. The candidate for this degree comes to the school with 3 years of broad general education or with an academic baccalaureate degree. After 3 years of professional education, the person graduates as a beginning practitioner of nursing. This is a major difference from the Ph.D. in nursing or the nurse scientist doctorate. The Ph.D. in nursing further refines the specialization process.

The nurse who is interested in education at the graduate level should keep in mind that graduate

---

*Schlotfeldt, R.M.: The professional doctorate: rationale and characteristics, Nurs. Outlook **26:**302, May 1978.

study requires independent thinking and that although increasing numbers of programs are giving consideration to the individual student's needs, abilities, and previous educational backgrounds, the nurse must possess sufficient intellectual capacity to profit from graduate study. Graduate programs for the most part are conducted by departments within the graduate school of a university, and the applicant must first meet requirements established by the graduate school. Most universities have general rules such as the following:

1. The applicant must hold a baccalaureate degree from an accredited college or university, and one that is equivalent to the baccalaureate degree given by the university.

2. The applicant must show by previous record or other means the ability to satisfactorily pursue advanced study and research.

3. The applicant must have had adequate preparation to enter into graduate study in the field selected.

The individual department can then establish admission requirements that may be higher but never lower than those established by the graduate school. Following are common requirements for admission to graduate programs in nursing:

1. The applicant must be a graduate registered nurse.

2. The applicant must hold a baccalaureate degree in nursing from an approved college or university. In addition, the majority of programs require that this degree be awarded by an NLN-accredited institution, and all programs require that the applicant must have had an acceptable upper division major in nursing at the baccalaureate level.

3. The applicant must give evidence of scholastic ability (usually a minimum grade point average of 2.7 to 3.0 on a 4.0 scale).

4. The applicant must demonstrate satisfactory achievement on a qualifying examination.

It is understood, of course, that while in the program, the graduate student in nursing will maintain scholastic standards acceptable to both the graduate school and the department in which he or she is studying. Since all graduate schools have

somewhat different requirements, it is wise for the prospective graduate student to examine carefully the bulletins and catalogs of the school being considered.

Although it is impossible to project the length of time required to complete the doctoral degree, most master's programs require from $1\frac{1}{2}$ to 2 years. Many nurse educators believe that the master's program in nursing should take only 1 year to complete and that in-depth study in nursing should take place at a postmaster's or doctoral level. Almost as many educators believe that since the master's degree may be the highest professional degree attained by the majority of nurse teachers and administrators, the programs should be broad and comprehensive. Regardless of the validity of each argument, the majority of programs currently being offered are longer than 1 year.

With the rapid increase in the number of health care agencies and the increasing need within the total health care system for individuals prepared to meet specific needs, the nurse will find unlimited employment opportunities. To be prepared to function fully in the future in view of the changing health care scene, the student in basic nursing should now begin to formulate goals that will eventuate in graduate study in nursing.

TRENDS IN NURSING EDUCATION

Since 1969, and with great vigor since 1972, much discussion has taken place on the career ladder approach to nursing education. Some leaders believe that no one should be penalized for not entering nursing through a top educational program, that schools should develop their curricula in such a way that elements are taught to all practitioners in a similar manner, and that it should be easy for a nurse to move upward to the highest degree possible. Some universities are experimenting with this approach. The theory is that students should be able to stop at an appropriate time and enter the field of nursing and practice until they decide to resume their education to gain the next level in the practice of nursing.

This approach requires much thought and innovation. It is an exciting, creative idea and would allow for more flexibility on the part of the student, who would then not be punished for having had a limited career goal at the age of 18.

Some schools are doing extensive experimentation in curriculum implementation. For example, some are allowing the student more freedom in determining what is to be learned and by what method. Nursing faculties formerly had been very rigid in curriculum planning and implementation; however, some are now discarding old course titles, strengthening nursing approaches, easing rigid schedules, and allowing students to have opportunity for nursing course electives, to be involved in curriculum changes, and to make their own decisions as to their laboratory experiences. Curricula are being shortened in diploma programs and lengthened in baccalaureate programs. Objectives of the various types of programs are beginning to be different. All of this indicates an exciting decade ahead for nursing education.

One particular activity in schools has been the students' freedom to make decisions about their own learning. With schools having autotutorial laboratories fully equipped with slides, films, tapes, and patient care equipment, students can learn at their own time and speed. They are given the behavioral objectives of the course and can determine in which patient care setting and under what circumstances they will best learn the objectives. Students also are able to choose the sequence of courses that best suits them.

Faculty members are using their time in motivating students to learn rather than simply giving facts. This demands more from the faculty, since teaching is more on a one-to-one basis and certainly more relevant. Nursing educators are using all the modern equipment at their disposal and taking advantage of the skills nursing students are bringing with them from previous educational experiences.

Although articulation from one program is desirable, another philosophical issue arises. Can vocational education be the base for professional education? The purist believes that for professional education to take place, a liberal education must be the base. The pragmatist believes that as a person's goals change, the liberal education can be gained as it is needed to support new levels of nursing to be achieved.

Nursing education and the entry to practice issue will be forced into decision. Either the profession's pronouncement will become a fact or there will continue to be four approaches to becoming an RN: the traditional three and the nurse doctorate.

However, that education issue cannot be laid to rest until there is agreement that a "nurse is a nurse," or better said, until functional redundancy is eliminated. When the right to practice nursing rests solely with *one* basically prepared individual, then the education issue will fall into place.

SUMMARY

Registered nurse education can be obtained in three types of programs: junior colleges, hospitals, and universities. There are limitations to the scope of education in each. Although each program has similar objectives to "prepare a nurse to practice nursing at the bedside," each accomplishes this differently.

In addition to RN education, there is practical nurse education. The practical nurses are limited in education and skills. They must work under the direction of the RN.

Graduate education in nursing can be achieved throughout the United States. Master's degree and doctoral degrees in nursing can be found in senior universities. Nurse researchers, educators, administrators, and direct care givers need increased knowledge and skills with which to address the complex concerns of nursing.

Discussion questions
1. Discuss the difference between postsecondary education and higher education in the general scheme of education.
2. Discuss the differences among vocational, technical, and professional nursing education.
3. Discuss the need for educational mobility in nursing.
4. Discuss the issue of professional education and the

relationship to meeting the needs of an occupation or a profession.

5. Discuss whether two levels of nursing education are needed or one that provides only for a highly skilled, technologically prepared professional nurse.

SUGGESTED READINGS

Associate degree education, Nurs. Outlook **25,** Aug. 1977 (entire issue).

Bridgewater, S.C.: Organizational autonomy for nursing education, J. Nurs. Ed. **18:**4-7, Jan. 1979.

Brower, H.T.: Potential advantages and hazards of nontraditional education for nurses, Nurs. Health Care **3**(5):268, 1982.

Bullough, B.: The associate degree: beginning or end? Nurs. Outlook **27:**324-326, May 1979.

Dustan, L.C.: Needed—articulation between nursing education programs and institutions of higher learning, Nurs. Outlook **18:**34, Dec. 1970.

Editorial: the baccalaureate degree, Nurs. Outlook **25:**369, June 1977.

Frank, S.C.M., and Heidgerken, L.: Perspectives in nursing education, ed. 3, Washington, D.C., 1968, The Catholic University of American Press.

Future directions of doctoral education for nurses, Bethesda, Md., 1971, U.S. Department of Health, Education and Welfare.

Grace, H.K.: The development of doctoral education in nursing, J. Nurs. Ed. **17:**17-27, April 1978.

Hawken, P.L., and Reed, S.B.: Preparing for accreditation, Nurs. Outlook **26:**761-765, Dec. 1978.

Ingles, T., et al.: A proposal for health care education, Am. J. Nurs. **68:**2135, Oct. 1968.

Kelly, L.Y.: Open curriculum—what and why, Am. J. Nurs. **74:**2232-2238, Dec. 1974.

Kramer, M.: Credit for competency, Am. J. Nurs. **70:**793, April 1970.

Matheney, R.: Can nursing live with open admissions? Am. J. Nurs. **70:**2561, Dec. 1970.

Montag, M.: The education of nursing technicians, New York, 1951, G.P. Putnam's Sons, Inc.

Montag, M.: Community college education for nursing, New York, 1961, McGraw-Hill Book Co.

Nursing Outlook **18:**21-58, Sept. 1970 (entire issue devoted to nursing education).

Pellegrino, E.D.: Rationale for nursing education in the university, Am. J. Nurs. **68:**1006, May 1968.

Ramphal, M.: Rethinking diploma school and collegiate education, Nurs. Outlook **26:**768-771, Dec. 1978.

Reed, C.F.: Selecting a graduate program, Am. J. Nurs. **71:**100, Jan. 1971.

Reed, F.C.: Education or exploitation, Am. J. Nurs. **79:**1259-1261, July 1979.

Scheinfeldt, J., and Palmer, S.R.: Expansion: new youth in nursing, Am. J. Nurs. **70:**1713, Aug. 1970.

Schlotfeldt, R.M.: The professional doctorate: rationale and characteristics, Nurs. Outlook **26:**302-311, May 1978.

Schwairen, R.M., and Gortner, S.L.: How nursing schools predict their successful graduates, Nurs. Outlook **27:**352-358, 1979.

Slaninka, S.C.: Baccalaureate programs for RN's, Am. J. Nurs. **79:**1095, June 1979.

Styles, M.M.: On nursing: toward a new endowment, St. Louis, 1982, The C.V. Mosby Co.

Walker, D.J., and Hungler, B.P.: A proposed approach to the education of nurses, Nurs. Outlook **16:**24, Aug. 1968.

Wozniak, D.: External degrees in nursing, Am. J. Nurs. **73:**1014, June 1973.

CHAPTER 7
Professional nursing practice

JOANN HOLT
MARY FISHER
NANCY KILBANE
MARIANNE CRAWFORD

OBJECTIVE: On completion of this chapter, the student of nursing will be able to discuss seven factors influencing nursing practice today.

There are a number of variables that influence the practice of nursing, some of which are quality assurance, patient classifications, cost containment, external influences, support services, computerization, and nursing research. The professional nurse and the technical nurse become involved with these variables within a variety of settings and organizational structures and differing direct care roles, systems for the delivery of care, and staffing and scheduling.

Basic to the practice of nursing is the nursing process. Professional practice of nursing is a high level of problem solving within which alternative decisions are made in order that appropriate nursing interventions occur. Technical nursing utilizes the nursing process in making decisions based on predictable data. Problem solving is basic to the nursing process.

It is the intent of this chapter to provide a broad spectrum of those areas that influence the professional practice of nursing. The student will want to read Chapter 13, Professional Nursing, for an understanding of what a profession is, as well as other factors that impinge on the professional practice of nursing.

QUALITY ASSURANCE

Many external forces demand that we measure the quality of patient care. The federal government with the passage of the Social Security Act of 1972 directed the Department of Health, Education and Welfare to develop a program to ensure the necessity, quality, and cost-effectiveness of care financed by the federal government. This resulted in the formation of professional standards review organizations (PSROs) and audit systems to review and evaluate patient care. Because of the tremendous increase in health care costs, third-party payers (insurance companies and businesses) are scrutinizing the quality of the care they finance. Accrediting bodies, such as the Joint Commission on Accreditation of Hospitals (JCAH), require measurement of quality. To maintain accreditation, hospitals must comply with the JCAH quality assurance standard.

Quality assurance is described as the continual process by which the outcomes of care can be measured, evaluated, and monitored for excellence. Throughout the years nurses thought they could describe quality nursing care. This description was based on nurses' opinion, education, experience, and values. The problem with this approach was that outcomes were not measured, and subjective evaluation varied with each nurse. In recent years, nursing has implemented internal audits that monitor nursing practice. Presently a system of nursing diagnosis is evolving with which to measure quality care.

Hospitals and community health programs are responding to external demands with organized quality assurance programs. Written plans are prepared by each agency. There is usually a quality assurance committee with overall responsibility for monitoring the quality of care in the institution. This committee, reporting through the administration and the medical staff, is accountable to the board of trustees.

A staff nurse should expect to become involved in the quality assurance program in his or her place of employment. In many institutions, staff nurses are members of the nursing quality assurance committee. A staff nurse can offer valuable insight into the identification and resolution of problems that affect the quality of patient care.

Just as quality assurance programs have developed and nursing diagnoses were identified, a classification of patients began to take form.

PATIENT CLASSIFICATION

Grave concerns about staffing and justification for nursing budgets precipitated development of a number of systems that in effect measure quantitatively the amount of nursing care a group of patients require over a given period of time. The systems have been termed *patient classification systems, management systems for staffing*, and *acuity systems*. These systems are present in hospitals that have developed their own methods as well as in private corporations that have developed classification packages that can be purchased by hospitals.

Utilization of nursing personnel is more timely and efficient with the use of patient classification systems. All these systems begin at the patient unit level when a nurse places a numerical value on patients' needs from standards previously devel-

oped and approved by the nursing staff. Therefore the amount of staffing is no longer determined by the number of patients on a nursing unit but rather by the level of nursing care required by a group of patients. These systems provide nursing services with an objective method of projecting staff requirements at any given time. Many hospitals have placed their systems on computers, providing yet another move toward automation of a once very subjective task.

COST CONTAINMENT AND PRODUCTIVITY

Uppermost in the health field in the mid 1980s is cost containment. Dramatic changes are predicted in the delivery of health care in order to drive the cost of health care down or at least remain at the status quo. Nursing services are a major factor in the cost of health care. Personnel costs are the largest portion of the nursing budget. For these reasons, when the reduction of health care costs is an issue, nursing is directly involved with cost-cutting measures.

Staffing and scheduling constitute the area in nursing practice where the most scrutiny exists because of the labor intensity of the budget. Great efforts are being made to reduce such costs as overtime and sick time. When that fails, nursing frequently has to accept a reduction in the number of persons assigned to work on a unit.

Patient classification systems assist in the justification of nursing budgets. Before patient classification, nursing productivity was frequently measured by hours per patient day. Productivity measurement related to patient days erroneously assumes that all patients need the same amount of care. Advanced patient classification systems are now being used as a measurement of productivity and do take into account the differences in individual patients' needs.

The national concern over health care costs will indeed force all health care workers to find more efficient and less costly ways of getting the job done. Major concern is being voiced by nursing leaders that the quality of care issue is being ignored. In November 1983 the ANA was awarded a grant from the Health Care Financing Administration to study diagnostic related groups (DRGs) for nursing care. See Chapter 1 for a discussion of DRGs and the resultant cost-containment expectations.

Reimbursement for nursing care

Even though nursing services are a large portion of any hospital budget, they have been included in room and board charges in most patient billing systems. Examples of ancillary services that are part of room and board are housekeeping and dietary. Other services that appear on patients' billings as separate costs include respiratory therapy, radiology, and laboratory.

In recent years the nursing profession has preferred that nursing services be separated from room and board charges. Some advantages of this concept are as follows:

- Patients would understand the cost of nursing care and therefore develop a better appreciation for the profession.
- Formal recognition would be given to the amount of revenue that nursing provides for a hospital. This direct attention from the consumer would assist the nursing professional in becoming more accountable for patient care.

With patient classification systems, some hospitals have the ability to charge patients for nursing care. The charges have been billed using the classification system given. Billing separately for nursing services is an ideal situation. Some hospitals have a nursing billing process built around specific services, for example, starting an intravenous infusion. Patients are billed only for care received. Presently, many hospitals average patient charges for all patients, whether acutely ill or moderately ill. This means that those needing less care pay for those requiring more care.

EXTERNAL INFLUENCES ON PRACTICE

Cost containment is a major external influence on nursing care, however, boards of trustees, administration, medical staff, and employees in an organization have significant influence and power. These groups may be viewed as internal to an organization, but it is important to realize that they are external to the nursing profession.

The influence that these groups have on nursing practice can be lessened. Political savvy by staff nurses and all other nurses in the agency becomes more important daily. Staff nurses must realize that the competence with which they perform and the knowledge they possess of the whole organization will determine the status of nursing for the future.

The nurses' role is becoming more politically important to health care organizations. The rising concern that organizations have about their public image puts the bedside nurse in the position of projecting a caring image to the public. Patients and physicians often choose hospitals based on excellence of nursing care.

Because of rising health care costs, legislators, third-party reimbursers, and industry have greatly influenced health care. See Chapter 1 for a discussion of the Tax Equity and Fiscal Responsibility Act (TEFRA) of 1982 and Diagnostic Related Groups (DRG). The TEFRA amendment and Medicare legislation have dramatically changed reimbursement for hospitals and physicians. Third-party reimbursers are beginning to follow government's lead. Industries are joining together to reduce health care costs. Industry recently has placed key figures on hospital boards of trustees in an effort to control and reduce hospitals' organizational and capital costs.

Due to these major impacts, new graduates must realize that hospitals may no longer have the financial ability to respond to the needs of all persons. Although it may be desirable for patients, health care organizations may no longer be able to afford luxury items.

SUPPORT SERVICES IN NURSING

One characteristic of any profession is that avenues of support are provided for its members to continue to grow, expand their scientific knowledge base, and improve services to clients. The following sections discuss such support services and their place within the practice of nursing.

Nursing administration

All institutions are made up of human resources and a physical plant. However, in a service organization, employees deal directly with the patient and are the most important aspect of patient care. A nursing administration that maximizes people's talents by helping them develop problem-solving skills, assume responsibility, and participate in decision making will achieve the primary goal of excellent patient care and a secondary gain of a stable and involved staff.

Nursing administration also has a responsibility to evaluate the staff to assure their growth. It is vital that each employee's self-respect be maintained while the employee is helped to face mistakes realistically. A climate for growth also can be facilitated by establishing a clear-cut definition of responsibilities, allowing freedom to perform, welcoming ideas and opinions, appreciating efforts, and nurturing creativity. Beginning nurses find support from their head nurse and nursing supervisor for difficult clinical decisions. This is especially important to remember when working evening or night shifts. The nursing supervisor serves as a resource person with broad clinical background and should be called on in times of difficulty.

Staff development

Staff development departments exist to close the gap between the skeleton of a nurse's basic educational preparation and the body of knowledge necessary to practice in the rapidly changing technology of America's health care industry. Staff development must create an environment that fosters lifelong learning and helps nurses adjust to changes in patient demographics and practice roles. America is aging. Educational levels are rising. These two factors heavily influence the chronicity of illnesses that are seen and the share in decision making that patients expect from health care workers. There is also a trend toward greater specialization

and variety of health care personnel with which nurses must interact.

Ever-changing governmental controls and requirements of accrediting agencies also make staff development vital. Nurses must be updated on the legal constraints under which they practice and ways of improving productivity and quality control. New funding legislation for Medicare programs imposes ever-tightening cost containment on the industry. The JCAH requires that every accredited agency provide orientation for employees covering care standards, job duties, personnel policies, institutional regulations, electrical safety, and fire regulations.

Because staff development faculty assist the learning of adults, they must be aware of the special learning needs adults demonstrate. Most adults are very pragmatic learners. They define a problem and gear their learning to that need rather than taking a subject-centered approach. Adults generally are goal-directed, active, and autonomous learners and require a more supportive, less directive approach than traditional students. Because a group of nurses may come from widely divergent experiences, educational preparations, clinical focuses, expertise, and interests, they are considered to be a heterogeneous group to teach. The staff development instructor therefore must be able to draw from group members and acknowledge their contributions to the learning process. Audiovisual aids help adult learners to reinforce learning, resulting in better understanding and longer retention of information.

There are several distinct services that staff development can provide within an institution:

General orientation provides new employees with content necessary to their successful adaptation to the new work setting. The institution must be assured that each nurse possesses adequate clinical skills to be a safe practitioner by evaluating the nurse on procedures and policies. Additional information frequently included in the orientation includes personnel policies and benefits, discipline and grievance procedures, union contract provisions, charting procedures, report protocols, laboratory requisitioning, and emergency procedures.

Specialty orientation is necessary for nurses to safely enter new specialty fields in nursing. Examples of formalized specialty orientations include critical care, obstetrics, neonatal, and psychiatric nursing courses. Generally these are formal classes with successful completion of a posttest and supervised clinical practice required.

Some new graduates prefer the glamour and excitement of critical care to a more general assignment and seek first positions in critical care units. Institutions differ in their policy on new graduates working in specialty units, and they also differ in the length and quality of their specialty orientation courses. Generally, one could expect 2 to 4 weeks of class and a more prolonged period of clinical orientation than the general medical-surgical orientation.

The controversy over employing new graduates in specialty units has two sides. Proponents suggest that new graduates are needed, are more energetic and enthusiastic, and have a fresher formal knowledge base to draw on than older nurses. They are used to caring for only one or two patients and can easily adjust to a more in-depth application of familiar concepts. There are more support personnel available in specialty units because staffing on the evening and night shifts, when most new graduates work, is generally better than on general floors.

Opponents cite the lack of experience and skills as being unsafe for patients when immediate assessment and action are required. New graduates have not gained confidence in their role as nurse before being confronted directly with numerous decision-making situations in a highly stressful environment.

In-service education is ongoing in all health care institutions and refers to skill development for the direct care givers. Because of rapid changes in medical technology, new products, equipment, and procedures must be presented to everyone in the institution to ensure uniformity and safety of care. This type of service is offered on all shifts and to all levels of personnel as appropriate.

Continuing education refers to ongoing formal programs that are designed to maintain the current practice of nursing. Some states legally impose on RNs the requirement to continue their education in order to ensure safe practice to the public. This is termed *mandatory continuing education* because the nurse's eligibility to obtain a license renewal is tied to attendance at continuing education unit (CEU) offerings. One CEU is equal to 10 contact hours of class and is awarded by state nurses' associations when programs meet specific requirements. Many states require 15 contact hours per year. Approved continuing education programs must be made available if mandatory. In some instances this has forced employers to make adequate time and money available for continuing education and thus has aided nursing. The controversy in the mandatory continuing education issue is the question of whether forced attendance will change the mind set or behavior of nurses who have not internalized a professional role model.*

In other states, continuing education is voluntary and regulated within the profession. This must be a preferable model to any profession, that is, to internally control professional practice rather than have nonmembers intervene.

There are many ways an adult learner can update professional knowledge in addition to the formal classroom situation. Self-study modules may soon be accredited for CEU endorsement by having nurses send their posttests to the accrediting body for evaluation.

Management training should be offered by staff development to prepare nurses to assume leadership roles within the institution. Baccalaureate education in nursing does not presume to prepare managers but is sometimes the only educational prerequisite to employment at the head nurse or supervisor levels. Managers require skills in communications, disciplining, conflict resolution,

---

*Stevens, B.J.: Mandatory continuing education for professional nurse relicensure: what are the issues? Staff Development **1:**82-86, 1975.

budgeting, scheduling, union contracts, time management, and theories of motivation, management, and leadership.

Organizational development refers to efforts within the institution to program change. Examples of programs for organizational development include the following: changes in patient care delivery systems, efforts to unify the nursing process, and computerization of nursing documentation. Staff development provides the vehicle to start these new systems and the support services necessary to formalize the changes and thus develop the organization.

Preceptor programs use key nursing personnel to work directly with new nurses in a buddy system where the two share an assignment for a specific period of time. The preceptor introduces the new nurse and eases adaptation to the culture of the unit and its physical facilities. The preceptor also serves as a role model by example and by encouraging the new nurse to establish priorities, learn to delegate, and make meaningful rounds and reports.

Biculturalism programs have been developed in many institutions in an effort to ease the disparities between school values and work values of new graduates as described by Kramer and Schmalenberg.* Conflict results when the nurses see practices that are inconsistent with principles learned in the educational process (reality shock). Burnout, the term used to describe the nurse who cannot make the needed role transformation by accepting positive aspects from both cultures, results in nurses dropping out of the profession.

Kramer and Schmalenberg advocate a biculture training program with three components:

1. The affective component consists of seminars with other new graduates 6 to 8 weeks after hiring to clarify issues, establish a climate of trust, and increase self-awareness and acceptance.

2. The cognitive component involves reading *Path to Biculturalism* and performing self-learning exercises.

3. The behavioral component 4 to 5 months after employment includes conflict resolution workshops and role playing.

Research results indicate that nurses will be better prepared through this program to cope with the stresses of nursing and will be less likely to leave the profession as a result of reality shock.

Assertiveness training is offered by many institutions to help nurses deal more directly with problems in communication that arise in their daily practice. Role playing, critique of videotape vignettes, and feedback from actual work situations are techniques that are frequently used to help nurses actively use and internalize the concepts.

COMPUTERIZATION

Computerization of many standard nursing tasks is already a reality throughout the country in future-thinking institutions. Physician orders are easily and simultaneously transmitted to all the necessary departments with only one command instead of having to send several pieces of paper all over the institution or having to make several phone calls. Nursing care plans are on-line, allowing automatic updating and printing for use during shift report. When medication orders are entered into the computer, the pharmacy automatically dispenses drugs to the unit. The pharmacy can then compare dispensed drugs with those charted for change purposes and thus decrease charting errors and loss. Supplies are automatically reordered as used so adequate stores are assured and use of outdated materials is prevented.

Computers aid in research by organizing and sorting information according to any desired parameter. Patient acuity systems are linked closely to the computer and provide a rationale for staffing assignments. State of the art use of computers in nursing includes charting of nurses' notes and monitoring systems with dysrhythmia detection and trending in the coronary care unit. These tools can

---

*Kramer, M., and Schmalenberg, C.: Bicultural training and new graduate role transformation, Wakefield, Mass., 1978, Nursing Resources, Inc.

decrease charting time and overtime costs for the institution, resulting in more efficiency.

Nurses have voiced concern that computers will foster impersonal care. An additional ethical concern is patient privacy. In balance, however, the benefits of providing more time for nurses to spend at the bedside must outweigh concerns over potential problems.

NURSING RESEARCH

Research supports nursing practice by serving as a basis for professional practice. Nursing no longer can justify perpetuating old practices without evaluating their effectiveness in relation to alternative models. The ultimate outcome of nursing research will be the development of clinical protocol based on new knowledge. Patients will be the direct beneficiaries. As more nurses with master's and doctoral preparation are available to serve as leaders for research efforts and to help other nurses pursue their clinical questions, a research culture will develop in nursing and research will become the norm rather than the exception. It is the research in clinical nursing that will make the difference in professional nursing practice. See Chapter 12, Research in Nursing, for a more complete discussion of this topic.

VARIABLES INFLUENCING NURSING PRACTICE
Settings for practice

A variety of opportunities for practice are available to the new graduate nurse. The most basic choice centers around the decision to work in a traditional acute care hospital setting or in a community health care agency. The choice takes on more complexity when one examines the differences in hospitals related to size, community versus university setting, and teaching versus nonteaching status.

The very small community hospital may have only a few patient care units. Generally, there is no resident house staff coverage. Each patient care unit provides care for clients with a variety of prob-

lems; thus the nurse must have a broad knowledge base to deal with different patients' needs. The nurse is required to exercise a high level of assessment skill and independent decision making in determining when the private physician should be contacted and informed of changes in patients' conditions.

Larger hospitals, particularly those affiliated with universities, often participate in nursing and medical education programs. Resident physicians and nursing students are part of the health care team. Educational programs are often based on the medical model with focus on specific body system failures. These factors contribute to specilization and clustering of patients on nursing units based on specific physiologic problems. Residents are available to work closely with nursing staff 24 hours per day, assessing changes in patient status and implementing rapid intervention.

Both public and private community home health care agencies operate throughout the United States to meet the health care needs of clients in the home environment. Nurses employed by these agencies visit clients' homes regularly to provide health teaching, referral information, and direct "hands on" care. These nurses too must possess a broad knowledge base to deal with the variety of needs and conditions experienced by clients in their homes.

As health care agencies increase in size and specialization, the demand for leaders with specialty expertise increases. The organizational structure often reflects the complexity of roles and functions in the agency.

Organizational structures

People and groups make up organizational structures. They work together to fulfill the mission of the agency. Success or failure of an organization depends on how well this group of people works together. Persons and groups are interdependent in their efforts to achieve success and fulfillment of the primary goal.

Structures are called *organizational charts* when

drawn pictorially. The charts diagram the relationship of positions in the overall structure. They also reflect status, influence, and authority within the organization. Accountability and lines of authority are identified using organizational charts.

Structure is built around programs and functions. Nursing structures have for years been hierarchical in nature. They are designed as flat, horizontal structures or tall, vertical ones.

Tall structures are most frequently found in large teaching hospitals where the nursing organization has diverse and clearly defined programs and several levels of management to carry out the programs.

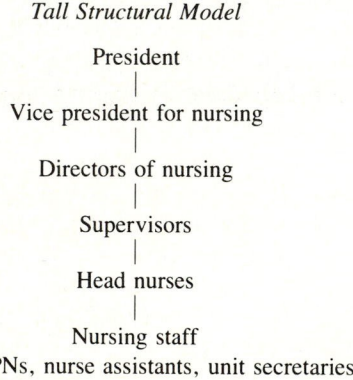

Tall Structural Model

President
|
Vice president for nursing
|
Directors of nursing
|
Supervisors
|
Head nurses
|
Nursing staff
(RNs, LPNs, nurse assistants, unit secretaries)

Tall structures, which are pyramidal in design, are used when change within the organization is rapid and centralized coordination of the change is necessary.

Communication is rapid in this environment, but more attention is paid to communication with superiors than with peers. Decision making takes less time because decisions are made by a few people at the top of the structure. The major problem with

the vertical structure is lack of understanding between the lower and higher levels of the organization. Communications may become distorted because of the numbers of people transferring information up the chains of command.

Flat structures provide fewer levels of supervision, as reflected in the horizontal lines that characterize them (see below). This minimizes the distortion of communication. Success of the flat structure is believed to occur because of high employee morale from their direct involvement in decision making. It is more democratic than the authoritarian style of a tall structure. However, flat structures provide fewer promotional opportunities than tall structures.

Staff nurses should be cognizant of the position of the most senior nurse administrator in the organization. Nursing autonomy in the organization may depend on this person's title and reporting relationship. The nurse administrator who holds a vice president position and reports directly to the president will exercise more direct influence on decisions made by the president and board of trustees. Close examination of the organzational chart may suggest the amount of control exercised by nurses over nursing practice.

Structure has thus far been discussed as formal organizational models. Nurses also must be aware of the informal organization in the institution. This informal organization does not appear on the chart, but it does affect nursing practice. Communication flows quickly in the informal organization, but problems of accuracy exist with this "grapevine." The informal organization is a social one and can be a negative or positive force.

Hospital administrations recognize the need of

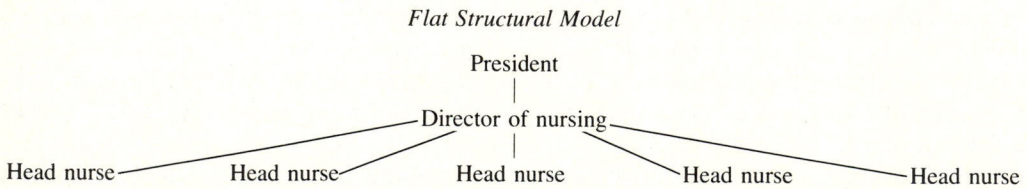

Flat Structural Model

President
|
Director of nursing
|
Head nurse — Head nurse — Head nurse — Head nurse — Head nurse

nurses to participate in decision making regardless of structure. Staff nurses may become involved by participating on hospital and nursing committees. Committees are a consistent part of all nursing organizational frameworks. Nurses are frequently involved in policy, procedure, quality assurance, nursing practice, staff development, and staffing committees. These committees make recommendations for change through the formal system. Sometimes staff nurses contribute to general hospital and medical staff committees. It is important for staff nurses to participate in committees in order to provide input from all levels of nursing and to allow the nurses to mature in their understanding of how to effect change in a large organization.

Many organizational changes have been noted in the literature in the past 10 to 15 years. Some have occurred through efforts of nursing service and nursing education to work more closely. Other structures try to facilitate collaboration between physicians and nurses. Nursing is striving toward a position of autonomy equal to that of the medical staff in hospitals. Other structures support the need for nursing, medicine, administration, and other hospital disciplines to interface efficiently for the sake of improving patient care. The following discussion focuses on recent organizational models developed to facilitate this interface.

Matrix organizations

The matrix organization is one of the first structures to recognize that it takes a team effort to provide care for patients. It is derived from both flat and tall structures to provide a grid effect at the patient care level. A team is formed consisting of the nurse, attending physician, social worker, dietician, physical therapist, and other care providers. The team is led by the nurse whose primary responsibility within the matrix is coordination and communication regarding patient care. The team represents the flat structure previously described and has the authority to plan and implement changes in patient care. The vertical or tall structure

remains in place to carry out other formal functions of the organization.

Collaborative models

In 1970 the Lysaught report recommended that joint practice committees be formed on a state, local, and institutional basis. The committees would involve the major disciplines (i.e., nursing and medicine) along with other health management executives and allied health personnel. The purpose of the committees (commissions) was to "join in planning for optimum working relationships and concerted role performance that will assure the best delivery of care."* For this concept to become a reality, demonstration projects were financed by the W. Kellogg Foundation in the late 1970s.

Joint practice models are used in ambulatory care settings with nurse practitioners. This model calls for six concepts to be in evidence before joint practice can be implemented:

1. Commitment of medical staff and nursing to a primary care delivery system
2. Reward system for clinical excellence
3. Clinical competence of the nursing staff
4. Collegial relationship between medicine and nursing
5. Administrative support of quality patient care
6. Nurses' acceptance of each other as professionals

Joint practice models for improved collaboration between physicians and nurses is a positive move for nursing. The nurse and physician work as peers, each with their own expertise, caring for a case load of clients. Organizational structure need not be changed to implement this model.

The *unification model* binds together nursing service and nursing education. Nurses working in hospitals in university settings that share the same board of trustees are likely to experience this or another form of collaboration. The dean of nursing in this model is responsible for both the quality of

---

*Lysaught, J.: An abstract for action, New York, 1970, McGraw-Hill Book Co.

nursing education and the quality of nursing practice. This model allows nurses to practice in both an educational and clinical setting, thus providing clinical role models for staff.

Hospitals not falling under the unification model have also achieved education and service collaboration. Hospitals and universities are providing qualified nurses with joint appointments. Nurses in this role spend a portion of their time in education and a portion in service. Adjunct faculty appointments (noncompensated teaching positions) are being offered to qualified nursing staff.

Some universities are now requiring faculty to maintain their clinical skill levels to remain in the academic setting. Hospitals are helping faculty achieve these goals by offering flexible hours and intermittent schedules compatible with the academic calendar. Results of collaboration using these methods have been most positive. These efforts should continue until nursing education and practice work together in concert.

Shared governance

Shared governance as developed at Rose Medical Center in Denver, Colorado, achieves a nursing staff structure equal to that of the medical staff structure. The entire nursing staff are members of a nursing congress, receiving their power from the board of trustees that approved their by-laws. The nursing congress provides the mechanism for input and makes recommendations for practice, salaries, benefits, and working conditions. This approach eliminates the necessity of utilizing a third party (union) for negotiation and representation purposes.

• • •

The organizational structures discussed provide some ways of achieving improved collaboration, patient care, and a more autonomous position in the organization. Nursing should continue to reorganize toward structures in which recognition and rewards are possible.

GROWTH IN DIRECT PATIENT CARE ROLES

For many years, nurses who worked in health care organizations had little or nor opportunity for advancement if they chose to remain at the bedside with patients. Advancement occurred only through staff development or nursing management positions. Reward systems were not present for nurses to do what they had been taught, that is, to give care to patients. Job dissatisfaction because of lack of promotional rewards for good nursing care created a shortage of nurses interested in caring for patients.

CLINICAL LADDERS

During the late 1970s and early 1980s, many systems were developed by hospitals to address the need to reward those who care for patients. These systems of promotion were generally called *clinical ladders*. Ladders differ depending on the organization, the organization's preferences, and the goals that organization wishes to achieve for staff nurses with a clinical ladder program.

Ladders are built with two to five levels through which a nurse may practice and be clinically promoted. Reporting relationships on clinical ladders systems vary. Some have the lower level clinician reporting to higher level clinicians. Other systems continue having the clinician reporting through the management structure. There are a limited number of positions available for each clinician level in some institutions, while others continue previous staffing patterns without regard to the number of clinicians achieving each level.

Financial reward systems associated with clinical ladders vary. Some systems have management and clinical ladders equal in pay and authority. Others continue to be separate even to the degree that it takes the highest level clinician to reach the bottom level management pay scale. Promotion methods vary for clinical ladder systems. Some hospitals have built ladders primarily based on educational preparation of the nurse. Others have set standards and competency levels that a nurse must attain before moving up to the next rung on the ladder. A third model shares a combination of the two. Certification also plays a role for advancement in some ladders. Most clinical ladders are voluntary programs. Nurses are not forced to enter this promotional tract if they do not wish to participate. However, most nurses do enter the system because financial rewards and professional recognition arise from such systems.

The structure and function of clinical ladders are not important. It is important that nurses are rewarded for excellent nursing care and have the opportunity for clinical career advancement.

CERTIFICATION

A number of nursing organizations also have seen the need to recognize excellent nurses. The American Nurses' Association, Emergency Nurses' Association, and the Critical Care Nurses' Association are three groups that have developed certification programs. Certification is a method outside the place of employment where a nurse can gain recognition for expertise in practice through passing a national examination. Nurses should try to achieve this recognition, both for personal professional growth and for advancement of the profession as a whole.

EXPANDED ROLES FOR NURSES

Two expanded roles are those of nurse practitioners and clinical specialists. Preparation for these roles varies. Nurse practitioner programs can be entered without regard to previous education preparation in nursing. Clinical specialist programs are on the graduate level and normally require a B.S.N. for entrance into the program.

Nurse practitioners most often function in the ambulatory setting. Their major area of expertise is in physical assessment. They work under fixed medical protocols in serving well patients or those with stable chronic conditions.

Most clinical specialists find positions in large medical centers or university hospitals. Their ex-

pertise includes knowledge of pathophysiology and nursing care protocols for a defined clinical population. They serve as role models through their expertise in the nursing process, through research, and in staff development.

SYSTEMS FOR DELIVERY OF NURSING CARE

The profession of nursing has responded and reacted to society while trying to move toward a goal of professional status. Functional nursing was a reaction to the scientific revolution, and the case method was a response by the profession to patients needing one individual for their care. Team nursing, a post–World War II system resulting from the nursing shortage, and primary and modular primary nursing are the profession's current answer to care of the total patient. Both reflect the profession's ongoing reach for quality in its patient advocacy role. It is hoped that the profession will continue to strive toward a more autonomous professional role through developing delivery systems to meet ever-changing needs. Society's push to decrease health care costs may indeed be the major force against that goal. A summary of the nursing delivery systems of the twentieth century follows.

Functional nursing

Functional nursing is task oriented, utilizing all skill levels of nursing personnel. One person may give medications, another may do all the vital signs, and another do patient baths. This assembly line concept of getting work accomplished is very efficient but impersonal. Patients may become confused about the variety and number of personnel who affect their day.

Case method: total patient system

The total patient system recognizes the needs of patients to relate to fewer individuals. In this approach, RNs have responsibility for all patient care functions. This continues to be a method of assignment when teaching student nurses. The system also recognizes levels of care required. For instance, acute care patients or those with complicated treatments are assigned to nurse assistants. The major concern is that even less acutely ill patients deserve to have an RN coordinate their care.

Team nursing

Team nursing, a response to a nursing shortage, incorporates LPNs, LVNs, and nurse assistants through delegation of work by RNs. Geographical distribution is usually a major factor in assignment and does not address patient needs. Team nursing removes RNs from direct care functions and places them in charge of a group of care givers. All patients are at least indirectly cared for by an RN who leads the team, making team nursing superior to functional nursing.

Primary nursing

Primary nursing represents a trend toward more professional practice. It was first implemented using an all-RN staff and has been the delivery model in community health agencies for years. Specific patients are assigned to primary nurses from admission to discharge. An RN frequently is the primary nurse for 5 or six patients. On another primary nurse's day off, she is also an associate nurse for the other nurse's primary patients. This system can use nurse assistants and LPNs for lower level and very defined tasks. Primary nursing provides a limited span of control and comprehensive individualized care to a limited group of patients. RNs are accountable for planning, coordinating, and implementing patient care within this system.

Modular primary nursing

Modular primary nursing developed at the same time as primary nursing. It combines team nursing and primary nursing. The modular system results when hospitals choose to continue to use LPNs and nurse assistants for patient care but want their nurses to assume greater accountability and to provide direct physical care and health education for patients. This system gives the RN the responsi-

bility and authority for total care using the nursing process. Geographical distribution of patient assignments continues as in team nursing. The modular primary nurse serves as an associate nurse for patients from another module when their nurse is not working.

• • •

Even though the nursing profession has moved through these different delivery systems, it must be recognized that all these systems continue to be practiced. Although the literature and current professional leaders believe primary nursing is the preferred system for the delivery of care, members of the nursing profession are slow to change. It is indeed a paradox. A new graduate should not be surprised to work in a hospital that continues to use the functional model.

STAFFING AND SCHEDULING

Nurses, whether they work in community nursing settings or hospitals, consider unit staffing and scheduling the variable in nursing practice that affects them the most. Professional nursing staff must care for patients 24 hours a day, 7 days a week. Many community health agencies such as visiting nurses' associations and home care programs also have nurses available for weekend, evening, and night coverage.

New graduates find that daylight positions are sometimes available in community health settings. It is uncommon for hospitals to have daylight positions available. Therefore new graduates commonly have to choose among working evenings, nights, or a rotation of days to evenings or days to nights. Many hospitals schedule at least every other weekend off, but other hospitals continue to provide only every third weekend off.

During the 1970s, because of the shortage of nurses and the need to respond to nurses' concerns about the impact of scheduling on their life-style, a number of new scheduling patterns and methods were offered to nurses. Some examples of flexible scheduling follow.

Every other weekend off. A weekend is defined as Saturday and Sunday for 7 to 3:30 and 3 to 11:30 shifts but ordinarily means Friday and Saturday for the 11 to 7:30 shift. Schedules with every other weekend off are in a cycle that tends to repeat itself so that days off are predictable. One concern with the every-other-weekend-off pattern is to assure that nurses do not work more than 5 days in a row.

Option 12. A nurse can choose to work two 12-hour shifts on a weekend and receive 36 to 40 hours of pay. This is possible because hospitals are willing to provide premium pay (time and a half) to secure the necessary staffing help on weekends. Paying premium wages for weekend work has been questioned because of cost-containment restrictions. In the 1980s this option may not continue to be possible due to cost to hospitals and reimbursement restrictions. Increasing the availability of nurses may eliminate the need to use option 12.

Baylor plan. Option 12 was an offshoot of the Baylor plan, at Baylor University Medical Center in Dallas, Texas. When a nurse is employed, there are two full-time options. A nurse can work two 12-hour shifts on the weekend or choose to work Monday through Friday. This program is not presently considered to be cost-effective. At the time of its implementation, however, it answered an immediate need for enough staff to care for patients.

Four-day week, 10-hour day. Many hospitals attempted the 4-day week in the 1970s. This schedule provides more personnel for patient care than the traditional 5-day, 40-hour workweek. Once again this pattern may not be used as much in the 1980s because of the added cost of extra personnel. Where work-load statistics can indeed show that a 10-hour shift is helpful to patient care, the practice will continue. One of the main reasons this schedule may be used less is poor utilization of personnel time during the overlapping hours and the decrease in continuity of the nurse-patient relationship over the nurse's 3 days off.

Seven-seventy. The 7-70 approach to scheduling provides nurses with 7 days off alternated with 7 days of work. One of the problems frequently discussed with this scheduling is maintaining continuity of care. Overtime and sick pay decrease with 7-70 scheduling. Some hospitals pay for 70 hours of work with this schedule, while others offer 80 hours of pay.

Supplemental agencies

During the last 10 years, the number of nurses employed by supplemental agencies has increased as a result of acute nursing shortages in some areas of the United States and the desire of nurses to be more independent. The rapid rise in nurses working for these separate corporations has been in response to the nurses' needs for flexible schedules and higher wages.

The use of agencies increases the cost of nursing services because hospitals must pay both the nurses' salaries and an agency fee. Hospitals are responding with float pools, groups of nurses employed by the hospital that are set up to eliminate the need for supplemental agencies. A float pool nurse may be asked to work in a variety of clinical units to fill vacancies, cover for persons on vacation, or help the hospital to deal with a fluctuating census or changes in patient acuity levels.

It is not recommended that a nurse's first position be with a supplemental agency. Experienced nurses have less difficulty adjusting to different hospitals and different nursing units because of their experience and nursing confidence. New graduates would not receive an adequate orientation to each facility to allow them to adjust to these variations.

NURSING PROCESS: BASIC TO NURSING PRACTICE

Throughout this chapter a number of variables have been presented that influence nursing practice; however, the greatest influence for change occurred when nursing process was introduced into the education/practice arena. Nursing process is a way of thinking through a problem and making decisions regarding appropriate nursing interventions.

Nursing process has become the most valuable

approach to improving quality and consistency in nursing practice. Often it is viewed as tedious and confusing, but in fact its potential for assuring organization, productivity, and satisfaction is extremely valuable. There are several steps within the process: assessment, nursing diagnosis, planning, implementation, and evaluation.

Assessment, the first step, includes the collection of data about the patient's condition. This function resembles the activity of old television detectives who declared ''just gimme the facts.'' Both subjective and objective facts must be gathered from every potential source including the patient, family, history, physical examination, and laboratory data.

Nursing diagnosis, the second step, begins with analysis of the data and leads to identification of a nursing diagnosis. When beginning the process of completing a jigsaw puzzle, one examines all the pieces and picks out the blue pieces to form a picture of sky and then the green pieces to form the grass. In formulating a nursing diagnosis, nurses use the detective approach by examining the facts to see which pieces fit to form a picture (nursing diagnosis). The nursing diagnosis must flow logically from the data base, and the data must support the diagnosis. This diagnosis is basically the statement of a patient problem, need, or concern. It may reflect teaching or learning needs, emotional concerns, or physical problems. Statement of the nursing diagnosis always includes a phrase that reflects possible causal or contributory factors from the data base. The diagnoses are then listed in order of priority according to how seriously they affect the patient's status.

Planning, the third step, includes establishing patient-centered objectives in collaboration with the patient and identifying nursing interventions that will help to achieve each objective. If the nurs-

Table 1. The nursing process

Assessment data	Nursing diagnosis	Patient-centered objective	Nursing interventions	Evaluation
Clothes too tight Average of seven meals/day Average of 4300 cal/day Numerous rolls of excess adipose tissue Minimal activity No stair climbing; elevator only SOB† when walking and talking Weight 30 lb over insurance table recommendation	Overweight related to excess intake and inadequate exercise	Short-term: patient will demonstrate 5-lb weight loss by 1 mo from today Long-term: patient will demonstrate 30-lb weight loss by 6 mo from today	Limit caloric intake to 1200 cal/day Increase activity by walking briskly 1 hr/day Eliminate between-meal snacks Eat only at table Establish reward for each 5-lb loss (not to include food)	Patient has lost 6 lb after 1 mo of plan; continue plan*

*If the evaluation proved that the patient had lost only 2 lb after 1 mo, the process would begin again. The nursing process is the logical approach for nurses to identify and resolve patient care problems and measure the effectiveness of patient care. While evaluation of individual patient care is important, evaluation of overall care is also a serious concern for health care agencies.

†Shortness of breath.

ing diagnosis identifies the patient problem, need, or concern (a desirable state), the patient-centered objective should describe an improved state related to that diagnosis. It must be stated in behavioral, measurable terms. Each objective is followed by a list of nursing actions by priority that will help the patient to accomplish the objective. Table 1 gives an example of the process.

Implementation, the fourth step, entails putting the plan into action. All nursing interventions are carried out in order of priority to best assist the patient to achieve the objective.

Evaluation (modification), the fifth and final step, may be the most important step of all. It may also be the first step in repeating the entire nursing process. At this point the nurse must determine whether each patient-centered objective has been achieved. This is the most important consideration, since each objective represents an improved status for the patient problem (need or concern) identified in the nursing diagnosis statement. If the objective is achieved, the problem is resolved. If not, three questions should be asked. First, is the initial data base valid or should patient status be assessed again? Second, is the objective realistic? If not, it should be changed in collaboration with the patient. Third, if the objective is realistic, what should be added or changed in the nursing interventions so that the objective can be achieved? The answer to these questions may result in modification of the nursing care plan.

While nursing process is based on the age-old scientific method, its practicality causes it to be used commonly but unconsciously in daily life. Consider the process experienced in deciding to diet (Table 1).

SUMMARY

Nursing practice has evolved partly in response to changing societal needs but also from direct action by nurses seeking advancement for the profession. Strengthened by adherence to the nursing process and commitment to quality patient care, nursing has sought increased status among the health care professions.

Numerous variables influence the practice of nursing today. Practice depends on organizational structure, models of delivering care, expanding roles for nurses, staffing patterns, and external factors. The beginning nurse must analyze these factors to select a work setting that will be compatible with the nurse's value systems.

Discussion questions

1. Describe the steps of the nursing process and illustrate their use.
2. Describe five models of delivering nursing care.
3. Discuss five ways that staff development can assist nurses in their professional growth.
4. Discuss the 24-hour need for nursing services and its potential impact on the individual staff nurse.

SUGGESTED READINGS

Aherns, W., and Norris, B.: Expanded roles in critical care: nurse practitioner or clinical specialist? Dimensions Crit. Care **2**(2):98-101, 1983.

Arndt, C. and Huckabay, L.M.: Nursing administration: theory for practice with a systems approach, ed. 2, St. Louis, 1980, The C.V. Mosby Co.

Baker, C.: Moving toward interdependence: strategies for collaboration, Nurse Educator, pp. 27-31, Sept.-Oct. 1981.

Blazek, A.M., et al.: Unification: nursing education and nursing practice, Nurs. Health Care, pp. 18-23, Jan. 1982.

Cason, C.L., and Beck, C.M.: Clinical nurse specialist role development, Nurs. Health Care, pp. 25-26, 35-38, Jan. 1982.

Cooper, S.S.: Continuing education: yesterday and today, Nurse Educator, pp. 25-29, Jan.-Feb. 1978.

Edwardson, S., and Anderson, D.: Hospital nurses valuation of quality assurance, J. Nurs. Admin., pp. 33-39, July-Aug. 1983.

Everson, S.J.: Integration of the role of clinical nurse specialist, J. Contin. Educ. Nurs. **12**(2):16-19, 1981.

Garvey, J.C., and Rohet, S.: Expanding the hospital nursing role: an administrative account, J. Nurs. Admin., pp. 30-34, Dec. 1982.

Gassert, C., Holt, C., and Pope, K.: Building a ladder, Am. J. Nurs., pp. 1527-1530, Oct. 1982.

Gillies, D.A.: Nursing management: a systems approach, Philadelphia, 1982, W.B. Saunders Co.

Hanson, R.C.: Management systems for nursing service staffing, Rockville, Md., 1983, Aspen Systems Corp.

Happ, B.: Should computers be used in the nursing care of patients? Nurs. Management **14**(7):31-35, 1983.

Huey, F.L.: Looking at ladders, Am. J. Nurs., pp. 1520-1526, Oct. 1982.

Knauss, P.J.: Staff nurse preceptorship: an experiment for graduate nurse orientation, J. Contin. Educ. Nurs. **11**(5):44-46, 1980.

Kramer, M.: Reality shock: why nurses leave nursing, St. Louis, 1974, The C.V. Mosby Co.

Kramer, M., and Schmalenberg, C.: Bicultural training and new graduate role transformation, Wakefield, Mass., 1978, Nursing Resources, Inc.

Lee, A.A.: What computers can do for you . . . and what they're already doing for the lucky few, RN, pp. 43-44, Sept. 1982.

Magula, M.: Understanding organization: a guide for the nurse executive, Wakefield, Mass., 1982, Nursing Resources, Inc.

Moyer, M.G., and Mann, J.K.: A preceptorship program of orientation within the critical care unit, Heart Lung **8**(3):530-534, 1979.

Murphy, J.G., and Schmitz, M.: The clinical nurse specialist: implementing the role in a hospital setting, J. Nurs. Admin. pp. 29-31, Jan. 1979.

Nurse-physician-administrator relationships, Nurs. Admin. Q., vol. 7, no. 4, 1983.

Payss, A.S., and Vivenzo, K.M.: Should new nursing graduates be used in critical care, Dimensions Crit. Care Nurs. **1**(1):44-49, 1982.

Prescott, P.A., et al.: Supplemental nursing services: how and why are they used? Am. J. Nurs., pp. 554-557, April 1983.

Reeves, D., et al.: Mount Sinai's distinctive nursing department, Nurs. Admin. Q., pp. 12-22, Spring 1982.

Ritter, H.: Nurse-physician collaboration, Conn. Med. **45**(1):23-25, 1981.

Schmad, J.C.: Quality assurance: examination of the concept, Nurs. Outlook, pp. 462-465, July 1979.

Stevens, B.J.: Mandatory continuing education for professional nurse relicensure: what are the issues? Staff Development **1**:82-86, 1975.

Sultz, H.A., et al.: Nurse practitioners: a decade of change. II, Nurs. Outlook, pp. 216-269, July-Aug. 1983.

Tarnow, K.G.: Working with adult learners, Nurse Educator, pp. 34-40, Sept.-Oct. 1979.

Woldum, K.M., et al.: The professional development program: an alternative to clinical ladders, Nurs. Admin. Q. **7**(3):82-93, 1983.

Zielstorff, R.D.: Computers in nursing, Rockville, Md., 1982, Aspen Systems Corp.

CHAPTER 8
Nursing leadership

NANCY KILBANE
MARIANNE CRAWFORD
MARY FISHER
JOANN HOLT

OBJECTIVE: On completion of this chapter, the student of nursing will be able to discuss the concept of leadership as it is applied to the role of the nurse.

In the profession of nursing the function of leadership is often considered to be the responsibility of those holding official supervisory or management positions. At the very least, some assume one must be acting as team leader to exercise leadership. Actually, nothing could be further from the truth. This chapter emphasizes that all nurses providing patient care use leadership skills daily as they interact with patients, families, staff members, physicians, and other departments or agencies.

Definitions of leadership vary from source to source. However, one basic theme emerges consistently: leadership is the process of influencing the behavior of others. Only with a clear understanding of this concept can one appreciate that leadership is a function exercised by every practicing nurse who influences the behavior of individual patients, their family members, and other members of the health care team.

Leaders emerge whenever group activities occur. During an interaction between two individuals, one may emerge as the leader because of personal influence or positional power exerted over the other. Similarly, in group activity, individuals emerge as leaders to influence activities of the group.

The staff nurse providing direct personal care to patients is definitely viewed as a leader, an expert in what is best for their recovery and their healthy life-style. Most often the patient follows the nurses' instructions on how to transfer from bed to chair, how often to cough and deep breathe after surgery, what restrictions to observe at home, when to contact the physician, and so on. In hospitals and community health care agencies where primary nursing is practiced, it is common for all patients to call "their nurse" for guidance following discharge. Family members routinely seek out the patient's nurse for instructions on how they should handle the patient at home as well as in the hospital. This influence on the behavior of others is a serious responsibility experienced by nursing students, new graduates, and veteran nurses alike.

Whether they are functioning as team leader or team member, staff nurses influence the behavior of other members of the nursing team as well. Assisting or instructing the nurse assistant to safely and effectively transfer a specific patient from the bed to a chair is a simple example of the influence exerted. The team leader's influence on behavior may be more formal and obvious as assignments are made, instructions are given, outcome expectations are clarified, and progress reports are received from various members of the nursing team. Head nurses and supervisors exercise leadership most visibly as they influence staff members' behavior to accomplish objectives of the unit or agency. This may be on a broader scale, but it is no more or less significant than the leadership exhibited by the staff nurse.

Various theories related to personality, physical characteristics, knowledge, expertise, interpersonal style, official position, group size, environment, and training are cited in the literature as factors contributing to the emergence of leaders and to successful leadership behavior.* Each student of nursing as well as each nurse may profit from self-analysis to increase awareness of personal characteristics that influence success or failure in leadership endeavors.

LEADERSHIP STYLES

As surely as leaders emerge, either naturally or by appointment, the development of leadership styles will follow. A review of the literature on leadership reveals numerous styles, including participative, consultative, and paternalistic. However, three classic styles have been acknowledged over the years and remain basic today. These are autocratic, democratic, and laissez-faire.

The *autocratic leader* decides unilaterally and imposes the decision on the work group without their input. This is most appropriate in an emergency situation such as managing a cardiac arrest, but it probably leads to discontent among workers in daily operations, since they have no input or control over their own work.

The *democratic leader* seeks input from all parties involved before making a decision. Sometimes the group members actually make the decision. This provides the members with a higher level of satisfaction and responsibility for the decisions

---

*Tappen, R.M.: Nursing leadership: concepts and practices, Philadelphia, 1983, F.A. Davis Co., pp. 39-62.

made and often evokes greater commitment to accomplishing the task by group members. However, the process of reaching group decisions may be extremely time consuming and frustrating. There will always be individuals holding opinions in the minority who will be unhappy with the outcome of such decisions.

The *laissez-faire leader* allows group members a great deal of autonomy and self-direction in decision making and in daily operations. This may work well when all group members have a clear and consistent understanding of the required outcome and when communication among members is efficient. When group members are not strongly self-directed or when communication is not efficient, it has potential for creating a chaotic environment with minimum productivity.

Each of these basic styles has positive and negative aspects, and each may be more or less effective depending on the situation in which it is used. Most often leaders find themselves using a variety of styles depending on the situation, the needs of the people involved, and the outcomes desired.

AUTHORITY, RESPONSIBILITY, AND ACCOUNTABILITY

Those persons who demonstrate leadership behavior do so because they possess authority. The *New York Times Everyday Dictionary* defines authority as "the power or right to do something; also, a person . . . with power or expert knowledge." Certainly the professional nurse is viewed as a person with expert knowledge who therefore possesses the power or right to exercise authority in interaction with patients and colleagues. But rights always go hand in hand with responsibilities. Thus one cannot exercise authority without accepting responsibility for the outcome of that action. Nor can one assume responsibility for an outcome unless one also possesses the authority to influence or control the outcome. Possessing this authority increases in importance when one is accountable or answerable to another, particularly when the other has the power to evaluate one's performance or influence one's career. In providing nursing care, the nurse is accountable to the patient, the family, the physician, the nursing supervisor, and all other nurses in the profession. The importance of controlling one's practice cannot be overemphasized; thus every action taken must be within the nurse's authority as allowed by license. Only then can the nurse be responsible and accountable for the results of his or her action.

ASSERTIVENESS

Maintaining control of one's practice is not always an easy task. Patients, families, physicians, and even nursing supervisors may hold inappropriate expectations of the nurse's performance. The new graduate nurse who must call the attending physician about a patient at 2 AM can easily be intimidated by an angry response. The demands of a nursing supervisor or the requests of a patient or family member can present a similar dilemma. An assertive response in these situations is one that is calm rather than aggressive. A response based on communication of objective facts about the situation rather than defensiveness can be very helpful in resolving the conflict.

It is important for the student to recognize and practice the difference between assertive and aggressive behavior. Assertive means to maintain, to be firm, and to stand for what is fact, whereas aggressive is to attack, to encroach, and to be pushy, obtrusively energetic, or indifferent to others' feelings.

Assertiveness is an extremely beneficial skill that must be studied and practiced to be used effectively. Whenever possible, students of nursing should include assertiveness training in their basic education, participate with practicing nurses in continuing education, or attend hospital in-service classes to perfect the skills of assertive communication.

POWER AND CONTROL

Power, although similar in definition to influence and authority, is derived from various sources. The head nurse may possess formal power, but the staff nurse may emerge as the group leader as a result of informal power awarded him or her by virtue of personality, charisma, educational credentials, knowledge, or clinical expertise. On occasion, the veteran nurse assistant may possess more informal power than anyone else. Each nurse must develop the ability to recognize the use of power personally and in other members of the nursing team.

Professional nurses must value the formal power they possess because of their education and expertise. Exercise of this power, of course, includes the responsibility and the right to control the quality of nursing care given under their guidance. Whether nurses function as primary care givers with the aid of nurse assistants or as team leaders with other RNs and auxiliary staff reporting to them, the power to control the quality of care is theirs. The *right and responsibility* of the RN to set goals for patient care, to demand certain levels of performance and quality, and to hold team members accountable cannot be challenged.

BEGINNING NURSE AS A LEADER

The nurse, as the professional care giver, is expected to be the leader of the group of nursing personnel who administer patient care. This is often a difficult task for new nurses who struggle to organize elements within their own practice before being able to lead others. The number of tasks to be accomplished by the nurse each day presents a real challenge for organizational skills. Time constraints must be considered in deciding which needs should be met first. The laboratory test that must be sent by 8 AM, the insulin that must be given by 7:30 AM, and the patient who must be ready for surgery by 8:15 AM all influence how the nurse organizes his or her work. The logical, orderly flow of work or the influence of one procedure on another may make certain organizational approaches necessary. Certainly the diabetic patient's fasting blood test for glucose should be drawn *before* breakfast rather than after. Basic knowledge and experience help the nurse grow more secure in these organizational skills each day. That security is necessary before one can begin to provide instruction and leadership for other members of the nursing team.

Leadership skills cannot be perfected in an educational setting. Competency for new graduates in the leadership role is gained from observation, imitation of other nurses, and experience. The new graduate can become a strong leader under the guidance and example of a competent head nurse.

Priorities of nursing care

After a thorough assessment to identify needs, the nurse begins to set the priorities for action. The overall process should address patient, team, and unit needs. The most critical needs must be met first. Initially the new nurse may have to choose a method and concentrate on setting priorities. Eventually the priority-setting process becomes automatic and internalized in the nurse's practice.

There are various approaches that can be used to set priorities. One such method might consider the seriousness (life-threatening nature) of the situation. For example, the LPN/LVN reports to the nurse that a patient has chest pain at the same time that the laboratory is calling with a urinalysis report for a preoperative patient. Although all needs are important, the potential seriousness of the chest pain for one patient is greater than getting a laboratory report for the other. The nurse, considering the seriousness of both situations, cares for the patient with chest pain before calling the laboratory back to get the report. Another method of priority setting is to use a hierarchy of needs approach. Maslow's hierarchy is most frequently used. According to Maslow, basic physiological needs for food, comfort, and elimination must be met before higher level needs such as self-esteem can be achieved.* A nurse using this method to set priorities would administer medication to relieve a patient's pain before attempting to teach another pa-

*Maslow, A.: Motivation and personality, ed. 2, New York, 1970, Harper & Row, Publishers, Inc.

tient how to change his or her dressing when at home. After determining the priorities of the work to be done, the nurse must delegate some tasks to other members of the nursing work group.

Delegation

It is impossible for the nurse to provide all of the nursing care needed by a group of patients. The nature of the role requires that the nurse delegate work to others. Delegation is described as a process through which the nurse can get the work done with the assistance of other people. Before delegating tasks, it is important to consider the skill level of each member of the nursing work group based on education, experience, and job description. The job description will become the most used document to determine if the task is an allowable delegated function. Assigning the nurse assistant to regulate a patient's intravenous infusion would be inappropriate based on these criteria.

Delegation is more than the process of assigning tasks. Leaders must control their attitudes and fears in order to develop the skill of appropriate and effective delegation. The new nurse faced with delegating work has many questions that need to be answered. Some typical questions might be:

- What tasks can I safely delegate?
- Can I trust that person to do it correctly?
- Do I feel comfortable in delegating some of the work for which I'm responsible?

These questions will be answered as the nurse begins to delegate and finds that the tasks have been performed correctly. It is important to understand that although the nurse delegates work to others, accountability for this work is retained. The delegation process is not complete until the nurse evaluates the performance of the work that was delegated.

Evaluation of other personnel is often difficult for a new nurse because many of the ancillary personnel are older or more experienced within the institution. An evaluation of how the team members performed the tasks, the feedback received from patients and other staff, and the nurse's comfort with the situation all help the nurse to analyze whether the delegation was appropriate. This evaluation process also assists in developing skill for future delegation. The ability to communicate effectively and the ability to motivate individuals are skills that also are required to be successful in delegation. Although persons must be self-motivating, the proper use of positive reinforcement and reward for work well done may encourage them to perform better.

Role modeling

The nurse working in an institutional setting is continually being scrutinized by patients, families, physicians, nursing management, peers, and subordinates. It is important to realize that each nurse is a role model representing professional nursing. Many factors contribute to the image of nursing conveyed to our many audiences. In addition to clinical skill, the nurse's appearance, posture, gait, facial expression, and tone of voice can indicate the nurse's level of self-confidence, professionalism, and sense of caring.

The nurse can be a model for desired behavior in many situations. The new nurse often observes behavior by long-term employees in the nursing work group that seems unacceptable in relation to the nurse's education and experience. It is intimidating and probably unwise to confront this behavior immediately. Investing time in establishing one's credibility as a competent nurse is often a necessary first step to correcting the undesirable behavior of others. The nurse should take advantage of opportunities to demonstrate clinical skill to these nursing personnel. Consistent performance of quality nursing care provides a model for other employees and establishes the nurse's personal competence and authority. Often this recognition provides the new nurse with the security to confront others and to explain that their performance does not meet acceptable standards and therefore must be improved. The importance of maintaining high-quality nursing practice is vital because many people look to the professional nurse as a model.

Evaluation

Not all persons perform equally in the work environment. Individual motivation to work also varies. It is important to realize these factors in assigning and evaluating employee performance. Therefore employees should not be evaluated in comparison to each other but in comparison to standards of performance found in the job description. The professional nurse as a responsible leader should contribute to the formal evaluation of various nursing employess. This is particularly true during evening and night shifts when nursing management personnel are not always available on each nursing unit. The nurse is the person who assigns the employee, observes performance, and evaluates the overall quality of the work. It is important for the nurse to remember that employees who report to the nurse need ongoing feedback regarding their performance. Feedback should include positive as well as negative input, given in a calm, objective manner.

Conflict management

Whenever people work together in any organizational setting, there are times when conflict will occur. The nurse, whether experienced or new in the role, will be expected to resolve the conflict. This is particularly true on the evening and night shifts where many new nurses are assigned. It is important for the nurse to develop a problem-solving approach to conflict resolution. Using the steps of the nursing process, a creative, acceptable, and realistic resolution of the conflict can be achieved. For example, the nurse makes an *assessment* that two nurse assistants on the unit are constantly in conflict. They refuse to help each other, and often they refuse to speak to each other. Sometimes they are overheard in loud, angry arguments. The nurse continues the assessment, a part of the nursing process, to resolve this problem. The nurse collects additional data by speaking with each person individually to determine his or her perceptions of the problem. The assessment is now complete. The assistants are asked to meet with the nurse to analyze the data and to develop conclusions *(nursing diagnoses)* identifying the actual problem. Once the root problem is identified, the nurse can work with the nurse assistants to *plan* short-term and long-term objectives for their performance. Then specific steps or interventions necessary to accomplish the objectives can be identified. After a short period of time, with both nurse assistants working on *implementing* the plan, all three meet again to *evaluate* whether or not the plan is working. If objectives are being met, the plan may be continued. If not, modification of the plan should be made. Ongoing evaluation of the work relationship must continue.

The foundation of leadership skill is being built first from the initial experiences of a new graduate nurse and then through daily activities. Each experience, whether frustrating or rewarding, should be viewed as a challenge and a learning opportunity. Planning ahead for the type of career desired helps one to use each challenge to the best advantage. Because numerous factors influence health care today, a broad scope of experience will better prepare the nurse for advancing leadership positions.

Other factors influencing nurses in leadership roles

In addition to understanding leadership theories and the staff nurse's role as a leader, it is essential for every nurse to have a concept of other factors that influence nurses' leadership roles. Leadership positions within health care organizations are found in either line or staff positions.

Persons in *line* positions have direct responsibility for the operation of the organization or for accomplishing the objectives of the organization. Under this definition, staff nurses exercise line authority, since they supervise other employees and delegate authority to achieve the objective of optimum patient care. However, in some situations, tasks that are normally considered line tasks may not be carried out by staff nurses. For example, a staff nurse may counsel an employee working under the nurse's supvervision, but formal written disciplinary action would occur through the head nurse with the staff nurse's input. Other persons who exercise line authority include the head nurse, supervisor or coordinator, director of nursing, vice president for nursing, and the president of the hospital. When problems arise, resolution of the problems should occur at the lowest possible level in the organization. Therefore staff nurses are involved with problem solving in areas that directly affect their patients' welfare. Policy issues with more general applicability, however, are more appropriately resolved at higher levels.

Persons in *staff* positions, in contrast, assist the line managers to work effectively to accomplish the primary objectives of the organization. Staff positions are by nature advisory, consultative, and informational. Staff persons can merely make recommendations. It is the line managers who must decide whether to accept or reject the recommendations. Similarly, hiring, firing, and disciplinary functions are restricted to persons in line positions. Therefore the power of any staff position lies in the expert knowledge and interpersonal skills of the individual staff person. Examples of staff positions include infection control nurse, nutrition support nurse, staff development faculty, clinical nurse specialist, and nurse recruiter.

Promotions may advance in either line or staff tracts and depend on the individual nurse's educational preparation, personality, motivation, clinical expertise, and experience. Line promotions lead either into the management hierarchy or through a clinical career ladder. Staff promotions occur in nursing education, research, clinical specialization, or other support positions.

Career-minded nurses should identify long-term goals early in their career and then set about achieving intermediary steps necessary to reach their final goal. It would be unrealistic for a staff nurse to expect to be promoted immediately to a director of nursing position. However, a nurse with this long-term goal should carefully select job experiences, promotions, and educational experiences that would provide the necessary knowledge base to prepare the nurse for an eventual director of nursing position. This type of plan could be used to achieve any nursing career goal, whether practice, education, research, or management area is sought. Because advanced nursing education tends to become more specialized, nurses must be careful not to become narrowly educated or too specialized in a direction that will be contrary to their eventual goal. This discussion of career development illustrates the necessity for nurses to have a clear idea of their ultimate career direction.

The career development plans outlined here may not be appropriate for everyone. Because the majority of nurses are women, many choose to pursue intermittent careers while meeting family obligations. Those nurses may want to focus their efforts on maintaining current knowledge and developing skills necessary to perfect their present practice. This is often achieved through continuing education.

Certain personality traits and interpersonal skills are necessary for success, no matter what career path is chosen. The ability to work positively with others, communicate effectively, and accomplish the objective of one's job with self-direction are essential factors that influence nurses' actual leadership advancement.

POLITICAL INVOLVEMENT

Hospitals differ from most other formal organizations in that hospitals have authority arising from three distinct groups rather than a single pyramidal structure. Legal responsibility for legislating broad policy is the charge of the board of trustees. Physicians' claims to policy making arise from their status as medical experts and the fact that they are the true consumer of health care provided by the hospital. A hospital would have no patients without physicians who admit patients to the facility. Finally, the persons who are responsible for

the operation of the organization (i.e., the administrative personnel, which includes nursing management) also claim policy-making privileges. Because the three groups interact formally and informally in the daily operation of the institution and possess differing perspectives, there are many opportunities for conflict and power struggles to arise. Conscious efforts to improve communications and interdisciplinary involvement in decision making must be ongoing to prevent misunderstandings and hostilities.

Where does this reality put nurses? In a very difficult position, for nurses also believe they should set policy for nursing practice. It is not unusual to find nurses in the middle of the conflict. Nurses interact daily with physicians who direct patient care efforts and also with nursing management who represent hospital administration. At times nurses find themselves being pulled in different directions. Ultimately it is the administration who signs the nurse's paycheck. Therefore the nurse needs to support nursing administration and may be best advised not to be placed in the middle of political struggles. This neutral position will best serve the patient and will allow the nurse to interact with both parties in a positive manner. Avoiding unnecessary conflict will enable the nurse to maintain an optimum political position for effecting change. There are times, however, when nurses must make personal decisions to become involved in conflict when issues are important to the nurse or when patient welfare warrants such involvement.

Political action does not merely occur in the work place. Nurses are making their collective voices heard on federal, state, and local governmental levels through exercise of their right to vote and political activism involving health care issues. There are nurses who hold offices on all three levels. Such involvement should be supported by all members of the profession. Nursing organizations have channeled political power in support of candidates and issues that affect the health care industry. Staff nurses should seek opportunities to become involved in political issues that affect their practice or the welfare of their patients.

SUMMARY

Leadership is a quality that nurses must demonstrate for success at every level of nursing. Although scope of leadership responsibility varies with position, all nurses interact with a variety of persons to coordinate patient care. Organizational skills are therefore central to the leadership role. The nursing process serves as the basis for rational decision making, priority setting, and conflict resolution. Since the nurse cannot perform all aspects of patient care because of time constraints, the ability to delegate successfully must be perfected. No delegated task is complete without evaluation of the work performed and the patient's response.

Leadership requires development of assertiveness as part of the professional role. Assertiveness skills can be acquired through an active, participative educational program where nurses practice the skills in a controlled environment. In a similar manner, conflict management can be learned.

Nurses must become more astute about internal and external politics affecting health care and must plan their careers with a vision toward the future.

Discussion questions

1. Discuss the benefits and disadvantages of the three classic leadership styles.
2. Give examples of the staff nurse in a leadership role.
3. Describe a method for setting priorities to be used by a staff nurse.
4. Discuss the difference between line and staff authority.
5. Explain how nurses are accountable to all other nurses in the profession.
6. Who is the true consumer of hospital health care?

SUGGESTED READINGS

Arndt, C. and Huckabay, L.M.: Nursing administration: theory for practice with a systems approach, ed. 2, St. Louis, 1980, The C.V. Mosby Co.

Booth, R.: Conflict resolution, Nurs. Outlook 30(8):447-453, 1982.

Calabrese, R.: Interaction skills for nurse managers, Nurs. Management 13(5):29-30, 1982.

Chartier, M.R.: Clarity of expression in interpersonal communication, Nurs. Admin. pp. 42-46, July 1981.

Chopra, A.: Motivation in task-oriented groups, J. Nurs. Admin. 3(1):55-60, 1973.

Dudjak, L.: A staff nurse's guide to leadership, Nurs. Management 12(10):26-27, 1981.

Gambacosta, S.: Head nurses face reality shock, too! Nurs. Management 14(7):46-48, 1983.

Gilles, D.A.: Nursing management: a system approach, Philadelphia, 1982, W.B. Saunders Co.

Gleeson, S., Nester, O., and Riddal, A.: Helping nurses through the management threshold, Nurs. Admin. Q. 7(2):11-16, 1983.

Kepler, T.L.: Mastering the people skills, J. Nurs. Admin. pp. 15-20, Nov. 1980.

Lewis, J.: Conflict management, J. Nurs. Admin. 6(10):18-22, 1976.

Magula, M., editor: Understanding organization: a guide for the nurse executive, Wakefield, Mass., 1983, Nursing Resources, Inc.

Marriner, A.: Line-staff relationships, Supervisor Nurse 8(11):27-32, 1977.

Maslow, A.: Motivation and personality, ed. 2, New York, 1970, Harper & Row, Publishers, Inc.

Nyberg, J.: The role of the nursing administrator in practice, Nurs. Admin. Q. 6(4):67-73, 1982.

Oncken, W., and Wass, D.: Management time: who's got the monkey? J. Nurs. Admin. pp. 26-30, July-Aug. 1975.

Phippen, M.L.: Winning through communication, AORN J. 34(6):1043-1049, 1981.

Schachat, R. and Anastasi, J.: How to break down communication barriers between you and your co-workers, Nurs. Life, pp. 17-23, Sept.-Oct. 1982.

Stevens, W.F.: Management and leadership in nursing, New York, 1978, McGraw-Hill Book Co.

Tappen, R.M.: Nursing leadership: concepts and practice, Philadelphia, 1983, F.A. Davis Co.

Veninga, R.: The management of conflicts, J. Nurs. Admin. 3(4):13-16, 1973.

Volante, E.: Mastering the managerial skill of delegation: the techniques of nursing management, Wakefield, Mass., 1975, Nursing Resources, Inc.

Wlody, G.: Effective communication techniques, Nurs. Management 12(10):19-23, 1981.

CHAPTER 9
Nursing ethics—commitment in action

LEAH CURTIN

"No matter how trifling the matter on hand, do it with a feeling that it demands the best that is in you . . ."
Sir William Osler

OBJECTIVE: On completion of this chapter, the student of nursing will have an appreciation for the need to include nursing ethics as a way of life for the professional.

Marie Smith* is 37 years old, she has cerebral palsy, and she wants to die. Specifically, she wants to starve herself to death and she demands that the physicians, nurses, and other personnel working in the hospital help her to do so. She refused to go home, and she refused to be transferred to another facility. When the health personnel refused to comply with her demand, she hired an attorney who took her case to court. The court denied her petition and, in fact, ordered her to be tube fed if she refused to eat.

Were Ms. Smith's rights violated? All accounts indicate that she is rational. She has a long-term, chronic debilitating disease that inevitably leads to death. She has weighed the pros and cons of her life—and chosen death. She chose how she wanted to die, that is, by starvation, and whom she wanted to help her die, that is, the physicians and nurses caring for her in a particular hospital. They refused, on the grounds of professional ethics, to help Ms.

Smith starve herself to death. Was their conduct ethical or unethical?

ETHICS AS A DISCIPLINE

When people become concerned about ethics, they usually do so because some difficulty is threatening their peace of mind. Wellman's definition supports this proposition: "Ethics is a discipline in which one attempts to identify, organize, analyze and justify human acts by applying certain principles to determine the right thing to do in a given situation."* However, professional ethics are not built solely around the problems a professional faces. Even though contemporary health professionals confront enormous problems, these are not the essence of professional ethics.

All approaches to ethics are founded in some form of philosophy, or beliefs about how human

---

*A pseudonym.

*Wellman, C.: Morals and ethics, Glenview, Ill., 1975, Scott, Foresman & Co., p. 317.

beings relate to one another and to their world. The behavior that flows from these beliefs is called ethical. Put in another way, ethics is the practical arm of philosophy; the method by which ideals are translated into the real world of action.

Generally speaking, philosophical approaches to ethics can be roughly divided into two schools of thought: deontology and teleology. Teleological approaches concentrate on developing principles (guides to action) that help people choose actions that produce the most desirable (or least undesirable) results. What constitutes desirable results may be determined by (1) ascertaining which action produces the greatest amount of good for the greatest number (utilitarianism) or (2) determining which action results in enhancing what is truly human (natural law).

Deontological approaches concentrate on developing principles that help people choose actions that most clearly conform to duty. What constitutes duty may be ascertained by determining which action is most in keeping with (1) the commitments one has made, (2) the role(s) one has assumed, and/or (3) the obligations attached to the general concepts of human rights.

All approaches to professional ethics are deontological; that is, they center on the duty of the professional to (1) the patient or client, (2) the patient's or client's family, (3) other professionals and the profession itself, (4) the institutions that employ professionals, and (5) the society that sustains the profession. Although grounded in general philosophical ethics, professional ethics concentrate on the added duties voluntarily assumed by the professional.

PROFESSIONAL COMMITMENTS

To ascertain our ethical obligations as professionals, then, we first must examine the commitments we have made. At rock bottom a professional's commitments are inextricably tied to the nature of a profession. The word *profession* is rooted in the Latin word *profitere*, which literally means "to promise publicly" that you will do something.

Centuries ago, this word was applied to certain occupations whose practitioners were required to make public promises. These occupations were singled out because their practitioners provided services that were *vital* to mortal and spiritual well-being. Clearly, if the services provided were *vital*, those who would provide them must be distinguished by their excellence. Thus those who would practice a profession were required to promise publicly that they would be master craftsmen, the very best they knew how to be, and that this commitment to excellence would be lifelong. Just as clearly, if the services provided were vital, those who needed such services were vulnerable; that is, they could be easily exploited. Thus those who would provide vital services to a vulnerable population were required to promise publicly that they would maintain an extraordinarily high standard of conduct toward those who sought or received their services. The essence, then, of a professional's commitment is the promise of excellent practice combined with the promise of a high degree of altruism.

The word *promise* itself infers a very special set of obligations and privileges. The philosopher J.L. Austin made a now famous distinction between two kinds of statements; one descriptive and the other performative (or promissory).* Descriptive statements describe, transmit, or reveal some reality in this world, but they do not change anything. For example, "it is sunny outside" or "grass is green" or "you have cerebral palsy" or "your child was born with a condition called meningomyelocele." Such statements do not change what is: they merely describe, transmit, or reveal it. However, performative statements or promises actually change what is by introducing an ingredient that would not be there apart from the statement. Promises alter reality: they change the nature of relationships and alter people's experience of their lives. The implicit

---

*Austin, J.L. as quoted in May, W.: Normative inquiry and medical ethics in our colleges and universities. In Smith, D., and Bernstein, L., editors: No rush to judgment: essays on medical ethics, Bloomington, Ind., 1978, Indiana University Foundation, p. 356.

or explicit promise of aid, in itself, changes the nature of the relationship between professionals and patients; it becomes a fiduciary relationship.

At the basis of all professional practice is "a significant interpersonal relationship that involves some of the most personal concerns human beings have, life, liberty, knowledge and the like. . . ."* The moral question, then, for the professional is not so much the telling of descriptive truths (although there is that too) but rather being true to the promises (implicit and explicit) of the profession. The promises a professional makes, and whether or not he or she keeps them, significantly change how people experience their lives. That is, professional practice, properly undertaken, *changes* people's lives. That change, and whether or not it is produced, is *the essence of the profession*. Everything the professional does, every action undertaken, is an ethical act.

This sounds very esoteric, but some examples may bring this statement down to earth. A man who has suffered a stroke enters the hospital. He is partially paralyzed on his left side. Whether or not nurses undertake the simplest task, for example, appropriately positioning his paralyzed leg, can considerably change this man's experience of his life. If they do not properly position his leg, he may never walk again, or at the very least, he will have to undergo far more extensive and painful rehabilitation. If they do properly position his leg, their actions will speed his recovery and he may return to a near normal life.

A woman is referred to an outpatient department for treatment of her diabetes mellitus. If the nurse takes the time to teach her about her diabetes (i.e., how to test her urine, how to give herself insulin, how to regulate her diet), she will regain control of her own life again. While the physician's therapeutic act consists of controlling her acute symptoms, the nurse's therapeutic act consists of restoring her autonomy. If the nurse fails to teach

---

*Wasserstrom, R.: Lawyers as professionals: some moral issues, Human Rights **5:**2, 1975.

the patient, the disease rather than the person controls her future.

ROLE OBLIGATIONS

Every profession arises from a need in society: a need that the practitioners promise to fulfill. Thus the ethical obligations of any one profession are built around the specific promises it makes to the public. Clergy do not promise to protect people from the power of the state, lawyers do not promise to lead people to eternal happiness, teachers do not promise to cure disease, physicians do not promise to educate the young, nurses do not promise to create a just society, politicians do not promise to help the ill regain their health, and so forth. Although all professionals are linked by the promises of excellence and altruism, their specific duties are determined by the particular role each one's own profession fills in society. For this reason, subcategories of professional ethics emerged. Subcategories, such as medical ethics, legal ethics, or nurses' ethics concentrate on the role obligations of the persons in those professions.

The profession of nursing has made certain promises to the public, and these promises make up our contract with society. Specifically, nurses have promised (1) to help the ill regain their health, (2) to help the healthy maintain their health, (3) to help those who cannot be cured to realize their potential, and (4) to help the dying to live as fully as possible until their deaths. These promises outline the role obligations of nurses. They define the scope of practice and create the structure of nurse-patient relationships. The profession's standards of practice and code of ethics articulate this outline. Standards of practice define what it is we do (in general and in specific areas) and at what level we do it. They deal with our functions and with the level of excellence demanded of the practitioner. They define our ethical, and often legal, obligations to patients, families, employers, and society. Codes of ethics deal with our relationships to and with patients or clients, their families, our colleagues and employers, and society. Although codes of ethics usually are written in terms of "do's and dont's,'' they are not merely lists of prescriptions and proscriptions. Rather a code of ethics embodies those *values* that the practitioners of the profession find fundamental in practice.

Simply defined, values are matters of such importance that people (consciously or unconsciously) live by them. They can be both individual and shared. That is, they can be unique to one person or shared by a group or even a society. Professional values, then, are those ''matters of importance'' that define the nature and scope of professional relationships. They flow naturally from the commitments we have made, the role we have assumed, and the standards for which we are held accountable. Even though a professional may choose to actualize one value rather than another in a specific situation, all the values articulated in the profession's code of ethics are obligatory (i.e., they are not optional and one may not sacrifice one value to another). When these values conflict or when one or more professional values conflict with the values held by individuals or by society, the professional faces an ethical problem, perhaps even a dilemma.* By and large, these problems or dilemmas are the subject matter of ethical analyses in the professional context.

HUMAN RIGHTS

To refer back to the situation presented at the beginning of this chapter, Marie Smith demanded that the nurses help her to starve herself to death. How the nurses might feel about the demand, while not entirely irrelevant, is not a legitimate basis for action. Indeed, many nurses may sympathize with her desire to die; others may feel that she is being cowardly; still others may be angry becaue she is trying to impose her will on them.

Nurses, as human beings, have the same obligations that other people have to respect individuals' human rights. Moreover, because they deal

with people who often are quite vulnerable, they have added obligations to protect the rights of their patients. Marie Smith's demand places the nurses in a position of conflict. Helping someone to starve herself to death (1) is not within the scope of the profession (some may even see it as a violation of the profession's contract with society), (2) violates the Code for Nurses (specifically, article 3: the nurse acts to protect the patient from the unethical or illegal conduct of any person, which presumably could include the patient herself), and (3) is contrary to standards of practice.

Nonetheless, a large body of nursing literature urges nurses to act as patient advocates, that is, to help patients exercise their legal and human rights. The courts said that Marie, at least in this set of circumstances, does not have a legal right to starve herself to death. However, does she have a human right to take action to kill herself? If so, are the nurses faced with a conflict of duties, that is, a conflict between their obligations to fulfill their social contract (to practice in keeping with the Code for Nurses and standards of nursing practice) and their obligations to respect Marie's human rights?

Obligations attached to human rights

More often than not, the ethical problems professionals face involve some aspect of human rights and the obligations attached to those rights. The concept of human rights emerged over the centuries from observations of what is needed for human beings to be human. Fundamental subsistence rights derive from those things necessary for survival—food, water, air, and protection from those elements (animate or inanimate) that could kill us. Because fundamental human rights derive from fundamental needs, they are universal. That is, they do not depend on time, social customs, laws, or personal values. Whether one lived 1000 years ago or today, whether one is Oriental or Caucasian, man or woman, child or adult, Christian or Hindu, Eskimo or Bantu, one needs food, water, air and protection. The term *universal* means that fundamental human rights are universally applicable—

---

*By definition, a dilemma is a choice between equally unfavorable alternatives. It is not a synonym for ''problem.'' Problems have solutions; dilemmas do not.

not universally recognized, accepted, or respected. Human rights exist even where they are violated because the need exists whether or not it is met.

As knowledge of human beings has grown, so has the concept of human rights. Thus the need to know became a right to learn, the need to initiate activity became a right to be free, and so forth. In short, the concept of human rights is not static but evolves with our knowledge of human beings. Precisely what rights attach to the human needs we discover often is a matter of debate. For example, we now know that human beings need love, but how is love to be defined? Is being loved automatically owed to one by virtue of existence, or is it a privilege one earns?

The human right in question in Marie Smith's situation is a right to die. At best, this is a debatable claim. How is this right to be defined? Does it include a right to commit suicide? If so, does it include a right to demand that others help you commit suicide?

By and large, in the Western world, the right to refuse treatment has been established (philosophically, at least) based on the right to self-determination. However, the right to self-determination does not necessarily include a right to coerce others. If there is such a thing as a right to die, the exercise of such a right would not be unlimited.

In short, even human rights, although universal, are not absolute. Even the most fundamental right is circumscribed by the rights of others. That is, even though I have a right to be and remain alive, I may not exercise this right by demanding from others what they need to live. It is not that I have lost my right but that my exercise of that right is shaped or diminished by the rights of others. Likewise, if I have a right to die, that right also is limited by the rights of others.

Each right has duties attached to it, duties that impinge on oneself as well as on others. The duties imposed on me by my right are called the duties of *moral correlativity,* that is, the duties of me to me. Usually, they require some positive action on my part. For example, if I claim a right to be and remain alive, I impose on myself a duty to take reasonable precautions to protect and preserve my own life. If I claim a right to die, I impose on myself a duty to take reasonable steps to hasten my own death.

The duties imposed on others by my rights are called the duties of *logical correlativity.* Usually, these duties are negative; that is, they require others to refrain from doing something. Thus if I claim the right to be and remain alive, other people have a duty to refrain from killing me. On the other hand, if I claim a right to die, I impose on others, at best, a duty to refrain from saving me. Marie Smith, by refusing to go home or be transferred to another facility, tried to turn a negative duty to refrain from ''saving'' her into a positive duty to help to kill her.

Whether or not this duty can be translated into a positive duty (an obligation to protect my life or, in the latter case, to help take my life) is contingent on at least four factors:

1. The extent to which I am able to exercise the duties of moral correlativity. That is, the extent to which I can protect my own right. You have no duty to protect my right if I can protect it myself. Marie Smith tried to protect her right by using legal means to coerce staff, but she refused to take other actions (e.g., going home or transferring to another facility) to protect her right.

2. The extent to which my right infringes on the rights of others. That is, you have no duty to sacrifice your own rights to protect my rights. Although you are free to choose to sacrifice your rights to protect me, you have no obligation to do so. The nursing and medical staff also have rights among which is the right to freedom of conscience. Marie's right to die does not include a right to force others to violate their consciences. Health professionals are human beings, not robots programed to carry out the commands of others. Among the most important duties of all human beings is the duty to protect their own integrity. No person ever has a right to coerce another into violating his or her conscience.

3. The presence of a prior duty. Suppose two people claim aid; both are in equal need, and both are equally incapable of protecting their own right. I have the resources to help only one of them without infringing on my own rights. To whom is my duty? My obligation is to the first person who comes to me. This does not deny the need of the second person but rather recognizes that no one person can deprive another to fulfill his own needs. In the case of Marie Smith who wants to die by starvation, the health personnel had a host of prior duties, professional and legal, to help her to live and to reduce her suffering. Whether or not these duties are superior to her demand for death may be open to question, but their existence is not.

4. The presence of a higher duty. A person's obligations can be roughly divided into two categories: duties *in rem* and duties *in personum*. Duties *in rem* are the general duties of all persons to all other persons. Duties *in personum* are the duties of one identifiable person to another identifiable person or group of persons. Usually duties *in personum* take precedence in decision making (i.e., they constitute higher duties) over duties *in rem*, *unless* the general rights involved are of a more fundamental nature. For example, emergency room nurses have a higher duty to a newly admitted patient than they do to the general public. Thus, even if the patient is a convicted felon, the nurses have a duty to use the resources that society has provided to render him aid. However, if the patient is violent (i.e., is a clear and present danger to others), the nurses have a duty to restrain him even if he demands release. In short, the rights of unspecified members of the public to life and bodily integrity are more fundamental than the patient's right to freedom of action.

In the case of Marie Smith, and in the absence of any general consensus, legal or moral, on (a) the existence of a right to die, (b) the limit and scope of such a right, and (c) the legitimate role of the health professions in the face of such a right, the duty to preserve life or at least to refrain from deliberately taking life is a higher duty than is the duty to respect a patient's wishes. In fact, even if the nurses felt that Marie Smith was within her rights and even if they had no objection to participating in her suicide, any action they might undertake to assist her to commit suicide would be open to legal, professional, and ethical censure.

Although the health professional's role in society and his or her commitments to society infer a duty to render aid to those in need of service, health professionals have not promised to fulfill *all* human needs nor have they promised to sacrifice their integrity (moral or physical) to the will of others. Thus, for example, nurses may be justified in refusing to participate in procedures or actions that violate their consciences. As a matter of fact, law provides for conscientious refusal to participate in such procedures as sterilization or abortion. Nurses and physicians, although obliged to act in the best interests of their patients, have no obligation to submit to physical or even verbal abuse from their patients.

ANALYSIS OF ETHICAL PROBLEMS

When faced with a particular problem in practice, a professional analyzes that problem in light of (1) the promises of the profession, (2) the profession's standards of practice, and (3) the profession's code of ethics. To consider all aspects of the problem and to determine the best course of action, the professional:

1. Gathers all available information and ranks this data according to its *relevance* to the decision (problem, issue) at hand.
2. Determines the nature of the problem by ascertaining whether or not it has one or all of the following characteristics of an ethical problem:
   a. It is a problem of values rather than of fact; that is, it is not a scientific problem.
   b. It is inherently perplexing (Why should I prefer one person's rights to another? What

do I do if my duties conflict with the desired outcome? When values conflict, why should I choose one rather than the other? etc.).

  c. The answer reached influences many areas of human concern.

3. Considers the general and specific duties, rights, and values of all people involved in the decision (at this point, standards of practice, codes of ethics, and role responsibilities are identified).

4. Identifies all viable alternative courses of action and projects as accurately as possible the likely outcome of each option.

5. Moves to resolve the problem by balancing the rights and duties of the decision makers with the course or courses of action that produce the best possible outcome.

6. Plans and designs a strategy for accomplishing the desired resolution.

Although no method can guarantee that one always will make a "right" decision, careful analysis helps reduce the potential for error. Situations similar to Marie Smith's rarely result in happy solutions. However, such problems—carefully analyzed—can lead us to a fuller understanding of our professional roles, the limitations of patient's rights, and the legitimate exercise of our own rights. Watching a person die of a chronic, debilitating disease is a terrible thing, but helping to kill that person, even at his or her request, is perhaps worse. Health professionals, by the very nature of their work, come into contact with a great deal of human suffering. Although they are expected to practice compassionately, they are not—for very good reasons—expected to allow their emotions to determine the course of their actions. Careful, logical analysis of the situation and a dispassionate weighing of the rights and responsibilities of *all* involved are imperative. In most circumstances we are making decisions that affect other people's lives more than our own; thus we dare not operate solely on our own value systems or our own feelings.

Perhaps the most important thing to understand about professional ethics is that it is founded in philosophical ethics but grounded in professional practice. All professional activity is based on the promise or promises of the profession. Thus ethics are not reserved for "problems" alone: they give life and meaning to the professional's every action and interaction.

SUMMARY

"Ethics is a discipline in which one attempts to identify, organize, analyze, and justify human acts by applying certain principles to determine the right thing to do in a given situation."[*] Although there are two schools of thought in the philosophical approach to ethics, professional ethics are deontological in their approach. The duty of the professional centers around (1) the patient or client, (2) the patient's or client's family, (3) other professionals and the profession itself, (4) the institutions that employ professionals, and (5) the society that sustains the profession.

In developing one's obligations to the profession, commitments made by the professional must be met. These are promises, which in turn become a commitment that infers certain actions. Obligations to patients, the profession, and to society become explicit as the nurse practices. These obligations set the scope of practice and create the structure of nurse-patient or nurse-client relationships.

As the professional encounters ethical problems an analysis must be made in light of the promises of the profession, the profession's standards of practice, and the profession's code of ethics.

Discussion questions

1. Discuss the definition of ethics in relation to the application of certain principles.
2. Discuss the difference between deontological and teleological approaches to ethics and why the deontological approach is used in professional ethics.

[*]Wellman, C.: Morals and ethics, Glenview, Ill., 1975, Scott, Foresman & Co., p. 317.

3. Discuss the professional commitments in relation to the promises made by the profession.
4. Discuss the kinds of situations which may arise in practice that threaten human rights of patients.
5. Discuss the three standards used to analyze ethical problems.

SUGGESTED READINGS

Bandman, B.: Option rights and subsistence rights. In Bandman, E.L., and Bandman, B., editors: Bioethics and human rights, Boston, 1978, Little, Brown & Co.

Barnes, W.H.F.: Intention, motive and responsibility. In Aristotelian society, supplemental vol. 19, London, 1945, Methuen & Co., Ltd.

Codes of the health care professions. In Reich, W.T., editor: Encyclopedia of bioethics, New York, 1978, The Free Press.

Curtin, L., and Flaherty, M.J.: Nursing ethics: theories and pragmatics, Bowie, Md., 1982, Robert J. Brady Co.

Ellery, J.B.: John Stuart Mill, New York, 1964, Grosset Dunlap.

Foot, P.: Euthanasia, Philosophy Public Affairs 7:1, 1977.

MacIntyre, A.: How virtues become vices: values, medicine and social context. In Englehardt, H.T., and Spicker, S., editors: Evaluation and explanation in the biomedical sciences, Dordrecht, Netherlands, 1975, D. Reidel Publishing Co.

Ramsey, P.: Basic Christian ethics, New York, 1950, Charles Scribner & Sons.

Wasserstrom, R.: Lawyers as professionals: some moral issues, Human Rights 5:2, 1975.

CHAPTER 10

Collective bargaining in nursing

MARIANNE CRAWFORD
MARY FISHER
NANCY KILBANE

OBJECTIVE: On completion of this chapter, the student of nursing will be able to discuss the involvement of nurses in collective bargaining.

The onset of collective bargaining for nurses represents one of the most controversial developments in the profession. Collective bargaining is a formalized decision-making process between management and labor representatives concerning salaries, work environment, and conditions of employment. Nurses must become familiar with facts surrounding collective bargaining so they can form opinions without undue influence from others.

HISTORICAL OVERVIEW

Throughout American history, the interactions between labor and management have been wrought with conflict. The classic struggle between the "haves and the have nots" goes on as "the rich get richer and the poor get poorer." Management obviously holds the role of the "rich haves" while labor is relegated to the "poor have not" position. Historically, mine workers, factory workers, and tradesmen have fought bitterly with owners to secure a just wage, decent working conditions, and adequate benefits. Resistance by owners has been vigorous as struggles to increase profit margins and accumulate wealth continued. This conflict has contributed to an adversarial relationship, a total lack of mutual respect and trust between management and labor.

In the health care industry, this same struggle exists, although it surfaced later than in industrial settings. In the nonprofit health care agency, the focus may be on increasing operational gains rather than profits in order to finance future operations. Nonetheless, this focus by management contributes to the basic adversity between labor and management in the hospital setting. Many hospital workers have organized in order to negotiate more effectively with their hospital managers. This discussion will focus on nurses who organize and the impact of this activity of professional practice.

There is no question that over the years nurses attempted to negotiate with hospital administrators through representative committees of nurses selected by their peers. They sought to correct perceived deficiencies in wages, benefits, hours, working conditions, and practice. In some instances they were denied a forum for discussion with management. In other situations, administrators met with nurses, listened, and then effectively ignored the nurses' input. It must be acknowledged that in some instances the process worked effectively, with administrators implementing their nurses' suggestions. These experiences were certainly not universal. This response by administrators placed the health care industry in the same trap previously occupied by labor barons. The health care field was ripe for unionization by its workers, particularly nurses.

Enabling legislation

In 1935 the Wagner Act (National Labor Relations Act) assured unions freedom and federal protection during organization and bargaining. It identified certain management activity as unfair labor practice, and it established the National Labor Relations Board to judge the validity of union complaints against management. The original act excluded nursing, teaching, and medicine.

The Taft-Hartley Act of 1947 revised the Wagner Act by citing *union* activity that constituted unfair labor practice. This allowed management greater freedom to express views opposed by unionization and established mediation, fact-finding procedures, and cooling-off periods before national emergency strikes. Perhaps the most notable provision, at least for the health care industry, was exclusion of nonprofit hospitals from the obligation to bargain collectively with employees. During this revision the hospital association lobbied heavily against nursing being included in the Taft-Hartley Act. It was not until 1950 that hospital employees were included. The American Nurses' Association (ANA) was successful in securing the inclusion of nurses in the Taft-Hartley Act.

In 1959 the Landrum-Griffin Act required registration of labor organizations with the federal government. Additionally, it regulated the use and reporting of union funds and assured democratic control of unions by the membership.

Federal legislation in 1962 enabled employees of the federal health care institutions to participate in collective bargaining. The ANA was identified as the bargaining agent for nurses of the Veterans Administration Hospitals.

Finally, the Taft-Hartley Amendment of 1974 reversed the exemption for nonprofit hospitals, thus leading to the obligation for health administrators to bargain with all employees. Further, it defined and restricted the role and activity of supervisors in the work place. Each of these pieces of legislation has affected some aspect of today's interaction between hospital and labor.

Nurses and collective bargaining

The ANA is recognized as the primary professional organization for nurses. The organization has expressed long-standing concern over economic and general welfare of its members. A standing committee of the organization has fought for years to improve economic and general welfare in nursing. State nurses' associations serve as bargaining agents for nurses on the local level. From 1950 to 1968 a no-strike policy was adopted by the ANA. The right to strike has since been reinstated in an effort to strengthen nurses' bargaining position. Thus, since 1968, there have been increasing numbers of strikes among professional nurses in the United States.

MANAGEMENT'S PERSPECTIVE

The literature on collective bargaining is consistent in its declaration that the objective of a union is to negotiate job security and improved benefits for its membership. The intention is to secure more and more concessions from management despite their effects on productivity.

Professional nurses who organize through their professional organizations declare quite an opposite objective. They proclaim a primary concern for improving the quality of nursing practice and thus the quality of patient care. Interestingly, they propose to improve the quality of care by negotiating improved wages, benefits, and hours for nurses. There is seldom reference to the research of Hawthorne, MacGregor, or Herzberg, which implies that wages and benefits are not motivators toward increased productivity or quality.

Despite the fact that nurses claim a desire to improve the quality of nursing care as their motivation for collective bargaining, the available data are contradictory. Between 1960 and 1974, more than 600,000 RNs were employed in the United States. Twenty thousand were involved in some type of work stoppage during this period. Of 103 incidents 39% were demonstrations, 31% were strikes, and 30% were mass resignations. Data were obtained by questionnaires on the motivation of nurses involved in 80 of the total 103 work stoppages. Fifty-one percent cited wages; 14% cited working conditions; 15% cited representation; and only 5% cited quality of care.*

While it is understandable that nurses have opted to use collective bargaining and work stoppage as mechanisms to improve results in their dealings with management, it is unfortunate that the only example available to them has been the labor union. This results in nurses imitating the labor model of behavior at the negotiating table and on the picket line, and it subjects them to accusations of highly unprofessional behavior. Significant conflict results from using collective bargaining and work stoppage to achieve professional recognition when the expressed purpose of collective bargaining is to secure improved wages and work conditions. Trying to achieve professional recognition through collective bargaining is like trying to combine oil with water; they just do not mix.

Nursing administrators agree wholeheartedly that nurses should control nursing practice and quality of care. But in a large bureaucratic agency with numerous nursing employees, it is impossible for each individual nurse to decide every detail of how he or she will practice. Policies, procedures, rules, and regulations are imperative to ensure consistency, quality, and safety of care. For this reason nurses should expect and demand that their departments be administered by nurses.

The new graduate, while interviewing for a first position, should review the organizational chart to determine whether nurses hold key positions

throughout the organization. Special attention should be paid to whether the RN who holds the vice president position for nursing reports directly to the president of the organization. Reporting through an executive vice president with business administration or hospital administration credentials may dilute the vigor with which nursing concerns are presented to the president and the board of trustees.

Information should also be sought on how many nurses participate in hospital committees where policies and procedures are generated. Finally, the disciplinary process should be examined for a focus on corrective rather than punitive action. Due process should be provided for every hospital employee.

Maintaining an adversarial relationship between hospital management and organized nurses is necessary for survival of a union. Conflict and discontent must be kept alive in order for the union to be valued and supported by the membership. However, constant conflict is always disruptive to smooth operations and a pleasant work environment. In the past the director of nursing acted much like a union steward for nurses, representing their needs and fighting for their rights and benefits. Presently the nurse executive finds himself or herself resisting nurses' demands based on the adversity fostered by unionism. This divisiveness within the profession can only harm efforts toward professional recognition for nursing. Instead, nurses' efforts should be directed toward collaboration and affiliation between staff nurses and nurse managers to achieve maximum progress for quality professional nursing.

NURSES' PERSPECTIVE

A review of the factors influencing nurses' choices to organize into a collective bargaining group indicate that these factors are grouped around two themes: women's issues and bureaucratic structure. The nursing profession has been and still is primarily a female profession. Many of the issues that dominated the women's movement of the

*Miller, M.H., and Dodson, L.: Work stoppage among nurses, J. Nurs. Admin., pp. 41-45, Dec. 1976.

1970s are factors that influenced nurses' decisions to organize. Women are socialized from childhood into steryotyped roles that demand submissive, conforming, and subordinate behavior. Nursing is viewed by many as low status work merely because it is performed by women. It is common to see nurses depicted with characteristic sexist traits such as short skirts, high heels, and bright makeup. The image of being handmaiden to a male physician still haunts the profession.

"Equal pay for equal work" cannot be used as a battle cry against the low wages and minimum benefit packages available to nurses. There are few men within the profession with whom to compare wages.

"Garbage collectors get better pay" is a common slogan used by nurses. Nurses are frustrated with their poor economic conditions compared with male-dominated groups that require less education, responsibility, and accountability. Comparable worth surfaced in the 1980s as a new method to group different jobs into salary categories.

The bureaucratic structure of the hospital, where the majority of nurses are involved in collective bargaining practice, has contributed to the nurses' decision to organize. Nurses have experienced a sense of powerlessness because they have little influence over the bureaucracy in which they work. Many indicators of professionalism such as control over practice, voice in working conditions, and adequate compensation for education and responsibility do not exist in the health care agencies. Nurses join unions because managers fail to recognize and provide for nurses' needs regarding ". . . more individual job freedom, greater input by nurses in matters that affect their jobs, greater control over their work schedule, more enlightened supervision and top management, and more advancement and educational opportunities."*

Many hospital nursing structures offer no rewards for staff nurses. Nurses must leave the direct patient care role to reap rewards of better pay,

prestige, and professional recognition. Those who prefer the staff nurse role now feel they must try collectively to achieve the things they are unable to obtain individually within the structure.

Hospital management has often been the primary motivator for nurses to unionize. Nurses working in hospitals may be faced with paternalistic or maternalistic attitudes from their hospital administrators and nursing directors that indicate they are not valued as professionals. Traditionally male hospital administrators advised nurses to "trust me," while nursing directors protected "my nurses." Both approaches assume that nurses are less than responsible adults who can speak for themselves.

Physician-nurse relationships often have been credited with motivating nurses to unionize. Treatment of nurses as subordinates rather than colleagues, refusal by physicians to include nurses in the patient treatment plan, and criticism of nurses' organizing efforts may all contribute to nurses' decisions to unionize.

Numerous factors have been discussed that, added together, create an environment in which nurses are motivated to seek outside representation for their collective needs.

Choice of representation

After dissatisfaction and frustration lead nurses to desire union representation, they must determine who shall represent them. Nurses across the country have chosen representation by affiliates of the industrial labor unions, self-formed local unions, and the ANA.

The issue of "who shall represent" is almost as strong as the issue surrounding collective bargaining itself. There are important characteristics to be considered in determining the representative. Some of these are as follows:

- Who can best assist us to build a strong union?
- Which organization has sufficient resources, skill, and funds to successfully negotiate our needs?
- Who is willing and able to understand and fight for our professional issues?

*Emanuel, W.: Nurse unionization is dominant theme, Hospitals, p. 121, April 1981.

Nurses faced with this decision must have a clear understanding of their needs.

Economic conditions of the early 1980s resulted in large industrial layoffs and loss of union membership. These depleted labor unions are actively seeking to represent nurses. Choice of an industrial labor union might provide negotiating expertise and sufficient financial resources to meet nurses' needs. However, such an organization will be based on the industrial model. Union representation would be restricted to salaries, hours and working conditions and would provide little or no understanding of nurses' professional needs.

Some groups of nurses shun the idea of being part of organized labor. They choose to form their own independent unions. Choice of this route would ensure representation of the local unit's needs. However, limited expertise and available funds may affect the success of negotiations.

Selection of a state nurses' association (SNA; SNAs are affiliated with the ANA) would be more appropriate to meet the nurses' professional needs. SNAs claim to focus on the needs and concerns of nurses with control over nursing practice as a stated priority. There is some question whether the ANA has been able to successfully organize and represent nurses. To date, the SNAs have not had the resources or experience to bargain from a position of power equal to that of the industrial labor unions. Another consideration is the charge that bringing unionism into the professional organization has split nursing administrators and eduators away from the ANA. This lowers nursing's power base on many other issues unrelated to collective bargaining where nurses need to pull together as a whole. Regardless of the organization chosen to represent them, nurses should make sure that the group selected can effectively negotiate to meet their needs.

Problems within the ranks

The collective bargaining movement in nursing has been hindered from within the ranks. Many nurses view unionization and strikes as unprofes-

sional for nurses. These nurses respond to collective bargaining activity with apathy or antagonism because they do not accept it as appropriate for professionals.

Some nurses involved in collective bargaining activity feel the need to intimidate peers holding differing opinions. This militant behavior stems from the recognition that only through a united front can bargaining power be realized. The behaviors that on the surface compel ''sisterhood'' are, in reality, harassment and coercion. This type of behavior ultimately leads to separation and conflict between members rather than to unity and trust.

There are many important lessons to be learned if nurses are to be successful in their efforts to exert control over their practice. Problems within the ranks will have to be resolved before collective bargaining activity can be effective.

Lessons to be learned

Karen and Robert Veninga identified important lessons from the 1981 Professional Air Traffic Controllers Organization (PATCO) strike. These lessons may influence the position of nurses engaged in collective bargaining*:

1. ''The strength of a profession is directly correlated with the unity of its members'' The success of a profession seeking to strengthen its bargaining position will be determined by whether or not the members support one another.
2. ''The strength of a profession is directly correlated with the strength of its alliances.'' Establishment of working alliances with other professions increases the likelihood of their support when changes are proposed.
3. ''Never underestimate the power of an adversary.'' Two common errors that occur in negotiating a contract are underestimating and

---

*Veninga, K., and Veninga, R.: The PATCO problems and nursing: a comparative analysis, Nurs. Outlook, pp. 265-267, April 1982.

overestimating the adversary's power. Underestimation can result in loss of jobs if permanent replacement is used. Overestimation of the adversary's power can weaken the bargaining position and result in a less than adequate contract.

4. ". . . The importance of having the support of the public" cannot be overemphasized. Nurses must understand the importance of public support gained through use of the media and through professional and community relationships.

THE NEGOTIATED AGREEMENT

The written contract is a formal, legal document outlining the relationship between two parties that cannot be changed except by mutual consent. Certain items must be negotiated according to provisions of the National Labor Relations Act. Wages, hours, benefits, and terms and conditions of employment fall under this mandatory category. Labor or management may waive or trade away their right to bargain about any specific mandatory subject, but neither can be forced to do so. Provisions beyond the scope of the mandatory category are voluntary and require the desire by both parties to address such issues. Nonnegotiable items include those already regulated by federal or state law.

Clauses sought by management

Because management views the collective bargaining agreement as an express limitation on managerial discretion, the most important clause to include in any contract is a *management rights* clause to assure an atmosphere that allows effective management. Language to preserve management's right to require standards of performance, select and hire employees, make temporary transfers, establish staffing patterns, lay off employees, promulgate reasonable rules and regulations, and discipline, suspend, or discharge for just cause is essential.

An *open shop* clause that would prevent union membership from becoming a condition of employment may be sought in an effort to maintain individual nurses' freedom of choice and assure ability to recruit nurses. An *escape* clause that calls for a period of time during which nurses may resign from membership in the union without forfeiting their jobs is the very least that management should seek to protect nurses' rights. However, this provision would affect only existing employees so that all new nurses would have to join the union to maintain employment.

A *no-strike* provision that would serve to assure the community that health care would not be interrupted for the duration of the contract is another clause management frequently requests. The contract can be stabilized further by seeking a *zipper* clause, barring any attempt to reopen negotiations during the terms of agreement. Finally, management will want to maintain their right to compensate individuals for efficiency and excellent performance by introducing a *merit increase* clause. The union will see this as antiunion because they cannot control the awarding of merit pay.

Clauses sought by the union

A *closed shop* clause that binds the employer to hire and retain only union members in good standing is most beneficial to the union. Without a closed shop the union will want to protect its economic stability by insisting on the acceptance of an *agency shop* clause that requires all nurses who do not join the union to pay a fixed amount equal to organizational dues to the union's welfare fund or a specified charity. A *check-off* provision also serves to ensure the union's economic welfare and would require the employer to deduct dues from the nurses' paychecks either on written authorization from the nurse or as a condition of the collective bargaining agreement.

An *escalator* clause automatically ties wages to cost-of-living fluctuations based on the Consumer Price Index without reopening negotiations during the life of the contract. A *reopener* clause, on the other hand, states times or circumstances under which negotiations on economic issues can be reopened before the expiration of the contract.

The union seeks ways to strengthen its stand on ongoing issues by establishing a *grievance* clause. Generally a grievance procedure consists of progressive steps for handling complaints. The final step is usually arbitration. Arbitration introduces an impartial third party to decide the issue. On the surface this appears harmless, but it results in additional expense and a loss of decision making for both parties if the arbitration decision is binding. A *past practice* clause sanctions existing practices so that they become binding, although they are not specifically included in the agreement.

Unfair labor practices

Both management and the union are subject to provisions of the National Labor Relations Act, violation of which constitutes an unfair labor practice. Generally, there are five areas where unfair labor practices occur:

1. *Interference*. Any activity that interferes with, restrains, or coerces a nurse's right to bargain is prohibited. The enforcement by management of any rule or regulation that conflicts with the collective bargaining agreement also is a form of interference. Similarly, union activity that results in interruption of an agency's operation may be interference. Coercive behavior intended to influence a strike or authorization vote is illegal by either side. Finally, one union cannot propose contract language that affects other classes of employees without their union's negotiation.
2. *Domination*. Management cannot legally sponsor, control, or otherwise assist any labor organization except to furnish customary services if requested. Managers cannot represent union members in any negotiations.
3. *Discrimination*. Threats of discipline, transfer, or other reprisals against any employee because of collective bargaining activity constitute discrimination and are prohibited.
4. *Discrimination for testimony*. Coercion or promise of benefit in exchange for a vote against collective bargaining is also illegal.
5. *Refusal to bargain in good faith*. Once an exclusive representative is recognized, both parties must meet at reasonable times and confer in good faith with respect to mandatory items. This does not mean either side must agree to any proposal or make any concessions. However, progress in negotiations is expected, and each side must submit counterproposals when rejecting a plan from the opposition. Other aspects of good faith bargaining include the following:
   a. The representatives at the bargaining table must have sufficient authority to engage in meaningful negotiations. Boards of trustees and union members do have the right to determine the final contract vote but not necessarily to be involved at each intermediary step of the negotiations.
   b. Management cannot make unilateral changes in wages, hours, or working conditions without first negotiating the items to an impasse.
   c. Both negotiating groups must participate actively in deliberations so as to indicate a present intention to find a basis for agreement.
   d. Neither group can exhibit a take-it-or-leave-it attitude.
   e. Both groups should center their negotiations around the bargaining table and not in the news media or on the picket line.

If either party is judged to be engaging in unfair labor practices, the courts will issue a cease-and-desist order.

Strikes and lockouts

Because of the service orientation of the profession, nurses have a moral responsibility to maintain service to the public. This fact causes a moral dilemma for many nurses and a split in the ranks of staff nurses who want both economic security and a professional level of practice. Ultimately it must be an individual decision to strike or to cross the picket line to care for patients, a decision for which the nurse must accept responsibility and be willing to live with the consequences.

A strike is any organized work stoppage by a group of employees to express a grievance, enforce a demand for changes in conditions of employment, or solve a dispute with management. Such an action is generally followed by a lockout in which the employer refuses entrance to the work premises by the striking employees.

There are three basic categories of strikes. The *unfair labor practice strike* is most beneficial to labor. In this instance, management is accused of unfair labor activity, and labor responds by striking. If the National Labor Relations Board judges the accusation true, all striking employees must be unconditionally reinstated. An *economic strike*, in which labor stops work to secure economic gains, may be most beneficial for management. In this case, striking employees may be permanently replaced. An *unprotected strike* is instituted in violation of legal constraints that apply to striking hospital workers (e.g., 10-day notification to the hospital and to the Federal Mediation and Conciliation Service, or secondary boycott/sympathy strike). In the case of an unprotected strike, strikers may be discharged immediately. It is important to realize that while economic and unprotected strikes place strikers at risk of losing their jobs, the conversion principle may place management at a disadvantage. This principle may result in a change of strike status from economic or unprotected to unfair labor practice when management is found guilty of unfair labor activity during either negotiations or the strike.

DECERTIFICATION

When a group of nurses believes the union is no longer meeting their representation needs or that they no longer need a third party to communicate their needs to management, they may petition the National Labor Relations Board for a decertification vote. Signatures equal to 30% of the bargaining unit are necessary to petition. This process must be initiated and carried out solely by the nurses without interference from management. A decertification election is then held.

In decertification the National Labor Relations Board withdraws the union's official recognition as exclusive negotiating representative. Any existing contract immediately becomes void. A majority vote in the decertification election run by the National Labor Relations Board is necessary to decertify. There are only two times that the decertification process can be initiated: (1) 30 days preceding the 90-day negotiating period before expiration of the contract and (2) after the contract has expired.

DEAUTHORIZATION

Deauthorization is a process similar to decertification in which at least 30% of the nurses petition to establish an open shop. This process may occur at any time and requires a majority vote during the deauthorization election. The union's certification is maintained, but nurses have a choice as to whether they want to belong.

COLLECTIVE BARGAINING ISSUES
Collective bargaining and professionalism

A key issue in nursing has been and continues to be the relationship between collective bargaining and professionalism. There are two opposing views. One view considers collective bargaining incompatible with professionalism in nursing. This is related to the belief that collective bargaining activities erode the public's image of nursing as a service-oriented profession. If a negotiating session fails to end in a signed contract, a strike could occur. A strike by nurses is viewed as an unprofessional act that violates the nurse-patient contract for service. Patients could be neglected or harmed. On the opposing side of the issue is the argument that the term *professional* is used as a flag waved in front of nurses to prevent their collective action. Those who favor collective bargaining believe that it is a means of achieving professional status for nurses by assisting them to gain control over nursing practice and by providing fair compensation for work.

A related issue is the long-standing and often discussed question of nursing's status as a profession. In the minds of some, this issue remains unresolved as well. Many discussions have combined the two issues in attempts to present how collective bargaining has enhanced the professional status of nursing. This approach seems to illustrate that the road to professionalism is through collective bargaining. An occupational group may evolve into a profession through meeting recognized criteria. The number and description of criteria differ according to author. However, there is consistently a long period of specialized education, public service orientation, compensation for service, and autonomy. This refers to the idea that the members of a profession have self-regulation and control of their functions in the work situation.

It does not serve a union's purpose to be concerned about the public need. Unions are big business with objectives and methods that are often at odds with the goals and expectations of those they represent and of the public being served. Unions legally represent their members. The public service criteria determining a profession would not be met through collective bargaining in the event of strike because services would be withdrawn.

Inherent in the concept of professionalism is the notion that professionals receive not only awards, honors, and prestige but also sufficient income for their services. Since the onset of collective bargaining with nursing, salaries have significantly increased. This could be interpreted by those in favor of unionism as indicating that collective action has advanced the economic component of professionalism. *Opponents* to collective bargaining often cite the increased cost of this activity to the agency and the employees. Union members are required to pay dues to their association. There also is potential loss of earnings during a strike. Costs to the agency for negotiations, legal fees, and grievance procedures are passed on to the patient and community. There is also an increased cost in providing staff coverage for the conduct of union activities. The costs incurred related to collective bargaining activity may prohibit any increased financial benefit for union members. Nor does a wage system that is determined by seniority compensate the individual according to professional achievements, education, or previous experience. In the area of professional rewards it cannot be demonstrated that collective bargaining has enhanced professionalism.

It is often stated that the true essence of a profession is control over the performance of practice by the professionals. *Proponents* state that collective bargaining can be an effective method for nurses to share in policy making and to exercise their professional responsibility for control over practice.

Cleland* describes a way for nurses to influence the character and climate of nursing practice by including three provisions in the negotiated contract. She suggests that managment and staff share the right to define the practice of nursing in an agency. This can be accomplished by establishing a nursing practice council. There also must be a provision for individual professional accountability through a peer review system and an approach to supervision that coordinates rather than controls. The problem with the shared governance model is that hospitals cannot legally relinquish authority, responsibility, or accountability for patient care. Hospitals' boards of trustees are legally accountable for the quality of care in a given institution. Therefore can there be shared responsibility without shared accountability?

It has not been demonstrated in the literature that nurses have gained control over their practice through collective bargaining. This results partially from the fact that hospitals do not legally have to

*Cleland, V.: Taft-Hartley amended: implications for nursing, the professional model, J. Nurs. Admin., pp. 17-21, July 1981.

bargain for practice issues under the National Labor Relations Act. It is unlikely that hospitals will negotiate and allow a contract provision on patient care issues because they do not believe these should be resolved at the bargaining table.

Collective bargaining and the professional nursing organization

Another key issue is the effect of the economic and general welfare program on the status of the professional organization. A professional association should provide for the expansion of professional knowledge, should represent as many members as possible, should be voluntary, and should advance both the profession and the professional. The ANA is the official organization of professional nursing and should speak for nursing. The economic and general welfare council proposes to negotiate economic security for its members as well as affording them an avenue for defining and controlling their practice. The ANA also expands professional knowledge through various seminars and educational programs. However, ANA collective bargaining activities have created a split between management and staff and threaten to destroy the professional association. Nurse managers often have been forced to resign from SNA offices because of the fear of management domination. Other nurse managers have been prohibited from continuing their membership by agency administrators. Some local association contracts mandate nurse membership, thereby violating the principle of voluntary membership. In both of these areas the ANA collective bargaining activity does not support the concept of professionalism. It denies managers the right to fully participate in the association. It requires them to financially support an activity in which they cannot participate or in which they may not philosophically believe. Managers are also denied the right to enjoy the educational benefits imparted by organizational activities, thus negating a basic and underlying philosophy of professional organizations.

Many nursing leaders have written proposals to address these problems and preserve the professional organizations. The suggestion has been made that the economic and general welfare (EGW) program be separated from the professional association. Only nurses participating in the EGW program would support it with their dues. All nurses could then be members, with the professional organization remaining unified.

Analysis of this issue results in the following conclusion: there is no documented evidence to indicate that collective bargaining in nursing has contributed to the professionalism of nurses. It does not provide for recognition of professional status and is in conflict with the public service orientation of a profession. Collective bargaining cannot legally mandate professional autonomy and cannot provide for a voluntary, equitable, fully participative professional association.

SUMMARY

This chapter traces the progress of nursing's involvement in collective bargaining. Legislation enabled nurses working in nonprofit institutions to participate in collective bargaining. However, bureaucratic structure and women's issues served as motivating forces to the collective bargaining movement for nurses.

Management and union perspectives toward collective bargaining for nurses differ. Administration seeks contract clauses that preserve their right to manage, limit disruptive influences on patient care, and assure the individual nurse's right to decide on union membership. Unions, on the other hand, concentrate contract language efforts on methods to preserve nurses' group rights, open the contract for ongoing changes, and preserve the union's economic welfare.

Numerous issues surround labor relations in nursing. The relationship of unionism to professionalism and the role of the professional organization in collective bargaining are important issues for nurses to consider.

Discussion questions

1. Identify the enabling legislation that provided for collective bargaining in nursing.
2. Describe four factors that influenced nurses to participate in collective bargaining.
3. List four clauses sought by management and four clauses sought by unions in contract negotiations.
4. Discuss the issues involved when professional nurses engage in collective bargaining.
5. Discuss the ethical, moral, and professional dilemmas surrounding strikes by nurses.

SUGGESTED READINGS

Adler, J.: When a nursing staff organizes: management rights and collective bargaining, Am. J. Nurs., pp. 1-12, April 1978.

Beletz, E.: Nurses participation in bargaining units, Nurs. Management **13**(10):48-57, 1982.

Bloom, B.I.: Collective action of professionals poses problems for administration, Hospitals, J.A.H.A. **51:**167-174, March 16, 1977.

Cannon, P.: Administering the contract, J. Nurs. Admin., pp. 13-19, Oct., 1980.

Castrey, B., and Castrey, R.: Mediation—what it is, what it does, J. Nurs. Admin. pp. 24-28, Nov. 1980.

Cleland, V.: Taft-Hartley amended: implications for nursing, the professional model, J. Nurs. Admin. pp. 17-21, July 1981.

Colangelo, M.: The professional association and collective bargaining, Supervisor Nurse, pp. 27-43, Sept. 1980.

Eldridge, I. and Leni, M.: Collective bargaining as a power resource for professional goals, Nurs. Admin. Q. **6**(2):29-40, 1982.

Emanuel, W.: Nurse unionization is dominant theme, Hospitals, pp. 121-128, April 1981.

Jacox, A.: Collective action: the basis for professionalism, Supervisor Nurse, pp. 22-24, Sept. 1980.

Johnson, L., Ray, K., and Shippey, S.: Union—yes or no? Nurs. Management, pp. 45-48, 1983.

Lieberman, N.: Before, during and after bargaining, Chicago, 1979, Teach'em Inc.

Lockhart, C.A., and Werthery, W.B.: Labor relations in nursing, Wakefield, Mass., 1980, Nursing Resources, Inc.

Luttman, P.A.: Collective bargaining and professionalism: incompatible ideologies? Nurs. Admin. Q. **6**(2):21-28, 1982.

Miller, M.H., and Dodson, L.: Work stoppage among nurses, J. Nurs. Admin., pp. 41-45, Dec. 1976.

O'Rourke, K. and Barton, S.R.: Nurse power unions and the law, Bowie Md., 1981, Robert J. Brady Co.

Shaffer, F.: The decertification process, Supervisor Nurse, pp. 55-57, Sept. 1980.

Veninga, K., and Veninga, R.: The PATCO problems and nursing: a comparative analysis, Nurs. Outlook, pp. 265-267, April 1982.

Zimmerman, A.: Taft-Hartley amended: implications for nursing—the industrial model, Am. J. Nurs. **75**(2):284-288, 1975.

CHAPTER 11
Power, politics, and the nurse

JANICE K. LANIER

"Politics in a real sense is the people who take the time to participate."
Senator Daniel Inouye

OBJECTIVE: On completion of this chapter, the student of nursing will have an understanding of why power and politics have become an important part of the nurse's role.

Power and politics will play important roles in defining nursing in the future. Nurses studying today must be ready to assume not only the traditional duties of the RN but also new duties more often associated with political activists than with health care professionals. This chapter will provide some insight into the political process so that the nurse of tomorrow can be an effective lobbyist for quality health care and the nursing profession.

According to Talbot and Vance,* there are over 1,000,000 RNs in the United States, 98% of whom are women. Any attempt to study politics and power in nursing must incorporate a study of women and their history. The evolution of the profession of nursing is closely intertwined with women's struggle to achieve autonomy.

Investigating the experiences of women through the past several centuries reveals distinct phases in their historical progress. "A dizzying variety of feminine images and female roles" fall into a pat-

tern that parallels the growth of the United States from a "peasant to a post-industrial society."*

Colonial femininity was noted as a time of subordination in a largely patriarchal society. Survival required both sexes to labor beside each other, but a secondary social status and political invisibility relegated women to a legally sanctioned dependency.

Women of the eighteenth century experienced the beginnings of sexual division of labor, which allowed a choice of alternative life-styles—"fashionable idleness, independent enterprise, or incarceration in an almshouse."†

In the nineteenth century, production was removed from the home. Women took on domestic tasks or low-status jobs in the work force that were viewed as "women's work." "The standard of femininity became nurturance—first of individual

---

*Talbott, S.W., and Vance, C.N.: Involving nursing in a feminist group—NOW, Nurs. Outlook, pp. 596-599, Oct. 1981.

*Ryan, M.P.: Womanhood in America: from colonial times to the present, New York, 1975, New Viewpoints, p. 11.
†Ryan, M.P.: Womanhood in America: from colonial times to the present, New York, 1975, New Viewpoints, pp. 13, 73.

families, and through the families all of society.'' The newly industrialized society deemed work a male prerogative and glorified women as ''mothers of civilization.''*

The suffrage movement of the early twentieth century represented an attempt by women to gain control of their destiny. Along with the right to vote, women gained a certain amount of new power when they took on the role of primary shopper for the items produced in the nation's factories. The industrially dependent society began to offer low-paying jobs to women, which added new dimensions to their role expectations. Two world wars and the depression were major events that altered the course of all history including women's history. Women began to perform ''men's jobs.'' The need to survive economically caused mothers to enter the work force. Despite societal pressures to do so, they did not leave their jobs once the times became less demanding.

The women of today can be described as fragmented—super wife, super mom, and super achiever—all things to all people. The support systems that women need from society to help them meet the demands of their new life-styles are still largely nonexistent. The development of programs that respond to the needs of women and families will be challenges in the next decade.

The knowledge of what has gone before and a sense of pride in accomplishments have made women aware of their potential for future achievement. The women of today are not the same as the women of the 1700s. Environmental influences both subtle and not so subtle have affected women in untold ways. These influences have made the role of women in society complex and full of contradictions. Despite the women's movement, political advances, and a growing public appreciation of the capabilities of women, the dichotomy of role expectations versus reality that has plagued women for centuries exists yet today. Only when women

can function as individuals first and women second will they be able to contribute fully to the betterment of society.

The nurses of today are the independent women of today. Forces at work in society that affect women have also affected the nursing profession. The nurse's professional world is a microcosm of society as a whole. The battles that women have waged to gain personal independence are mirrored in the confrontations between nurses and the power structures within the health care industry. The new role expectations of women (nurses) combined with societal and economic pressures have caused this struggle to intensify during the past decade. Women (and men) choosing nursing are more career oriented, more determined to define the limits of their profession themselves without outside interference. The repercussions of that attitude will have far-reaching effects on the entire health care industry.

Another important consideration is the health care industry itself. Growing corporate and public outrage at the inflationary spiral of health care costs has forced industry leaders to begin to reevaluate the services provided and the policies that govern those services. Who will care for patients, where, and for how long will be important considerations in the new cost-conscious environment. The health care industry that at one time could absorb new practitioners with no adverse effects for those already practicing can no longer offer limitless employment boundaries. ''Technicians'' will begin to impinge on the traditional roles of other health care providers. Rather than adjuncts to nursing care, technicians may become nursing substitutes. As more advanced professionals do everything possible to maintain their base of power, tasks previously delegated will be reclaimed and redefined so as to exclude other professionals, technicians, or paraprofessionals from care-giving roles they once controlled.

Future battles will most likely be fought not only within the confines of health care institutions but also before legislatures and in courts of law. An

*Ryan, M.P.: Womanhood in America: from colonial times to the present, New York, 1975, New Viewpoints, pp. 13, 73.

understanding of the forces at work (i.e., power and politics) will be vital if nurses (and women) are to be successful combatants.

POWER, POLITICS, AND THE NURSING PROFESSION

Politics and politicians are often associated with the legislative arena. To some, a politician is one who makes long-winded speeches, promises solutions to an assortment of problems, and runs for reelection on a regular basis. In reality, politicians are more than presidents and congressmen. They are the wise, wary, diplomatic, prudent, shrewd individuals who define problem areas, devise solutions, and determine policy both in the public and private sectors.

"Playing politics" describes the maneuvering that occurs in the halls of Congress, in the corporate board room, in a hospital administrator's office, and among health care workers struggling to have job responsibilities and rewards commensurate with their educational preparation. Politics is played everywhere, but it is played best by those able to manipulate the variables within the environment to their own ends.

Nurses are part of the political game both in their professional and personal lives. Too often they serve as pawns used by others rather than as a force that determines the final outcome of the game.

Playing politics implies control. Control implies power. Control is the means to the advancement of the profession of nursing. As long as others control the profession, it will be difficult to advance it. "Power is a positive force for creative change and is a central issue in nursing's struggle to define itself."* One cannot control unless one understands politics. Politics cannot be understood unless one understands power. The successful politician harnesses all power sources and is not afraid to use them to attain a desired goal.

"Power" comes from the Latin "potere," which means "to be able." In modern usage, power has become a value-laden word that holds for many an oppressive connotation.

In truth, power is neither good nor bad, It is most simply "the ability to make people do things they might not otherwise do or to stop people from doing things they might do."* Power is a relationship among people and is part of all forms of interaction.

What are the key elements in a power relationship?

1. *Legitimacy* The source of power must be valued and understood by those involved in the relationship. Authority lies in the right to expect *and* command obedience. Money is often equated with power in our society because it has become a desirable commodity not possessed equally by everyone. It is a valid base on which to build a foundation of power, and the majority of people do not question the validity of the claim.

2. *Consensus* There must be agreement among all those involved in the relationship. A person is not powerful unless perceived to be so by others.

3. *Acceptance* Those involved must accept the relationship and participate in it. If person A attempts to use power to bring about change while person B refuses to cooperate, the power relationship is altered.

4. *Consistency* The person with power must be both willing and able to affect others in the relationship. If an individual or group has the potential to bring about change (the requisite power base) but refuses for some reason to do so, the power base is eroded. Likewise, empty threats or promises do not prompt compliance.

5. *Extension* Power in one arena does not nec-

---

*Hendricks, D.: The power problem, Nurs. Managment, p. 23, Oct. 1982.

*Kalisch, B.J., and Kalisch, P.A.: Politics of nursing, Philadelphia, 1982, J.B. Lippincott Co., p. 3.

essarily carry over into another sphere. What is valued (or feared) in one community or society may not be appreciated elsewhere. However, the truly powerful person or group usually relies on more than one base of power to extend the realm of influence.

6. *Expense* What does it cost to tap a power source? Is the desired change worth the accompanying expenditure of resources? Will more be lost than is gained?

Power does not exist in a vacuum. Every element of power implies a relationship between two or more people. There are also varying degrees of power. Because one person or group has power does not mean others do not. Power in one situation does not necessarily translate into power in another. Person A may have great power over person B and less over person C. The Kalisches say that time and circumstances determine the degree of power in any given instance.

Nurses may have extensive power over the clients they serve by virtue of their expertise. That same expertise does not lend itself, however, to power over a hospital administrator.

Power, according to the Kalisches, can be called symmetrical if both parties have relatively equal strength; power is asymmetrical when one party controls a range of possible outcomes greater than another.

Power takes on many forms, for example:

1. Coercion
2. Persuasion
3. Manipulation

Coercion depends on force for its effectiveness. Fear of physical or psychological injury is a form of force. Labor strikes are another example of coercion. Persuasion involves the acceptance of arguments put forth by one person without threats or fear of retribution. Manipulation is the "con man" form of power. The power holder in a manipulative situation gains compliance without the power subject being aware of it. Ingratiation is one tactic used to manipulate the behavior of another.

Four bases of power have been identified by social scientists*:

1. *Reward/punishment* The ability to provide rewards if one agrees to act in a desired way or punishment if one does not comply.
2. *Expertise* The belief that one person is more knowledgeable than another about a particular subject.
3. *Referent* The ability of a recognized leader to exert influence over a variety of spheres because of the respect others have for that individual.
4. *Positional* The authority that is attached to the position one holds.

In addition, there are situational and personal power. Situational power stems from being in the right place at the right time. Personal power is the power that is based on unique characteristics found in an individual.

*Kalisch, B.J., and Kalisch, P.A.: Politics of nursing, Philadelphia, 1982. J.B. Lippincott Co., p. 17.

Power: The ability to influence the behavior of others

Form:	Manipulation	Persuasion	Coercion
Types:		Personal-situational	
Degree:	Symmetrical/ asymmetrical	Symmetrical/ asymmetrical	Symmetrical/ asymmetrical
Base:	Expertise—Positional—Referent—Reward/punishment		

Legitimacy

A look at nursing in relation to the elements of power reveals where nursing fits into the overall power structure. What legitimate source of power does nursing have?

1. Nurses provide a necessary service in the health care arena.
2. Nurses make up the largest segment of health care workers.
3. Nursing care is valuable to the health care consumer and is relatively inexpensive.

Only the second consideration has legitimacy in the larger power structure. Nursing's power lies in the number of nurses that are licensed to practice. The first consideration lacks validity because other health care workers have been employed to perform many of the tasks previously done by nurses. (The quality of care may be debatable, but the work itself is being done.) The value of nursing to the health care consumer, the third consideration, has not been reduced to dollars and cents evaluations. Nursing's claim to power based on the necessity and value of services is therefore not legitimate.

Consensus

A nurse's place in the health care hierarchy is not at the top. The general public as well as other health care providers do not perceive nurses as powerful instruments for change. It is only when nurses have used their numbers to organize for better patient care and better working conditions that their demands have been considered.

Acceptance

Nurses traditionally accepted their place in the health care power structure until the women's movement and an increased awareness of women's appropriate role in society made inroads in nursing's blind acceptance of the status quo. More men in nursing also forced a change in the ways nurses viewed their status and the ways nurses perceived nursing.

Consistency

Nursing's power rests with numbers, but nurses have been unable to speak in unison about many issues affecting the profession. Work stoppages, which are an example of a nurse's power to bring about change, are seldom undertaken because of the effect such stoppages are believed to have on patient care. Nurses may be *able* to organize but are not consistently *willing* to do so. The potential for power in numbers is further diluted when others, perceiving the hesitancy, disregard the nurse's potential to make things happen. Chapter 5, Issues in Nursing—an Overview, Chapter 6, Entry to Practice—Education, and Chapter 10, Collective Bargaining in Nursing, discuss the divisiveness and lack of consistency in the profession of nursing.

Extension

Nursing's lack of power in the health care arena is also evident in the amount of power the profession exhibits elsewhere. For example, nurses are seldom powerful sources for legislative change. They do not possess the tools of political power—the money, the contacts, and the know-how. The number of nurses able to bring about change in a single health care facility is seldom sufficient to bring about change on a larger scale. So far, attempts to organize nursing politically have been slow. Chapter 13, Professional Nursing, discusses participation in professional organizations.

Expense

What would it cost to tap nursing's power source? Is it possible to do so? What good are numbers without a common bond? Obviously, the potential exists for nurses to work together to reach desired goals. In the past, when the threat to practice was great enough, nurses showed remarkable resolve to work together regardless of cost. Recently, however, conflicts over educational issues and the extended role for nurses and other controversial matters have divided the profession. The cost of not working together may soon become great enough and obvious enough to force nurses in the future to tap the greatest power source they have, namely, each other, regardless of the cost to the individual.

If nursing's power is confined to the work place, it will not realize its full potential. Many decisions affecting the profession will be made in the halls of Congress rather than in hospital corridors. It is imperative that nursing's resources be targeted toward those that will have the greatest voice in determining the future of the profession. In summary, nurses must be aware of their resources and gain control of their profession through the responsible exercise of power at work, in the community, and in the legislature.

THE ROLE OF GOVERNMENT IN TODAY'S SOCIETY: NURSING'S ROLE IN THE GOVERNMENTAL PROCESS

"I don't want to get involved in politics." Think again. . . . Government doesn't mind getting involved in nursing.

Nevada Nurses Association

Although government has grown larger in the United States, fewer and fewer people have been active participants in determining who its leaders will be and what policies will guide their decisions. The people we elect and the policies they establish influence many aspects of daily living, yet in 1980 only 52.6% of the eligible population voted in the presidential election. Fewer still (34.5%) participated in state or local elections.* The majority of people cannot identify their federal, state, or local representatives. They have minimum knowledge about the legislative process and a limited awareness of how the system really functions. The vast size and the remoteness of the actual workings of government contribute to a feeling of ineffective-

ness among ordinary citizens. At a time when sophisticated communications networks bring lawmakers into the nation's living rooms, there seems to be an accompanying dissociation from politics and a growing cynicism toward the entire process. A failure to attract qualified people into the political arena and a waning of the individual's interest in the affairs of state do not bode well, especially considering the impact government has on daily activities.

More and more people are responsible for the very complex running of the vast governmental bureaucracy that has been created in the United States over the past 200 years. Those people who are politically astute (not just elected officials) can have an unprecedented influence on the path that government takes. Nurses or anyone willing to expend resources and make a concentrated effort to learn the political process could increase their effectiveness many times over.

Nurses were content for many years just to learn nursing. Little need for political awareness was felt by the profession, so little was taught about politics and power in schools of nursing. The last decade has seen that philosophy change. Nursing now sees the need for its practitioners to participate actively in the decision-making process both in the work place and the legislature. Individual nurses, however, often lack the expertise necessary to bring about the changes they seek. Inflexible work schedules and family responsibilities also prohibit active, effective involvement with legislators and governmental agencies.

Another consideration is the "personality" of the profession itself. Nursing is a nurturing kind of occupation that concentrates on the alleviation of stress and discomfort. Politics is full of controversy and strife between powerful individuals well-schooled in how to handle the unsavory aspects of the legislative process. Nurses are not readily attracted to that sort of fray and often cannot adapt to the emotional turmoil such confrontations invoke.

---

*Cook, R.: Have-not's surge to polls: major force in 1984 elections, Congressional Q., p. 1504, July 23, 1983.

Increased political participation has been described as "nursing's professional challenge."* If the political astuteness of the nurse is to be increased it will be necessary to build a formal organizational structure to support the political activities of the profession and to raise the level of political awareness of each individual practicing nursing.

Nursing's role in the governmental process is twofold. Nurses serve as *actor-participants* in the actual decision-making process and as *reactor/implementors* of the policies once they have been formulated. It is not enough simply to state that access to adequate health care is a right of every citizen. Programs must be developed, funding sources tapped, buildings erected, supplies secured, and people educated in order to make the philosophy a reality. There is an actor-reactor component to every step of the process. Nurses often become the logical implementors of governmental health care policies and programs by the very nature of their work. One is less likely to find a nurse functioning at the actor-participant level for the same reason. Nurses traditionally have been looked on as doers, not thinkers. Professional contacts have been with the patient or client rather than with policy-making networks. Particpation at the actor level has been an after-hours activity rather than part of the on-the-job expectation. Consequently, few nurses have been regular contributors to the decision-making process, and few policy makers have looked to nurses for their professional input.

Such apolitical behavior gives credence to political scientists who describe nurses as apathetic.

Four levels of participational political behavior have been defined†:

1. *Apathetic or apolitical*   These individuals are usually hourly wage earners with little time to devote to politics. They lack the economic resources needed to support political activities.
2. *Spectators*   These individuals vote but view the political process from the outside. They rely on television, newspapers, and magazines for their information. They may display candidates' signs and may adopt a party affiliation.
3. *Transitional*   In addition to participating at the spectator level, transitional participants donate money to campaign organizations and make direct contact with elected officials to communicate their opinions about specific legislation. These individuals may also campaign actively for the candidate of their choice.
4. *Gladiator*   These individuals are the most committed of all participants. In addition to acting at the transitional level, gladiators are candidates for office themselves. They may serve on boards or commissions as appointees of the president or governor.

It is obvious that the apolitical person cannot have a positive impact on the political scene. The apolitical posture, which many see as safe, can be (and often is) interpreted by those with power as satisfaction with things as they are. The interpretation may not be accurate, but without evidence to the contrary, it is accepted as fact. Apathy therefore loses its neutrality and becomes a negative factor often without anyone realizing it. The apolitical nurse must become convinced of the need to move into a more active political role. The profession must be willing to accept the risks that are associated with such a move.

Nurses at the spectator level can begin to increase their political effectiveness by intiating political discussions among themselves and by attempting to influence the votes of others through personal contacts and participation in petition drives.

Once at the transitional level, working in concert with nursing organizations to emphasize their numbers will enhance the impact nurses make in the political arena. One in forty-four registered female

---

*Omar, M.A., and Wyatt, G.: Political participation: nursing's professional challenge, Mich. Nurse, p. 3, May-June 1983.
†Omar, M.A., and Wyatt, G.: Political partipation: nursing's professional challenge, Mich. Nurse, p. 4, May-June 1983.

voters is a nurse. That fact alone, if well known, could force legislators to listen to the voice of nursing if the words were spoken in unison.

The nurse gladiator can have an enormous influence in the legislative process from the inside. The nursing profession could facilitate the successful candidacy of fellow nurses by working diligently to help elect those nurses willing to run.

Despite the advances made by women in employment situations, relatively few occupy seats in Congress or statehouses. Over the past 14 years, the number of women in state legislatures has more than tripled, but women still hold only 13% of the available statehouse seats. The Eagleton Institute of Politics has identified New Hampshire, Colorado, Connecticut, and Wyoming as the states with the highest number of female legislators. Mississippi, Louisiana, Pennsylvania, and Alabama have the fewest.

The number of nurses working on Capitol Hill has also tripled since 1979. In 1983, six nurses held responsible positions in the governmental bureaucracy. Those nursing leaders have begun to point the way for other nurses to follow. Nurses who use the resources of the White House to the advantage of the profession will only be imitating the behavior of other health care groups. "Ongoing relationships with the White House will give nurses the status and power other groups already enjoy."*

It is not necessary to work at the federal level to make a difference for nursing. Political scientists believe the balance of power has shifted from the federal government back to the states. It is at the state level that decisions are made that have the most direct effect on the health care industry. Regulation of professions is done by the states. Welfare and Medicaid programs and implementation of federal policy are the responsibilities of state government.

Nurses who have served with elected officials view such activity as an extension of their nursing skills rather than as an abandonment of their profes-

sion. Legislative internship programs at the state and federal levels offer opportunities for more nurses to become familiar with the political process and to meet the individuals occupying positions of influence and power. In addition, participating nurses can educate lawmakers about the role nursing could play in resolving the health care cost dilemma.

State nursing associations employing full-time lobbyists could offer graduate student internships that would enable students to participate in the political process in a semiofficial capacity. In this way the influence of the state nurses' associations would be expanded and a cadre of nurses developed who would be able to work effectively in the governmental system. Eventually, those experienced nurses would be able to lobby both formally and informally for the profession.

HOW DOES THE MYSTERIOUS LEGISLATIVE PROCESS WORK?

A knowledge of the legislative process is vital if nurses are to function effectively in the political arena. How does the mysterious legislative process work? How does a legislative idea become a reality? How does a bill become a law?

The steps need to enact a bill into law are learned in most high school civics classes. Unless individuals are actively involved with the legislative process, the "how to" is filed and gradually lost to memory. The procedure at most state capitals is similar to the one followed in Washington, D.C. (Fig. 3).

Although it is true that legislatures generally follow the same formal process, the actual enactment of a law includes much more than the steps shown in Fig. 3. This informal legislative process is often more important in determining which bills will be considered, by whom, when, and where. It is this "behind closed doors" activity that bears closer scrutiny.

As with any process involving people, individual personalities and personal relationships are more important to the process than the actual legislation

---

*Schorr, T., editor: Am. J. Nurs., p. 1205. Aug. 1983.

HOW A BILL BECOMES LAW

This graphic shows the most typical way in which proposed legislation is enacted into law. There are more complicated, as well as simpler routes, and most bills fall by the wayside and never become law. The process is illustrated with two hypothetical bills. House bill No. 1 (HR 1) and Senate bill No. 2 (S 2).

Each bill must be passed by both houses of Congress in identical form before it can become law. The path of HR 1 is traced by a solid line, that of S 2 by a broken line. However, in practice most legislation begins as similar proposals in both houses.

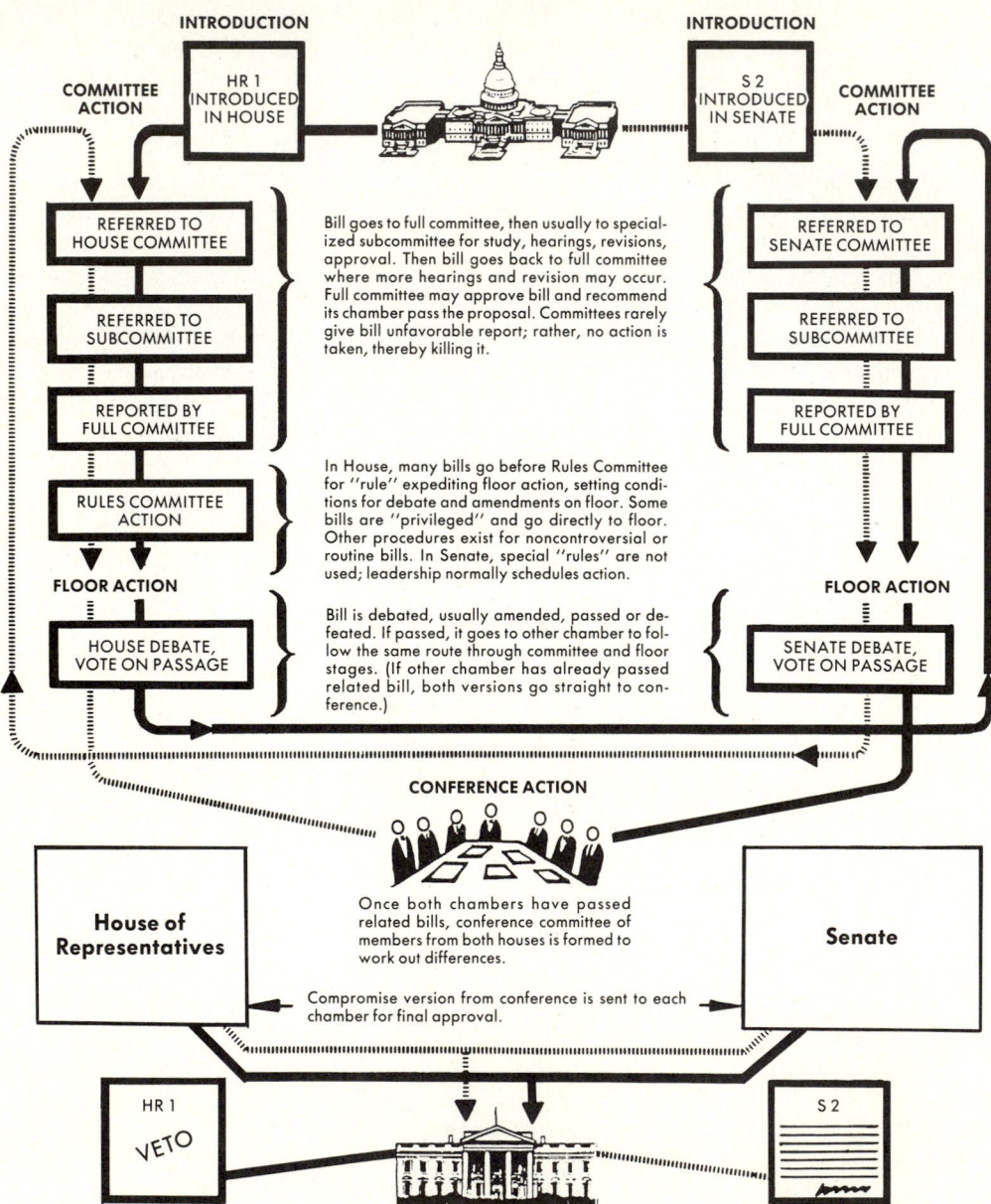

INTRODUCTION

HR 1 INTRODUCED IN HOUSE

COMMITTEE ACTION

REFERRED TO HOUSE COMMITTEE

REFERRED TO SUBCOMMITTEE

REPORTED BY FULL COMMITTEE

RULES COMMITTEE ACTION

FLOOR ACTION

HOUSE DEBATE, VOTE ON PASSAGE

INTRODUCTION

S 2 INTRODUCED IN SENATE

COMMITTEE ACTION

REFERRED TO SENATE COMMITTEE

REFERRED TO SUBCOMMITTEE

REPORTED BY FULL COMMITTEE

FLOOR ACTION

SENATE DEBATE, VOTE ON PASSAGE

Bill goes to full committee, then usually to specialized subcommittee for study, hearings, revisions, approval. Then bill goes back to full committee where more hearings and revision may occur. Full committee may approve bill and recommend its chamber pass the proposal. Committees rarely give bill unfavorable report; rather, no action is taken, thereby killing it.

In House, many bills go before Rules Committee for "rule" expediting floor action, setting conditions for debate and amendments on floor. Some bills are "privileged" and go directly to floor. Other procedures exist for noncontroversial or routine bills. In Senate, special "rules" are not used; leadership normally schedules action.

Bill is debated, usually amended, passed or defeated. If passed, it goes to other chamber to follow the same route through committee and floor stages. (If other chamber has already passed related bill, both versions go straight to conference.)

CONFERENCE ACTION

Once both chambers have passed related bills, conference committee of members from both houses is formed to work out differences.

House of Representatives

Senate

Compromise version from conference is sent to each chamber for final approval.

HR 1 VETO

S 2

Compromise version approved by both houses is sent to President who can either sign it into law or veto it and return it to Congress. Congress may override veto by a two-thirds majority in both houses; bill then becomes law without President's signature.

Fig. 3. How a bill becomes law. (From Government Relations Manual, American Nurses' Association, Division of Legislative and Governmental Affairs, Washington, D.C., 1981, p. 16.)

under consideration or the procedural rules established to guide deliberations. Political ambitions, party loyalty, personal loyalties, individual philosophies, promises made, and deals forged all play a part in determining how a lawmaker will finally vote. The ability of party leaders to control their caucus and the lengths to which these leaders will go to ensure loyalty are also important. Nurses with their educational preparation in interpersonal relationships, sociology, and psychology could find through studying the small-group dynamics of legislators the keys needed to successfully influence their deliberations.

Legislators will introduce a bill for a variety of reasons. Personal experience with a problem area or problems constituents bring to their attention often motivate the drafting of a bill. The fate of the measure depends on the legislators' own personal concern about the issues involved and the political effectiveness or expertise the elected official possesses.

If the matter is one the legislator believes must be addressed, everything possible will be done to see that the bill is considered by the appropriate committee in a logical time frame. Sponsors will ask their offices to arrange for witnesses to testify at committee hearings and will personally urge fellow lawmakers to support the proposal. Usually the chairs of committees to which bills are assigned take their cues as to how to proceed from the bill's sponsor. If a sponsor does not press for a hearing, a hearing will not be scheduled. If a legislator does not get actively involved in guiding a bill through the legislative process, the measure has slight chance for success.

Choosing a sponsor for a measure is a very important first step in devising legislative strategy. Majority party members are usually asked to be primary sponsors of bills because few measures sponsored by the minority party receive full consideration. If a measure is bipartisan in nature, minority party members may sign on as cosponsors once the bill has been introduced.

When seeking a sponsor for a bill it is advisable to present both the positive and negative sides of the question. An honest appraisal of the effects the bill will have will lessen the impact of any "surprise" opposition. Honesty between the bill's proponents and the bill's sponsor must be maintained. Legislators become identified with their legislation and do not like to appear uninformed. Their commitment to a proposal could disappear if they were to feel the bill's proponents had somehow misled them.

The chairs of the committees to which bills are assigned are also influential individuals. The chairs can singlehandedly affect the progress a measure makes through committee if they choose to do so. An unpopular proposal with unpleasant political consequences for the chair may never be scheduled for a committee hearing. A controversial bill with few political pluses may be assigned to a committee almost by default without regard for the subject matter of the bill or the expertise of the committee to which it is referred. Lack of interest on the part of the chair and other committee members could virtually guarantee the proposal no further attention. Legislation is more often ignored than defeated. Unless the bill receiving such treatment has popular support that is made apparent through skillful use of the media, or the support of a determined sponsor, it will not be resurrected.

Once a bill is before a committee, public hearings are scheduled during which proponent, opponent, and interested parties can testify. If a measure appears to be particularly troublesome, the committee chair can appoint a subcommittee to consider further testimony and to work on changes. The committee process is so unwieldy at the federal level that subcommittees are relied on regularly to do the hard work on a bill. Standing subcommittees receive bill referrals from committees in Washington, D.C., while state legislatures generally do not have permanent subcommittees in place. They are appointed on an ad hoc basis instead. If a committee chair wishes a bill to be killed in subcommittee or conversely wishes a measure to receive favorable treatment, the subcommittee appointments can reflect that preference. An alert public should watch this process and the interpersonal relationships at work for clues as to how the bill ultimately will fare in the legislative process. Timely letter-writing campaigns, attendance at committee and subcommittee hearings, and intervention with appropriate legislators can make a difference in the treatment afforded a bill in a committee or a subcommittee room. Too often these activites go unnoticed until it is too late to bring about changes.

Logistically the easiest place to have an impact on the legislative process is at the committee-subcommittee level. Relatively few legislators serve on any particular committee and they are usually well attuned to the subject matter handled by their respective groups. It is within committee that bills are rewritten, usually by the few individuals who take time to follow the proceedings and offer their suggestions in whatever capacity requested. Trying to influence the votes of an entire legislative body can be difficult and requires a very well-organized campaign. It can be done, but it takes time, dedication, and a willingness to aggressively pursue already established legislative goals.

To lobby means (1) to conduct activities with the objective of influencing public officials, especially members of a legislative body, about legislation or other policy decisions and (2) to advance or otherwise secure favorable treatment. Lobbying is done every day both inside and outside capital buildings.

The informal lobbying process involves individuals who either have social opportunities to provide legislators useful information or who meet regularly with a legislator to discuss issues. These individuals can be very influential in determining the mind set a legislator will bring to discussions about an issue. Many professional associations, including physicians, have initiated a program in which legislators are matched with a member of their profession. The professional makes regular contact with the legislator to establish an ongoing exchange of information.

The Congressional District Coordinators (CDC) project of the American Nurses' Association (ANA) is an attempt to put legislators in touch with nurses on a regular basis. Volunteers are assigned to key congressmen and asked to contact their representatives regularly. The CDC individuals also coordinate district-wide efforts to lobby their congressman when important legislation is being considered. State nurses' associations have initiated similar programs at the state level. It is important that legislators ask nurses about nursing issues and equally important that the nurses whom they ask respond professionally.

The formal lobbying effort is carried out by individuals employed and registered as legislative agents. Lobbyists may represent one interest group or may work on a free-lance basis for several clients. The ANA and many state nursing associations have lobbyists on their staffs who serve as liaisons between legislators and the nursing profession. These people are usually familiar with the legislators and the issues being debated. They are often asked to present a testimony and to be participants in the compromises that are negotiated between proponents and opponents. A legislator relies on lobbyists for factual information. The lobbyist in turn relies on the legislator for up-to-the-minute estimations about what is happening behind the scenes. Their relationship is delicate but vital if the interests of both are to be served.

Nursing's lobbyist also keeps nurses informed about the actions a legislative body has taken or plans to take. The lobbyist is a bridge between the profession and the politician. In the final analysis, however, it is not the lobbyist who has a pervasive influence over the final vote in the House or Senate. It is the nurse constituent who is the vital link in any successful legislative program. The lobbyist can set the stage, create the environment, ask the questions, and provide facts and figures, but individual nurses are the only people capable of convincing legislators that a particular bill either has or does not have the support of the people back home. This is the grass roots lobby.

The grass roots lobby writes letters, makes phone calls, and visits legislators to discuss specific issues. These lobbying efforts of individual constituents may be less visible than those of the professional lobbyist but are of far greater importance. These individuals do not have the ongoing, person-to-person relationship with a lawmaker, but they affect the votes cast, especially if their campaigns are well organized.

Letter-writing campaigns are the most common action taken by a grass roots lobby. Often the effectiveness of the campaign is diluted through the use of form letters that merely require the signature of an individual. Sheer volume of communications is not enough to convince a legislator that there is overwhelming public support either for or against a particular issue. Form letters can become a nuisance rather than an effective persuader. On the other hand, letters that represent the individual's personal opinion are believed to be representative of the opinions of many voters who did not take the time to write. The impact of that personal letter may be greater than the writer might suspect.

Grass roots lobbies can be organized by groups highly experienced in the use of persuasive tactics. They may include not only those individuals with a vested interest in the outcome of the legislative battle, but also other individuals who have been recruited to fill the ranks for various reasons. For example, legislation that affects nurses could also affect the health care consumer. An astute grass roots lobby would alert the public to the impact a particular bill would have on the quality or availability of care and ask their help to enact or defeat the measure. These less-structured groups can put together campaigns by alerting their members to the problem. In this way a cross section of people becomes involved, which gives the campaign a broader base of support. To maintain the necessary steady flow of communications expressing the lobby's point of view requires the dedication of everyone involved, often for months at a time.

In developing strategies for dealing with legislators it is important to consider the "shadow government" that has grown up around lawmakers at the federal level and is beginning to be felt in state politics as well. The shadow is the aide or advisor who conducts the research, defines the issues, drafts bills, and is generally the trusted confidante of the elected official. "They are the policy makers."*

Government is a multibillion-dollar business. To manage it, lawmakers have had to rely on the advice of specialists to fill gaps in their knowledge. Lawyers, accountants, and other experts serving in staff capacities are the most accessible and become the legislators' sounding board, advisor, consultant, and even substitute in some instances. The judgments of trusted aides are often relied on when a voting decision must be made. The impression a lobbying effort has made on the staff member can determine what information a legislator will receive in what kind of terms it will be presented. "By laying out options in a certain matter a staff member can lead a legislator to a predetermined conclusion."† Wise lobbyists are aware that they cannot afford to alienate the legislator's aides.

What influences a legislator to vote a certain way? Why does an aide listen to one group of constituents rather than another? Often the problems presented have no clear-cut, definitive solutions. A program that benefits one segment of the population could be disastrous for another. Why does one group win at the expense of the other? Power is the answer—power and the willingness to use that power to reach a desired goal. "Only power can get poeple into a position where they can be noble."‡

Various specialities have arisen within the nursing profession, for example, nurse practitioner,

---

*Sheler, J.L.: The "shadow government" operating on Capitol Hill, US News & World Report, p. 63, June 27, 1983.
†Sheler, J.L.: The "shadow government" operating on Capitol Hill, US News & World Report, p. 64, June 27, 1983.
‡Hendricks, D.: The power problem, Nurs. Management, p. 23, Oct. 1982.

nurse educator, nurse administrator, or nurse researcher. The title "nurse politician" might be added to the list to give recognition to those nurses who emphasize the political aspects of their careers. Few job descriptions actually mention the utilization of political action as a means to affect patient care. It is, nonetheless, a critical part of the nurse's role both inside in the health care facility and outside in the community. It is the nurse politician who will make the difference in the future for the nursing profession and the health care consumer.

SUMMARY

Politics is an inexact science that encompasses much of what is fundamental to the profession of nursing. Trying to generalize and make rules guiding participation in the legislative process will not guarantee success. Nursing education's special attention to the development of analytical assessment skills and the importance of planned intervention can be adapted to the legislative arena, however. The nursing process can serve as a foundation on which to base future legislative strategies of the profession.

Assess the people involved and the political climate

Plan strategies to take advantage of the prevailing mood of the legislature and the strengths of the profession

Implement the plan using all resources available

Evaluate the results and use that information in planning future strategies

"We will win some, and we will lose some, but whatever the outcome, we must return to play in the game again."*

---

*Archer, S.E., and Goehner, P.A.: Acquiring political clout: guidelines for nurse administrators, J. Nurs. Admin. p. 53, Nov.-Dec. 1981.

Discussion questions

1. Discuss the concept of power and identify the most powerful nurses in your state and in the nation.
2. Discuss the role of the lobbyist in the legislative process.
3. Discuss the need for a nurse politician.
4. Discuss the legislative process as it relates to a bill becoming a law.
5. Discuss power, politics, the individual, nursing, and the impact on nursing.

SUGGESTED READINGS

American Nurses Association, Division of Legislative and Governmental Affairs: Government relations manual, Washington, D.C., 1981.

Archer, S.E., and Goehner, P.A.: Acquiring political clout: guidelines for nurse administrators, Nurs. Admin. **11:**49-53, Nov.-Dec. 1981.

Curtin, L., editor: Political savvy, Nurs. Management, pp. 7-8, March 1982.

Hendricks, D.: The power problem, Nurs. Management, pp. 23-24, Oct. 1982.

Kalisch, B.J., and Kalisch, P.A.: Politics of nursing, Philadelphia, 1982, J.B. Lippincott Co.

Maraldo, P.: Politics, a very human matter, Am. J. Nurs. pp. 1104-1105, July 1982.

McTernan, E.J., and Leiken, A.M.: A pyramid model of health manpower in the 1980's, J. Health Politics, Policy, Law, pp. 739-751, Winter 1982.

Omar, M.A., and Wyatt, G.: Political participation: nursing's professional challenge, Mich. Nurse. pp. 3-5, May-June 1983.

Pinch, W.: Female attributes in a masculine world. Nurs. Outlook, pp. 596-599, Oct. 1981.

Ryan, M.P.: Womanhood in America: from colonial times to the present, New York, 1975, New Viewpoints.

Sheler, J.L.: The "shadow government" on Capitol Hill, U.S. News & World Report, pp. 63-65, June 27, 1983.

Storlie, F.J.: Power—getting a piece of the action, Nurs. Management, pp. 15-17, Oct. 1982.

Strickland, R.S.: Decisions: forging the missing link, Nurs. Management, pp. 44-45, July 1983.

Talbott, S.W., and Vance, C.N.: Involving nursing in a feminist group—NOW, Nurs. Outlook, pp. 596-599, Oct. 1981.

Walters, J.: Multiply your clout with a grassroots lobbying network, Assoc. Managment, pp. 57-61, April 1983.

CHAPTER 12
Research in nursing

It is most important to observe the symptoms of illness; it is, if possible, more important still to observe the symptoms of nursing: of what is the fault not of the illness, but of the nursing. Observation tells how the patient is; reflection tells what is to be done; training tells how it is to be done.''

Florence Nightingale

OBJECTIVE: On completion of this chapter, the student of nursing will have a realization of the need for an appreciation of research in nursing.

In all of Nightingale's wisdom she knew the gathering of data was the most important weapon to use in securing her position with a bureaucratic system. Her poignant statement "training tells how it is to be done" could very well be interpreted to mean that by researching the problem and examining the data collected, the hows, whys, where, and when will be answered. Observation is a skill the researcher must develop in depth, for the observation of any given activity should set off a whole chain reaction of thought. Thought can be at first ramdom in nature and become more select as the core of the problem is brought to focus.

Research in nursing and by nurses is a relatively young field. The thrust for research in nursing began in the early 1950s; momentum has increased since 1960. This chapter will provide a definition of research and describe types of nursing research, the importance of research, historical perspectives, publications related to nursing research, funding of research, the development of a research proposal, and the future of research.

DEFINITION OF RESEARCH

Research according to Webster is a "studious inquiry or examination." Adbellah and Levine define research as "an activity whose purpose is to find a valid answer to some question that has been raised. It is a purposeful activity."* Research is a formal, systematic study of a problem leading to conclusions.

Nursing research must have outcomes that provide meaning to the profession and the practice of nursing. Martinson states that "nursing research is the aspect of research related to the whole of nursing; nursing practice, nursing education and nursing service . . . [with] its primary aim to use the new knowledge as a means of effecting changes."†

Research in nursing practice is asking questions

---

*Abdellah, F.G., and Levine, E.: Better patient care through nursing research, ed. 2, New York, 1979, Macmillan, Inc., p. 703.

†Martinson, D.: Why research in nursing? Chaska, N.L.: The nursing profession—views through the mist, New York, 1978, McGraw-Hill Book Co., p. 156.

to validate if what is being done is accurate, to remove from practice a particular activity of nursing, or to add new knowledge. For example, in 1950, a usual practice for preparing a hypodermic syringe and delivering it to the patient was to draw up the medication and place the needle on a moistened alcohol sponge. In researching this practice it was determined that the needle became contaminated before it was used; in addition, the alcohol from the sponge seeped into the lumen of the needle, causing pain on administration. The procedure was changed as a result and has continued to change as new knowledge is gained on how best to transport a prepared syringe to the bedside. Changing nursing practice through research adds to credibility of the profession of nursing.

TYPES OF NURSING RESEARCH

There are many approaches to accomplish research. The approach utilized by any researcher depends on the problem to be solved and the level of sophistication and/or stage of development of the researcher. Some research will be done with highly technical instrumentation; other research will be done with people. All studies should be designed so that others can replicate them to determine validity.

Basically there are three types of research: historical, descriptive, and experimental. Best describes historical research as "what was," descriptive as "what is," and experimental as "what will be."* Nursing researchers use basic research and applied research. According to Martinson, basic research is "knowledge for its own sake" and applied is "practical application of theoretical or abstract knowledge."†

Nursing as a profession and nursing practice continue to be most often studied from a historical perspective. Historical studies are descriptive in nature and serve as a means of documenting the past. The historian utilizes libraries, personal documents of the time, and personal histories of leaders. Historical studies are valuable in presenting the past, giving a perspective that assists in predicting the future, and setting the stage for change.

Nurses who conducted historical research on Florence Nightingale, for example, have provided an insight to this woman who was heretofore much maligned. New respect for Nightingale and her efforts for nursing and health care can be gained by reading such authors as Palmer* and Barritt.†

Nursing as a profession is often the subject of the researcher. Much has been learned from such studies. The methodology used varies according to the problem being studied but involves either descriptive or experimental research. These studies have provided information about the type of individual who becomes a nurse, what knowledge nurses need, the nature of the profession, and whether nursing is a profession.

Nursing practice can be studied by using historical, descriptive, or experimental designs; however, it is more often experimental, requiring the use of human subjects. Armiger states:

Clearly, there are areas of research in nursing as in the biomedical and behavioral sciences in which living man is the necessary object of study. To establish the validity of findings in nursing practice research, investigations must be based on observations of human beings. The pivotal question for the profession at large and notable for nurse researchers concerns the ethical limits within which clinical research may be undertaken because research on the human person presents unique hazards, risks, and responsibilities. . . .

Emerging from the literature on the ethics of nursing research is a recurring theme: suprascientific values inhere in the individual dignified by human personality. A research perspective which honors human rights will nev-

---

*Best, J.W.: Research in education, ed. 2, Englewood Cliffs, N.J. 1970, Prentice-Hall, Inc., pp. 94, 116, 140.
†Treece, E.W., and Treece, J.W., Jr.: Elements of research in nursing, St. Louis, 1977, The C.V. Mosby Co., p. 5.

*Palmer, I.S.: Florence Nightingale, reformer, reactionary, researcher, Nurs. Res. **26:**84, March-April 1977.
†Barritt, E.R.: Florence Nightingale: her wit and wisdom, New York, 1975, Peter Pauper Press.

er widen the cleavage between the nurse's scientific and human values.*

Scientific research is a highly developed method of seeking new knowledge. In order to provide credence to clinical nursing, scientific research is done and is usually referred to as clinical research. Kerlinger defines scientific research as "systematic, controlled, empirical, and critical investigation of hypothetical propositions."† Empirical study is common among nurses since empiricism refers to gathering data directly through observation and use of our senses. Clinical research is a study of specific nursing problems with which a set of phenomena are observed and wondered about. As wonder becomes inquiry and inquiry becomes what if, the researcher begins to develop a set of questions to be investigated. The investigation begins to address the problem from a set protocol.

The nurse researcher must follow exact procedures and protocol, for, as Creighton says, "the legal aspect of nursing research should be consistent with the legal aspects of nursing practice. Because nursing research involves human subjects directly or indirectly, its activities should be guided by certain legal considerations."‡

Examples of clinical research accomplished or in progress are *Approaches to Alleviating Pain, Family Adjustment After Myocardial Infarction, Drug Interaction Among the Elderly, Preventing Post-Surgical Infarction, Understanding Obesity, Health Maintenance with Spinal Cord Injury, Screening for Cystic Fibrosis, Womb Simulation for Premature Infants, Preventing Corneal Ulcers, and Predicting Child Abuse.*§

Examples of historical studies are those on leaders of nursing such as Florence Nightingale and Stella Goostray.

Theories of nursing are developed through scientific research. Examples of these are Orem's theory of self-care and Rogers' theory of adaptation.

IMPORTANCE OF RESEARCH

Research in nursing will strengthen nursing as a profession, but, more important, it will change nursing practice to improve the quality of patient care. The American Nurses' Association (ANA) states, "research in nursing addresses the human and behavioral questions that arise in the treatment of disease and the prevention of illness and maintenance of health."*

As nurses gain expertise in research and study nursing problems, nursing gains in developing its own scientific base. For example, June Abbey, professor of nursing, has been studying "shivering" as a nursing problem. Through her studies she has determined there are different reasons for shivering to occur and relates these to the "shivering center." Abbey's research is on physiological activities of the body and what bioinstrumentation can be developed to provide improved nursing care. From her studies, a scientific base has evolved from which to develop the best nursing practice to prevent shivering or to care for a patient who is shivering.

Nightingale early described fresh air and cleanliness as needs for effective nursing care. These have been a part of the nursing theory since the late 1800s. In the 1980s these aspects of care have been researched, and although modification has occurred in maintenance of cleanliness, the underlying theory continues to scientifically support inclusion of this aspect of physical and environmental cleanliness as a base for nursing care.

*Arminger, Sister B.: Ethics of nursing research: profile, principles, perspective, Nurs. Res. **26:**335, Sept.-Oct. 1977.

†Kerlinger, F.: Foundations of behavioral research, ed. 2, New York, 1973, Holt, Rinehart, & Winston, p. 11.

‡Creighton, H.: Legal concerns of nursing research, Nurs. Res. **26:**337, Sept.-Oct.1977.

§American Nurses' Association: Research in nursing, toward a science of health care, Kansas City, Mo., 1976, The Association.

*American Nurses' Association: Research in nursing, toward a science of health care, Kansas City, Mo., 1976, The Association.

HISTORICAL PERSPECTIVE

Isobel M. Stewart, as head of the nursing department at Teachers College, Columbia University, New York, taught her students to answer questions by searching for reliable evidence through the findings of other experimenters. Stewart, as early as 1920, tried to establish an institute of nursing research in order that nurses would have a means of measuring safe nursing care. From 1932 to 1947, Virginia Henderson taught the course ''Comparative Nursing Practice'' as a means of introducing students to nursing research.

Before 1952, little was done to promote research in nursing. Nurses who were registered in universities for higher degrees were required to do master's theses and doctoral dissertations. These nurses were taught the skills of research. Through their efforts a scientific base for nursing began to evolve. Questions were being asked in nursing practice about nursing as a profession and the history of nursing. If nursing was to gain respectability as a profession, then clearly a scientific base had to be developed; this could only be done by research.

During the 1950s the ANA collaborated with other organizations on nursing function studies. This was an attempt to provide a scientific basis for efforts to improve nursing services and patient care. In 1955 Clara Harden authored the book *Twenty Thousand Nurses Tell Their Story,* which was the first complete publication on research regarding nursing functions.

The ANA as early as 1932 began yearly computation of published data and in 1952 established a Department of Research and Statistics. In 1954 to 1956 ANA established a standing committee on research studies to place, promote, and guide research and studies relating to the function of the association, and in 1955 the ANA established the American Nurses' Foundation (ANF) as a center for research. The ANF conducts research, administers funds for grants, and provides consultation to researchers.

In 1962 the ANA established a blueprint for research in nursing that outlined six categories of research to be used as long-range goals of the association. From 1965 to 1973 the ANA provided opportunities, through forums, for researchers to critique the work of nurse researchers. The ANA saw the need to develop and increase competence in nursing research and in 1970 established a Council for Research; in 1972 the council became a commission. The commission was to facilitate and disseminate research. The ANA Commission on Research in the 1970s established guidelines for schools of nursing as to what research skills should be taught in baccalaureate and graduate programs in nursing.

Simultaneous with ANA efforts, the National League for Nursing (NLN) also engaged in efforts to increase activity in research. The NLN in 1959 established a Research and Studies Department. This department conducts periodic surveys and collects data on student enrollment, graduations, and other factors. They have done studies on open curriculum, funding of nursing education, and student selection process. NLN research is of an applied nature and not clinically oriented.

The NLN Department of Baccalaureate and Higher Degree Programs has fostered the idea of research through the criteria established for the accreditation of baccalaureate and master's degrees. It is expected that research will be included in the curriculum and that it will be conducted by faculty.

Research conferences had their beginning in 1957 under the auspices of the Western Interstate Council of Higher Education for Nursing (WICHEN). The purpose of the conferences was to strengthen and expand effective research in the field of nursing. Following the WICHEN pattern, alumni associations, the ANF, the ANA, and Sigma Theta Tau now conduct conferences on research. Through these conferences new knowledge is disseminated and researchers have an opportunity to have their work critiqued, which in turn strengthens practice. Unless research is seen as a tool of science and is used as a means of developing substantive knowledge, the work of the researcher becomes lost. Conferences and publications are valued means of disseminating the results of research.

Various units of the U.S. government have been actively involved in research. The U.S. Public Health Service had three major thrusts from 1955 to 1976. From 1955 to 1968, the thrust was essentially developmental and dealt with the role of the nurse and the process and theory of nursing practice and nursing education. From 1962 to 1972, clinical nursing, which considered patient-client needs and services and the scientific assessment of the clinical aspects of patient care, was the major thrust, whereas outcomes of nursing care, which dealt with the evaluation of the effects of nursing practice on patient care, were studied from 1973 to 1976.

The Veterans Administration in 1960 incorporated nursing research into its activities of nursing service. The U.S. Department of Health, Education and Welfare fostered research as well as established rules and regulations governing the protection of human subjects. It was in the late 1970s that the National Commission for the Protection of Human Subjects of Biomedical and Behavioral Research was established.

In the summer of 1983 two ideas were generated from the Institute of Medicine study on nursing. One of the ideas became proposed legislation on establishing an institute of nursing under the National Institutes of Health. Representative Madigan of Illinois proposed such legislation. A second idea was, rather than an institute on nursing, a center for nursing research to be established within the federal government. The leaders of three organizations, (American Association of Colleges of Nursing [AACN], ANA, and NLN) discussed the proposals in regard to the National Nurse Training Act. Political ramifications and strategies to secure the best for nursing and nursing research were not clear; however, in the interest of securing nursing as a profession and a discipline, the leaders of the three associations left deliberations open.

In the late fall of 1983, Madigan introduced legislation to form an institute of nursing. It was passed by the House in November 1983.

Today in the late 1980s, medical centers, universities, major nursing services, and governmental and nongovernmental agencies are involved in nursing research with particular emphasis on nursing practice.

In the early history of research, nurses and nursing were more often studied than the practice of nursing. Sociologists and psychologists particularly found a fertile field in the study of nursing. Nurses were timid in their research. They, too, studied themselves rather than practice. Today, clinical research is evident. The reporting of results about ongoing research is done through nursing organization conventions, other related organizations, special conferences, major journals, and newspapers.

Doctoral programs in nursing emphasize research. Graduate faculty and students are engaged in research, all of which strengthens nursing as a profession and nurses as researchers.

PUBLICATIONS RELATED TO NURSING RESEARCH

Nursing Research, the first journal to be devoted to reporting research in nursing was established in June 1952. This journal celebrated its twenty-fifth anniversary of publication in 1977 by publishing a historical perspective of research in nursing. Thus the reader will find the 1977 issues of *Nursing Research* of particular interest in their treatment of development of research from surveys about nursing to the clinical issues of nursing.

New journals are appearing yearly to accommodate the publishing of the results of nurse-produced research in a referenced magazine. Examples of these are *Advances in Nursing Science* (Aspen), *Research in Nursing and Health* (Wiley), and *Western Journal of Nursing Research* (Pamela Brink, editor). Nurses are also reporting their research in allied discipline journals, depending on the thrust of the study. Sigma Theta Tau, the National Honor Society of Nursing, publishes *Image: the Journal of Nursing Scholarships*. This journal's express purpose is to promote and foster scholarly works as well as the ideal of the organization, which is research in nursing.

A few texts or references on research appeared in the 1960s, but a significant increase occurred in the 1970s. Among the first to publish such texts were Abdellah and Levine *(Better Patient Care Through Nursing Research*, New York, first edition in 1965, second edition 1979, Macmillan Company) and Simons and Henderson *(Nursing Research, a Survey and Assessment*, New York, 1964, Appleton-Century-Crofts). Later such authors as Treece and Treece *(Elements of Research in Nursing*, St. Louis, second edition, 1977, The C.V. Mosby Company), Polit and Hungler *(Nursing Research: Principles and Methods*, Philadelphia, 1978, J.B. Lippincott Company), Diers *(Research in Nursing Practice*, Philadelphia, 1979, J.B. Lippincott Company), Fox *(Fundamentals of Research in Nursing*, New York, 1970. Appleton-Century-Crofts, and Krampitz and Pavlovich *(Readings for Nursing Research*, St. Louis, 1980, The C.V. Mosby Company) brought nursing research as a discipline to the forefront of nursing.

THE DEVELOPMENT OF A PROPOSAL

Not every nurse is going to be a researcher; however, almost every nurse sometime in his or her career will be involved or contribute to someone else's research. Research is more than problem solving, and it is important for the nurse to know the difference. Every nurse who uses the nursing process has the rudiments of problem solving. In utilizing the five elements of problem solving the nurse can make decisions about care given on a day-to-day basis.

It is when on repeated inquiry the answers are not clear or the reasons why are not understood that one moves to develop a research idea. Developing an idea for a research proposal becomes the first step in the research process.

The research process includes statement of the problem and determining the significance of the problem, whether it is a researchable problem, the feasibility of the problem, and what use the data are going to be. From this process a research proposal is prepared.

The research proposal is a very tight document that provides the reader with enough information for understanding what, why, when, and for whom. A proposal will include several chapters. The first chapter will include a statement of the problem, definition of terms, research design, plan of study, delineations, and related literature.

The second chapter will be an extensive and exhaustive literature search. The literature search will address the theoretical framework, other research done on the problem, and related literature in and out of the field being studied. It is in the area of literature search that the researcher must be meticulous.

Literature search must locate references that are primary sources rather than secondary. Original sources often reveal data that are not transposed in the secondary source. There are many computerized on-line services to the student and researcher. Utilizing computer search is valuable if the right indexing of words provides the literature one wishes to read. Ready-made bibliographies are not always the most helpful. Once the article, book, monograph, or personal paper has been secured, reading and assimilating the data become utmost.

Reading occurs first to determine if any research has been done on the problem. If so, what relevance does it have to the study under consideration. If relevance exists, should the original study be replicated to determine the validity of the study. If there is no relevance, is there something within the study that will help further the study under consideration. The literature search also provides an opportunity to determine if others have had similar ideas but never pursued them further.

Reading also occurs for the theoretical framework and the research design to be chosen. Reading the literature helps the researcher to crystalize the concepts and place them into a researchable design.

The third chapter of the proposal becomes the

design and plan of execution. In this chapter the researcher decides what approach the study will take: descriptive, historical, or experimental. The research instrument will be selected and tested. This chapter becomes the guideline for collecting data. Time schedules, populations to be studied, limitations of the study, and procedures for protecting the human subjects all become necessary and are addressed in this chapter.

The three chapters of the proposal become the first three chapters of the final research project. Data collection and the results of the study and the recommendations derived from the study complete the process of the research.

You may never write a proposal; however, you will utilize the results of many research projects. Therefore knowing the steps of developing a proposal will help you be critical of a piece of research.

Professional researchers are constantly being critiqued in order to provide new knowledge. The most profound research project will mean nothing if the users of the outcomes do not critique and challenge the researcher. For it is inquiry that provides the researcher the avenue for questing new knowledge, which leads to new techniques and new nursing care approaches for the nurse to implement.

FUNDING FOR RESEARCH

To do research costs money, time, and effort. Often a research project requires many individuals beside the principal investigator. Equipment, staff, and space are needed. Funding becomes an important aspect of embarking on any research. The ANA, NLN, and AACN have consistently sought funding for research.

Major funding has been legislated by Congress through the Nurse Training Act and administered through the Department of Health, Education and Welfare. Grants can be awarded to individuals, groups, or agencies. A second major source is private foundations such as the Kellogg Foundation and the Robert Wood Foundation. A third source is the ANF and the Nurses' Educational Fund. Uni-

versities often have small amounts of money to offer the faculty researcher for pilot projects.

The ANF and the Nurses' Educational Fund derive their funds from contributions of individuals and smaller companies that wish to contribute to nursing research but cannot do so on a large scale. Nurses need to consider contributing to both of these funds.

The researcher is usually responsible for securing the funds to do the project. This requires that a research proposal (grant proposal) be written. The proposal describes the purpose of the study, the design, the anticipated outcomes, and the values that may be derived from the study. If human subjects are involved, then a description of what is involved accompanies the proposal when it is submitted for funding. The proposal must be approved by the appropriate body such as the Human Subjects Commission.

The skills of research must be learned before research is embarked on. Nurses graduating from most baccalaureate programs will have the beginning skills to conduct simple studies, whereas the graduate student will take several courses that give the methodology for designing and conducting studies. At the graduate level, nurses learn grant proposal writing, which helps to secure funding.

FUTURE OF RESEARCH

The future of research in nursing is bright and exciting. As more master's and doctoral programs in nursing are established and gain maturity, nurse researchers will become more visible. Financing of nursing research is the most crucial element to sustain the interest generated in the 1970s. As the economic status of the United States becomes more uncertain, funding will be more difficult. However, if the nursing profession continues to research problems as they relate to quality of care and life, foundations will provide money.

The future will see increased efforts in clinical practice, historical studies on individuals and their contribution to nursing, descriptive studies on the nurse's role, responsibilities, and accountability to the profession and public, and studies that provide data on the changing aspects of nursing, nursing service, and nursing education.

Research in nursing will provide a scientific base from which the professional will determine the appropriate nursing measures needed to promote health maintenance, prevent illness, and intervene in illness care.

All nurses at some time have said there must be a better way or asked "what if." Abbey was one such nurse who did this when faced with an obese patient who needed to be weighed several times a day. Two beds were required to accommodate the weight and size of the patient. There was no easy way to weigh the patient. Abbey said to her instructor, "There must be a way." The instructor responded, "If you're so smart, do it." A challenge was made, problem solving started, and 4 days later, Abbey had the beginning of a solution. Her idea became a patient scale to weigh people who could not get out of bed.

Research is an important phase of the development of nursing as a profession, for it is the scientific knowledge base from which practice evolves. The reason "just because" is no longer sufficient. Referring to Chapter 4 will assist the reader in understanding the value of research in nursing.

THE CHALLENGE

The challenge for nurses and nursing is to include the results of research in one's practice, teaching, or administrative role. If research is necessary to promote the profession in its quest for recognition, then nurses must make the reading of research articles and studies a part of their everyday practice in order to bring the patient, the student, and the staff the most up-to-date thinking. Research in nursing is only good if it becomes usable knowledge.

SUMMARY

Research in nursing was started with Florence Nightingale, who posited such questions as "What is not the fault of the illness but of the nursing?" This probing question laid relatively dormant until 1952, when nurses began to believe that research was necessary to develop a scientific base and a theoretical framework to nursing practice. The art of research gained momentum in the 1970s as more nurses were in graduate programs where research was expected as a part of their formal study. Nursing research has been done on nurses, the profession of nursing, nursing education, and the practice of nursing. It is with nursing practice research that changes will occur in the quality of nursing care patients receive.

Discussion questions

1. Discuss the differences between research and problem solving.
2. Discuss the value of research in nursing, about nursing, and on nursing.
3. Discuss the profession's need for research.
4. Discuss what a research proposal includes and how a researchable problem is determined.
5. Discuss the future of research and how research will assist nurses and those for whom nursing cares.

SUGGESTED READINGS

Abdellah, F.G.: U.S. Public Health Service's contribution to nursing research, Nurs. Res. **26:**4, 244-249, July-Aug. 1977.

Abdellah, F.G., and Levine, E.: Better patient care through nursing research, ed. 2, New York, 1979, Macmillan, Inc.

Armiger, Sister B.: Ethics of nursing research: profile, principles, perspective, Nurse. Res. **26:**330-335, Sept.-Oct. 1977.

Batey, M.V.: Conceptualization: knowledge and logic guiding empirical research, Nurs. Res. **26:**324-329, Sept.-Oct. 1977.

Carnegie, M.E.: A serious ommission, Nurs. Res. **24:**83, March-April 1975.

Christy, T.E.: Quality in research, Nurs. Outlook **23:**80, Feb. 1975.

Conway, M.E.: Clinical research: instrument for change, J. Nurs. Admin. **8**(12):27-32, 1978.

Creighton, H.: Legal concerns of nursing research, Nurs. Res. **26:**337-351, July-Aug. 1977.

Cross, E.D.: Nursing research in the Veterans Administration, Nurs. Res. **26:**250-252, July-Aug. 1977.

Davenport, N.J.: The nurse scientist: between two worlds, Nurs. Outlook **28'**28-31, Jan. 1980.

deTornyay, R.: Nursing research—the road ahead, Nurs. Res. **26:**404-407, Nov.-Dec. 1977.

Diers, D.: This I believe about nursing research, Nurs. Outlook **18:**50-54, Nov. 1970.

Dimond, M.: Research in nursing administration: a neglected issue, Nurs. Admin. Q. Summer 1978.

Elliott, J.E.: Research programs and projects of WICHEN, Nurs. Res. **26:**277-280, July-Aug. 1977.

Flynn, B.C., and Miller, M.H.: Current perspectives in nursing—social issues and trends, St. Louis, 1980, The C.V. Mosby Co.

Gortner, S., and Nahm, H.: An overview of nursing research in the United States, Nurs. Res. **26:**10-33, Jan.-Feb. 1977.

Hodgman, E.C.: Student research in service agencies, Nurs. Outlook **26:**558-565, Sept. 1978.

Hoskim, C.N.: Nursing research: its direction and future, Nurs. Forum **18:**175-186, 1979.

Jacox, A., and Prescott, P.: Determining a study's relevance for clinical practice, Am. J. Nurs. **78:**1882-1889, Nov. 1978.

Johnson, W.L.: Research programs of the National League for Nursing, Nurs. Res. **26:**172-176, May-June 1977.

Kalisch, P.H.: Weavers of scientific patient care: development of nursing research in the U.S. armed forces, Nurs. Res. **26:**253-269, July-Aug. 1977.

Krueger, J.C.: Utilization of nursing research: the planning process, J. Nurs. Admin. **8:**6-9, Jan. 1978.

Miller, J.R., et al.: Obstacles to applying nursing research findings, Am. J. Nurs. **78:**632-634, April 1978.

Palmer, I.S.: Florence Nightingale: reformer, reactionary, researcher, Nurs. Res. **26:**84-89, March-April 1977.

Polit, D.F., and Hungler, B.P.: Nursing research: principles and methods, Philadelphia, 1978, J.B. Lippincott Co.

Schlotfeldt, R.M.: Nursing research: reflection of values, Nurs. Res. **26:**4-9, Jan.-Feb. 1977.

See, E.M.: The A.N.A. and research in nursing, Nurs. Res. **26:**165-171, May-June 1977.

Spector, A.F.: Regional action and nursing research in the south, Nurs. Res. **26:**272-276, July-Aug. 1977.

Spector, A.F.: Research in the practice areas, Nurs. Res. **26:**177-221, May-June 1977.

Steckel, S.B.: If you want to make a positive difference in nursing become a nurse researcher, Nurs. '78 **8:**78-80, July 1978.

Stevens, B.J.: Theory, research and the scholarly paper, Res. Nurs. Health **1:**2, April 1978.

Williamson, J.A.: Current perspectives in nursing education: the changing scene, vol. 2, St. Louis, 1978, The C.V. Mosby Co.

Florence Nightingale   Live your life while you have it—life is a splendid gift. But to live your life you must discipline it. You must not fritter it away in fair purpose, erring act and inconsistent will.

The graduate of a school of nursing today has many responsibilities and opportunities to consider. During the senior year, students will begin to concentrate more definitely on career plans. Thoughts will turn to the procedure of licensure and the rights and obligations of the licensed practitioner. Students will analyze employment opportunities in nursing and determine what is best for them. They also need to know more about the responsibilities they will have in professional nursing.

Nursing will become a way of life for the majority of those who graduate from a basic nursing education program. According to Zen, in the Buddhist tradition, the bull represents life energy, truth, and action. According to Zen, a bull should not be confined and must always remain free and be continually sought after.

Leo Buscaglia, author of *Love,* has sought to understand life and has concluded that "life is an experience" and should not be harnessed with goals. If, however, goals or milestones need to be considered, it should be done creatively. Therefore, as students come to a milestone in life experiences (i.e., nursing education), they should be open to new experiences, be open to wondering about their surroundings and the situations in which they find themselves, and do it in joy, peace, and love.

Again, according to Zen, life is but a moment and each moment makes up an experience. We are not the same from moment to moment. As students embark on the next moment of their career in nursing, many decisions will need to be made. These decisions may give rise to feelings of insecurity. Every nurse stepping into the real world of nursing has experienced this anxiety. Every nurse from time to time undergoes new anxieties as new life experiences emerge.

The nurse must take time to think, to hear, to see, and to allow oneself to be in the state "of becoming." For we are always in the dynamic state of becoming. Nursing is a dynamic profession. The new graduate is the "way of the bull,"* full of life energy, truth, and action. Creatively use the basic knowledge of nursing to move forward.

A basic nursing education cannot begin to give all the knowledge and experiences needed. It can only pave the way for continued learning, for the development of interest in independent study, and for the desire to keep abreast of the new and the old in nursing. This section devoted to professional perspectives is designed to help the student assume professional responsibilities with more confidence.

---

*Buscaglia, L.: The way of the bull, Thorofare, N.J., 1973, Charles B. Slack, Inc.

CHAPTER 13
Professional nursing

OBJECTIVE: On completion of this chapter, the student of nursing will have encountered the concept of professional nursing and will have knowledge about professional and related organizations.

In the past 20 years much energy has been spent on the determination of whether nursing is a profession or a vocation; what is professional practice and what is technical practice; who are professionals and who are not. These questions are being asked throughout the world of nursing. American literature abounds with articles pertaining to the issue as does the literature of other nations.

Summer, in *Nursing Mirror* (Sept. 1982), responded to Mark Allen's farewell address on the paranoia existing within the profession. Klug, in *Canadian Nurse* (Feb. 1982), asked, "Is nursing a vocation or a profession?" Helga Dagsland, of Norway, addressed the issue in *International Review* (1981), and Tiffany asked the same question in Australia.

In examining the question of professional nursing it is the intent of this chapter to provide the student with an appreciation for the ongoing development of nursing and what it takes to "becoming" a profession. Nursing as a discipline is a way of life that provides life energy, truth, and action. If, according to Zen, we experience change from moment to moment, then nursing is experiencing changes from vocation to profession moment to moment.

DEFINITIONS

Webster defines profession as "a calling requiring specialized knowledge and often long and in-

tensive academic preparation; a principal calling, vocation, or employment; the whole body of persons engaged in a calling."

Webster defines professionals as "of, relating to, or characteristic of a profession; participating for gain or livelihood in an activity or field of endeavor often engaged in by amateurs; following a line of conduct as though it were a profession." He further defines professionalism as "the conduct, aims, or qualities that characterize or mark a profession or a professional person."

Styles gives a refreshing approach to defining and examining professional nursing in her book, *On Nursing: toward a New Endowment*. Styles introduces a new word, professionhood. She states "professionhood focuses on the characteristics of the individual as a member of a profession [while] professionalism emphasized the composite character of a profession."*

For the most part, persons who define a profession subscribe to six basic elements. Those elements, stated in Chapter 5, will be restated. A profession must have a strong scientific base, have a strong service orientation, be the recognized authority by the professional group with community sanction, have a code of ethics, have a professional organization that sets standards, and conduct on-

---

*Styles, M.: On nursing: toward a new endowment, St. Louis, 1982, The C.V. Mosby Co., pp. 8, 61.

going research. Some have included autonomy as a distinct element of a profession. Sociologists have studied professions and professionalism for decades. The issue becomes clouded for everyone when all who provide a service call themselves professional, which, according to Webster, would not be considered a profession.

PROFESSIONAL NURSING

Styles declares the following beliefs about the nature and purpose of nursing*:

I. I believe in nursing as an *occupational force for social good,* a force that, in the *totality of its concern* for all human health states and for mankind's responses to health and environment, provides a distinct, unique, and vital perspective, value orientation, and service.

II. I believe in nursing as a *professional discipline,* requiring a sound education and research base grounded in its own science and in the variety of academic and professional disciplines with which it relates.

III. I believe in nursing as a *clinical practice,* employing particular physiological, psychosocial, physical, and technological means for human amelioration, sustenance, and comfort.

IV. I believe in nursing as a *humanistic field,* in which the fullness, self-respect, self-determination, and humanity of the nurse engage in fullness, self-respect, self-determination, and humanity of the client.

V. I believe that nursing's *maximum contribution* for social betterment is dependent on:
   A. The well-developed *expertise* of the nurse;
   B. The *understanding, appreciation,* and *acknowledgement* of that expertise by the public;
   C. The organizational, legal, economic, and political *arrangements* that enable the full and proper expression of nursing values and expertise;
   D. The ability of the profession to maintain *unity* within diversity.

VI. I believe in *myself* and in my *nursing colleagues:*
   A. In our *responsibility* to develop and dedicate our

minds, bodies, and souls to the profession that we esteem and the people whom we serve;
   B. In our *right* to be fulfilled, to be recognized, and to be rewarded as highly valued members of society.

In stating her beliefs, Styles incorporates all of the criteria that are used to determine if a profession or a vocation exists. The student may wish to analyze the beliefs statement and determine if the statement meets the criteria of a profession.

Professional nursing is the practice of an art and a science. It is the upholding of standards set forth by the professional organization, adhering to a code of ethics; it is the utilization of specialized skills and knowledge; and it is being in control of the decisions to be made regarding client care. Further, it is a constant quest for new knowledge in providing care. It is the seeking of truth and placing into action the changes that occur through research. It is autonomy in directing and giving nursing care.

Professional practice standards have been identified and approved by the American Nurses' Association (ANA). The ANA has also approved a code of ethics with interpretive statements.

Autonomy of nursing practice provides the nurse with control of client care. In this area nurses must appreciate their own worth, be competent in knowledge and changing technology, and be lifelong learners.

The National Commission on Nursing, in *Nursing in Transition: Models for Successful Organizational Change* (1982), addressed the issue of professionalism among physicians, nurses, and other health care workers. In so doing, the commissioners identified characteristics common to professionals.

Characteristics common to professionals*

Professionalism has been defined in various ways but all the definitions imply control over a professional task

---

*Styles, M.: On nursing: toward a new endowment, St. Louis, 1982, The C.V. Mosby Co., pp. 8, 61.

*National Commission on Nursing: Nursing in transition: models for successful organizational change, Chicago, 1982, Hospital Research and Educational Trust, pp. 4-5.

(work to be done) and the immediate environment in which that work is to be performed. For individuals to have control over tasks, they must be members of a profession in which certain elements exist:

- Each professional possesses a specific body of knowledge and skills that serve as the basis for performing the task.
- The components or units of knowledge are translated specifically to the particular task that is to be performed. For example, both nursing and medicine use concepts from the fields of pathophysiology and psychology. However, nursing draws more heavily on psychology than does medicine.
- Professionals also use a logic that has been developed for their particular disciplines.
  —for physicians, the logic is used for the prevention of disease and the diagnosis and treatment of medical problems.
  —for nurses, the logic is used for diagnosis and treatment of patient's behavioral and physiological responses to changes in general health, illness and the treatment of illness.
  —for administrators, the logic is used for diagnosis and treatment of the health care institution's general viability and responses.
- Professionals develop language, jargon and symbols that are endemic to their own field. Some of the same words are used by different fields but their meanings or concepts often differ by profession. Individuals in nursing and medicine, for example, have encountered considerable misunderstanding over the use of words *joint* and *diagnosis* and the meanings attached to each word. Neither nurses nor physicians, in general fully understand concepts used by administrators, such as financial management and applicable mathematical formulas.
- Professionals are socialized in their profession's culture. The culture includes standards of behavior, dress, class distinctions, symbols, sanctions and rituals, a system of discipline and control.
- Included in the culture are written or unwritten oaths, prohibitions, rewards and codes of ethics.
- A system of legal sanctions, usually some type of licensing or universal credentialing system, is in place in most professions; professionals are credentialed by their peers who control the accrediting system.

These characteristics lead individual professionals to identify with their particular field. They possess a professional identity. They are knowledgeable of activities pertaining to their field and are aware of relationships that should exist among members in that field and with persons in other fields.

In conclusion, it is not a simple task to discuss professional nursing. The issue is complex; however, students are preprofessionals being socialized into a way of life, utilizing a set language, standards of behavior, and class distinctions that will set them apart from others. Admittance to professional nursing will be achieved when a liberal education and a body of knowledge regarding nursing have been achieved. Maintaining acceptance into professional nursing will occur through lifelong learning, through research and application to predictable and unpredictable situations. Professional nursing involves the adherence to a code of ethics and achieving the highest professional academic degree in nursing.

PROFESSIONAL AND RELATED ORGANIZATIONS

Participation in organized nursing activities is one way the nurse can demonstrate professional commitment. Nursing organizations are prolific in number and represent many vested interest groups. There are generally two kinds of organizations, the professional and nonprofessional.

According to Merton, ''A professional organization is an organization of practitioners who judge one another as professionally competent and who have banded together to perform social functions which they cannot perform in their separate capacities as individuals.''* For example, the ANA is the professional organization for RNs, since only nurses may join; whereas the National League for Nursing (NLN) is a nonprofessional nursing organization because people of many levels of nursing and nonnurses may join.

There are many organizations that nurses should know about because of their relationship to nurs-

---

*Merton, R.K.: The function of the professional association, Am. J. Nurs. **58:**50, Jan. 1958.

ing. Some of the organizations do not offer membership to nurses but still have a relationship to nursing. There are women's and men's business organizations that offer new sources to the nurse for being an active citizen through an organization.

National Student Nurses' Association

The National Student Nurses' Association (NSNA) is the preprofessional organization for all students enrolled in programs leading to a diploma or degree in nursing. The organization includes prenursing students of college or university programs and the RN who has returned to school full-time to complete an academic degree.

The purpose of the NSNA is:

a) to assume responsibility for contribution to nursing education in order to provide for the highest quality health care; b) to provide programs representative of fundamental and current professional interests and concerns; and c) to aid in the development of the whole person, his/her professional role, and his/her responsibility for the health care of people in all walks of life.*

The NSNA was officially organized in Cleveland in 1953 and incorporated in 1959. Before this time, students attended national meetings of the professional organization, had student sections, and had student organizations in many states. This was a common banding together to promote the welfare of the nursing student. In Atlantic City in 1952 the decision was made to form a national organization. The bylaws were formally adopted, and the first officers were elected in 1953 during the NLN convention.

The NSNA† has an executive director and other staff to handle the day-to-day activities of the association. The first executive director was Frances Tompkins, who served the association for 17 years.

Before 1964 there was no official organ of the association. In June 1964 the official magazine for the association became the *American Journal of*

Nursing. A newsletter was used as a means of communication to the membership; however, this newsletter was not sent to individual students and communication lagged. In January 1968 a new format for the newsletter was adopted. This newsletter became known as *Imprint*. It is published four times a year in February, April, October, and December. *Imprint* subsequently has become the official magazine of the organization. Each member receives a copy as part of the membership dues. The magazine is written and edited by students, and students are encouraged to submit original articles for publication. In addition to articles on clinical nursing, there are articles focusing on the association's activities as well as editorials dealing with important issues that involve the NSNA.

In addition to *Imprint*, communication is maintained between the NSNA, the state, and the school through *The N.S.N.A. News*, which is published seven times a year and contains news of an organizational nature and of board action.

Although the NSNA communicates with the ANA and the NLN and has opportunity to report to these organizations, it is financially and legally an independent organization. This was attested to in May 1968 when the statement, "shall be under the auspices of A.N.A. and N.L.N. Coordinating Council," was deleted from the bylaws.

The 1979 revised bylaws provide for consultants from the ANA and NLN. The consultants are "a) responsible for providing interchange of information between the Board of Directors of the A.N.A., N.L.N., and N.S.N.A., b) serve as resource persons consulting with the Board of Directors, members and staff, c) attend meetings of N.S.N.A."*

The ANA and the NSNA have a joint committee that meets to discuss and make decisions on common interests and goals. The first meeting was held in February 1967.

NSNA has had representatives on a variety of interdisciplinary student projects as well as in other

*From Getting the pieces to fit. IV. How to be an N.S.N.A. constituent, New York, 1979-1980, National Student Nurses' Association, Inc.
†Headquarters: 10 Columbus Circle, New York, N.Y. 10019.

*From Getting the pieces to fit. IV. How to be an N.S.N.A. constituent, New York, 1979-1980, National Student Nurses' Association, Inc., p. 23.

organizations, which has allowed for greater depth and understanding from a variety of sources. Examples of such involvement include NLN Advisory Committee on Open Curriculum; National Academy of Science–Study of Costs of Educating Health Professionals–Advisory Panel for Nursing; Over-the-Counter Drug Project; and National Student Health Organizations Liaison Committee.

Until 1974 the NSNA held its annual meeting just before the ANA or the NLN convention. In 1974 the NSNA held its first independent convention in Salt Lake City, Utah. It was an unquestioned success with over 2300 participants. The convention had 94 exhibitors, clinical nursing sessions, and business meetings.

The qualification for membership is enrollment in a state-approved program for the preparation of professional nurses. Students are encouraged to be members of the organization in order that they might be ready to assume the leadership of professional nursing at a later date. In addition to the professional reasons for belonging to NSNA, it is a way to make new friends and gain a broader understanding of the purpose of nursing.

Sally Forster, a former president of the NSNA, said, ''Our whole justification for spending thousands of dollars each year and using hundreds of hours of valuable student time on organization is to help the student make an easy and natural transition from the student association to the graduate professional organization.''*

The student associations are very active and are involved in promoting nursing. In 1979 the organization had as its major concern that of education for nurses. The delegates supported the need for federal legislation to support nursing research. *Imprint* summarized the NSNA policies regarding education in the following list of what the NSNA supports†:

---

*Forster, S.S.: NSNA's ten tall years, New York, 1963, National Student Nurses' Association.

†National Student Nurses' Association 1979: Where does N.S.N.A. stand on education issues? Imprint **26:**38-39, April 1979.

—The gradual movement of all programs preparing for practice as registered nurses to the baccalaureate level.
—ANA's first position paper on education for nursing.
—The development of pathways for career mobility for graduates of associate degree and diploma programs.
—The formulation of standardized challenge examinations for R.N.'s in B.S.N. programs.
—The Bill of Rights and Responsibilites for students of nursing.
—Voting representation by students on school governance committees.
—Clinical workstudy programs for nursing students.
—Investigations of educational entry level for nursing practice by state constituents and national organizations.
—The concept of mandatory continuing education for nurses.
—Student evaluation of nursing instructors.
—Recognition toward fulfilling requirements for course credits for participation in NSNA projects that meet curriculum goals and objectives.
—NLN accreditation of nursing schools as a primary criterion for eligibility for federal funds.
—Inclusion in the curriculum of:
  —Information on child abuse and family violence
  —Nursing Responsibility for care of rape victims
  —Operating room and emergency room experience
  —Health policy information
  —Health care needs of ethnic people of color.

Since the late 1960s, the association has given continued priority as well as financial support to a nationwide program called Breakthrough to Nursing. In 1971 this project received funding through the Division of Nursing, National Institutes of Health. There were five target areas: Phoenix, Arizona; Los Angeles, California; Denver, Colorado; Charlotte, North Carolina; and Columbus, Ohio. Student nurses throughout the country were encouraged to seek out experiences with minority students to assist them in entering nursing programs. Students worked in tutorial situations, and they actively recruited students and provided support in any way the minority student needed it. By 1973 there were 43 Breakthrough areas, with over 400 nursing students and 75 schools participating. It is estimated that the project has reached over

20,594 students and continues to serve the minority student in schools of nursing.

Nursing national honor society

Sigma Theta Tau, the only national honor society of nursing, was founded at Indiana University (location of present national headquarters) Training School for nurses in 1922. Six students founded the organization and chose the name Sigma Theta Tau to represent the initials of the Greek words, *storga, tharos,* and *tima,* meaning love, courage, and honor. October 5 is officially recognized as the anniversary date.

Membership is open to students enrolled in baccalaureate programs in nursing and to nurses matriculated for master's, postmaster's, doctoral, and postdoctoral study in nursing or in an area other than nursing. In addition, candidates may be selected from among nurses who have shown special interest in STT, have received a baccalaureate or higher degree, and have shown marked achievement in the field of nursing.

STT is a member of the association of college honor societies and is professional rather than social in its purpose. From a beginning of six members and one chapter in 1922, the organization has grown to more than 37,000 members and 94 chapters. New chapters are formed each year after much rigorous planning and meeting the criteria. Chapters develop appropriate programs and projects that contribute to the national commitment of STT. Chapters-at-large may be organized in an area where at least two schools form a cooperative honor society and meet eligibility requirements. New chapters are chartered after meeting the criteria set forth by STT. Membership is available by invitation through active chapters.

Following are the purposes of the society:
1. To recognize the achievement of scholarship of superior quality
2. To recognize the development of leadership qualities
3. To foster high professional standards
4. To encourage creative work

5. To strengthen commitment on the part of individuals to the ideals and purposes of the profession of nursing

A professional journal, *Image: the Journal of Nursing Scholarship,* is published four times a year, fall, winter, spring and summer. A newsletter, *Reflections,* is published five times a year. A media development program produces films and videotapes depicting historical and scholarly aspects of nursing.

National research conferences are scheduled at ANA and NLN biennial conventions. Many of the chapters sponsor annual research conferences. In addition, the national committees sponsor writers' seminars and regional conferences. Through its awards competition, STT recognizes the excellence of contemporary leaders in nursing. Small grants are made to qualified nurse applicants who have received formal preparation for research at the graduate level. Research reports are carried in *Image,* monographs are published containing papers presented at research conferences, and *Reflections* publicizes nursing research events.*

American Nurses' Association

The ANA was founded in 1896 as the Nurses' Associated Alumnae of the United States and Canada. Later the nurses from Canada withdrew, and in 1911 the name was changed to American Nurses' Association.

The development of the ANA has been based on the needs of the individual nurses throughout the country. As changes have been brought about by legislation and societal needs, the association has also made changes. In 1952 the functions of the ANA were restated, after an extensive study was done of the various nursing organizations in the United States. The function study required 13 years for completion. The function study started in 1939 but was slowed down during the war and did not gain impetus until 1945. The Raymond Rich As-

---

*Address: Sigma Theta Tau, Indiana University School of Nursing, 1100 W. Michigan St., Indianapolis, Ind. 46202.

sociates were employed to evaluate the needs of the ANA and all other nursing organizations in existence. All matters pertaining to the individual professional nurse were left to the professional organization. All matters pertaining to nursing were relegated to the NLN. The final decision for making two organizations out of six was voted on in San Francisco in 1952. The following years have been spent in strengthening the functions of both organizations.

During the function study, before 1952, the Rich Associates were asked to evaluate each of the nursing organizations: the ANA, the National League of Nursing Education, the National Organization for Public Health Nursing, the American Association of Industrial Nurses, the National Association of Colored Graduate Nurses, and the Association of Collegiate Schools of Nursing. The purpose of the study was to determine how organized nursing could best serve nurses and nursing. There was much confusion as to the need for six professional nursing organizations. Throughout the system there was much duplication of effort, often on the part of a few dynamic leaders in nursing.

The Rich Associates identified some basic structural principles:

1. Nursing should be unified in organized effort.
2. Every specialized nursing group should pursue its special interest.
3. Organization should make it possible for nursing to attack its problems on an efficient basis.
4. Individual members must be able to participate in the organization, thereby stimulating growth of new leaders.
5. Organization should facilitate cooperation and assistance from allied professions.

It was strongly suggested by the Rich Associates that there be one organization. However, there were three major points the six organizations could not agree on: nonnurse membership, special interests of individual nurses, and program emphasis. ANA President Pearl McIver asked the International Council of Nurses if the ANA could still belong to the council if there were lay (nonnurse) members in the ANA. The answer was not clear, except that nonnurse members could not be in control of the organization. It seemed definite then that ANA could not accept the one organization idea.

Because of these dividing factors, two organizations were proposed—the ANA and National Organization for Nursing Service, later called Nursing League of America and finally named National League for Nursing.

Throughout the 13 years of study many proposals were made and discarded. In 1950 a formal vote was taken by the six organizations to form two organizations to become effective in 1952. Both organizations were to have a common purpose. This was to develop the best possible nursing service for the people of the United States.

The bylaws and constitution of the old ANA became the nucleus of the new ANA, and the constitution and bylaws of the National League of Nursing Education became the nucleus of the NLN. The key difference between the two organizations was that the ANA was to be involved with the individual nurse standards of practice, standards of education, and economic and general welfare; and the NLN with nursing as it pertains to overall needs of service and education.

Before the reorganization in June 1952 in San Francisco, the American Association of Industrial Nurses voted not to become a part of the new NLN because the nurses believed it would not serve their interest. Two sections of the ANA, Federal Government Nurses and Men Nurse Section, disbanded and became part of the interest sections of the ANA.

The 1952 structures of the ANA and NLN called for a coordinating council of the two organizations. This was to safeguard against duplication and increase communications.

In 1958 many nurses still felt a need for one organization. A member of the House of Delegates at the 1958 ANA convention proposed one organization. Since it was not within the power of the ANA to act on such a motion, it was asked that a study be done to determine the need for two organizations. Both organizations, ANA and NLN, embarked on function studies. Each organization made a complete study of the 1952 structure; the ANA made changes in June 1966 and NLN in May 1967. The organizations determined that there were specific functions indigenous to the people they serve.

In 1962 the ANA House of Delegates amended the purposes and functions of the ANA to restate and add specific functions relating to nursing education and nursing service. In 1964 the House of Delegates instructed the Study Committee of the ANA to recommend in 1966 an organizational structure that would best fulfill these functions. The new structure allowed more freedom for district associations to function so that the individual nurse's needs were met. The House of Delegates in June 1966 voted to accept and implement a new structure.

The new structure placed more emphasis on the professional responsibility to economics and general welfare, nursing education, and nursing service. There were three commissions, one for each of the stated major areas. A fourth commission devoted to nursing research was approved by the House of Delegates in 1970. This move strengthened the premise that research was an important function of the association and was necessary for promoting the profession. Each of these commissions concerns itself with the specific problems related to that commission.

Individual nurse members also belonged to specific divisions of practice. The divisions of practice had as their major responsibility the advancement of various fields of nursing practice. The five divisions of practice were medical-surgical nursing, maternal and child health nursing, psychiatric and mental health nursing, geriatric nursing, and community health nursing. Until 1962 there was a provision in the ANA bylaws for individual membership. This permitted black nurses to have membership in the national organization if a district or state association denied them membership. As of January 1962 all state associations admitted black

nurses, and by 1964 all district associations in the United States provided for black nurses to become members, thus ending the need for individual membership at the national level.

The structure committee of 1962 proposed an academy of nursing, which was also suggested in the Rich report and discarded. The academy of nursing was to recognize those nurses who had contributed significantly to an area of nursing practice. It was to allow for implementation of goal 2 (see p. 200). In 1970 the American Academy of Nursing was approved by the House of Delegates and its *purposes* were stated to be "for the advancement of knowledge, education and nursing practice."* Members of the Academy of Nursing are to be those practitioners, known as fellows, who have been certified and endorsed by the division of nursing practice in which they have become qualified. In 1973 the ANA board of directors asked state associations and individual nurses to nominate those nurse practitioners who had made significant contributions to nursing to become the charter members of the academy. One hundred nominees were considered by the ANA board of directors, and 36 were chosen to be the first honored in March 1973. ANA President Rosamond Gabrielson said of the 36, "they symbolize the high degree of commitment of today's nurses to provide high quality health care."† Dr. Rheba DeTornyay was selected to be the first president of the academy. Dr. Faye G. Adbellah became president of the academy in 1974, and in February 1975, 26 new fellows were admitted.

In 1975 the purposes of the academy were restated to include the following‡:

Advance new concepts in nursing and health care; identify and explore issues in health, in the profession, and in society as they affect and are affected by nurses and

---

*American Nurses' Association: Article XVII of the bylaws, New York, 1970, The Association.
†The American Nurse, Kansas City, Mo., April 1973, American Nurses' Association.
‡The American Nurse, Kansas City, Mo., Oct. 1975, American Nurses' Association, pp. 3 and 14.

nursing; examine the dynamics within nursing, the interrelationships among the segments within nursing, and examine the interaction among nurses as all these affect the development of the nursing profession; identify and propose resolutions to issues and problems confronting nursing and health, including alternative plans for implementation.

Criteria for selection to the academy are based on the individual's contribution to the "advancement of knowledge, education, practice in nursing or to the profession of nursing."*

In 1968 the bylaws provided for a Congress for Nursing Practice with the following purpose†:

1. Establish the scope of nursing practice
2. Evaluate relevant scientific and educational developments and trends in health care practices for implication for nursing practice
3. Encourage and stimulate research on the practice of nursing
4. Formulate policy and recommend action concerning federal and state legislation related to nursing practice
5. Formulate, interpret and revise the Code for Registered Nurses
6. Study and advise upon the ethical and legal aspects of nursing practice
7. Plan and promote educational programs and guides for implementation of principles related to ethical and legal aspects of nursing practice
8. Provide continuing guidance to committees or councils on practice of state and district associations
9. Provide coordination of the work of the divisions to insure a reasonable uniformity in approaches to their defined responsibilities

In the early 1970s the ANA was one of the largest professional organizations in the United States. In addition to the national association, which takes care of those matters pertaining to all nurses throughout the United States, there were state associations that were known as the constituent associations of the ANA. The state associations had the same function as the national association. The structure of the state association was similar to that of the national organization.

The state organization was divided into districts, which were usually determined by geographical areas within the state. The district organization was the point at which membership started.

Between 1968 and 1970, a serious financial crisis engulfed the ANA. The crisis had been growing over a period of years. New programs were implemented, and activity on the part of the organization was increased to meet the problems confronting nursing. Whenever a dues increase was proposed, the membership balked. Instead of granting the full dues increase, the House of Delegates would grant only a portion of the proposed amount. In addition, the business practices in the office were archaic and unsound.

The 1970 ANA convention was a historic one in that the House of Delegates demanded and received an in-depth financial report. Once again individual nurses were against the full dues increase proposed by the board of directors. After lengthy debate, however, the dues increase was voted on and accepted.

To meet the financial crisis, the ANA decreased its staff to only those persons essential to the management. A new business manager was employed, and new accounting and controlling procedures were inaugurated. Office space not needed was leased, and furniture was sold. Also individual members sent in donations to help decrease the indebtedness. The House of Delegates also approved a move of the ANA headquarters from New York to Kansas City, Missouri. This move was effected late in 1972. The purpose of the move was to place the headquarters in a location that was more central for easier access by all nurses and that would be less expensive for overall operation.

For the first time in its history the ANA was unable to pay its dues to the International Council of Nurses; thus the stability of the council was affected.

The president from 1968 to 1970, Dorothy A. Cornelius, deserves special recognition. Through her leadership and the support of the officers during

---

*The American Nurse, Kansas City, Mo., Oct. 1975, American Nurses' Association, pp. 3 and 14.
†American Nurses' Association: Article XVII of the bylaws, New York, 1970, The Association.

this time, honest accounts were given to the membership.

The financial crisis was not the only concern at the 1970 convention; the convention was during the period of student unrest on campuses, the legality of the Viet Nam war was being questioned, civil rights were being implemented, and the nurses at the convention were an "involved" group in all aspects. One group of nurses calling themselves the Nurses for Society in Crisis promoted a change in the order of business to bring before the house social issues that involved nurses. Feelings were shown openly; anger was displayed and tears flowed. Caucuses were held and decisions were made. The 1970 report of the House of Delegates is a worthwhile document. Some of the resolutions passed at the 1970 convention were the following:

1. To make health career opportunities for the socioeconomically disadvantaged
2. To stimulate and develop effective systems of delivery of ambulatory care services
3. To be responsible for introducing legislation on national health insurance
4. To oppose utilization of persons other than RNs in leadership positions, for example, as team leaders
5. To help control the costs of health care
6. To work with groups to combat drug abuse
7. To intensify activities in defining the expanded role of the nurse
8. To study new approaches to the delivery of health care
9. To become involved in the quality of our environment
10. To promote remedial programs that prepare minority groups to enter nursing

Through the work of the ANA, nurses have received social security benefits, shorter work hours, monies for further education, and many other benefits. The functions, standards, and qualifications of various nurse positions such as general duty nurses, office nurses, and industrial nurses were defined. The Standards of Nursing Practice were approved in 1974 for medical-surgical nursing,

community health nursing practice, geriatric nursing practice, maternal-child health nursing practice, and psychiatric–mental health practice.

The organization not only examines the need of today but also anticipates future needs. To this end, three long-term goals had been presented to the ANA House of Delegates. In 1958 goals 1 and 2 were presented and adopted. Goal 1 was as follows: "Stimulate efforts by nurses and other specialists to identify and enlarge the scientific principles upon which nursing rests, and to encourage research by them in the application of these principles to nursing practice." Goal 2 was as follows: "Establish ways within the A.N.A. to provide formal recognition of personal achievement and superior performance in nursing."*

Goal 3 was presented to the House of Delegates in 1960 but was not adopted. This decision was made because of its widespread implications and the opinion that all nurses should have the opportunity to study goal 3 carefully. Goal 3 read as follows*:

To insure that, within the next 20-30 years, the education basis to the professional practice of nursing, for those *who then enter* the profession, shall be secured in a program that provides the intellectual, technical and cultural components of both a professional and liberal education. Toward this end, the A.N.A. shall promote the baccalaureate program so that in due course it becomes the basic educational foundation for professional nursing.

The ANA promotes many kinds of programs and has accomplished many improvements in behalf of the nurse and nursing.

In 1946 there was a great need to upgrade the economic and general welfare of the nurse. The Economic Security Program was adopted as a major program. Throughout the years this program has met opposition from those outside nursing and, in some instances, from nurses. Many people believed that nurses should not involve themselves

*American Nurses' Association: House of Delegates Report, 1960-1962, New York, The Association, pp. 28, 29.

with financial problems, but because nurses were not being recognized for their education and their worth, it was a much needed program. (For a more complete discussion of the program, see Chapter 15.)

The ANA has a specific responsibility to the health of the nation and therefore actively lobbies for social legislation. An example is the Medicare–Social Security amendments of 1965. In 1958 the House of Delegates voted to support legislation for health care for the aged through social security, mainly because many older nurses have been unable to provide themselves with adequate health care. Since nurses have not always had good salaries and good working conditions, they have not been able to provide for themselves. The ANA actively testified in behalf of this legislation, thus alienating those professional associations in the medical field that opposed its passage. The American Medical Association believed that this was the first step to socialized medicine. Many individual nurses did not support the ANA position and dropped their membership.

State and district nurses' associations assume leadership in offering refresher courses to the graduate who has been away from practice. Many workshops are held during each calendar year.

At ANA biennial conventions, clinical sessions have been provided to give assistance to nurses in increasing their knowledge. Thus the profession is actively engaged in offering programs to its members to promote better nursing practice.

It is a necessary function of a professional organization to define and enforce a professional code of ethics. The ANA revised its code in 1976. Congress for Nursing Practice prepared the code with an interpretive statement. State and district associations are responsible for taking disciplinary action if a nurse is found to be in violation of the code.

For the ANA to accomplish its goals, it is necessary for each nurse to be a member. Until 1968 there was a steady increase in membership. However, since then, membership in the organization

has fluctuated and has never achieved the strength of full membership. Some of the reasons given by nurses for not joining are as follows: "The organization does nothing for me." "The dues are too high." "I'm not a joiner." "I don't like the expectation or obligation to belong." "I disagree with the position of the ANA on education." "I disagree with the organization's stand on social legislation." "I disagree with the association's view on the economic and general welfare and its 'union' activities." Whatever the reasons for nurses not joining, the purposes of the organization remain relevant, and there is a need for all nurses to belong. Being a member of the ANA is one of the best ways for the nurse to become involved in the needs of nursing as a profession.

In 1978 the ANA elected its first black president, Barbara Nichols. The delegates reaffirmed the ANA's long-standing support of comprehensive national health insurance and the position that by 1980 two categories of nursing practice should be identified and titled and by 1985 the baccalaureate degree in nursing should be the minimum preparation for entry into professional nursing.

During the 1982 ANA convention held in Washington, D.C., significant changes occurred in the bylaws. No longer would individual nurses be members of the ANA. The organization became a federation of state nurses' association. State nurses' association would hold seats in the ANA House of Delegates. The functions of the organization were approved as follows*:

a. Establish standards of nursing practice, nursing education, and nursing services.
b. Establish a code of ethical conduct for nurses.
c. Ensure a system of credentialing in nursing.
d. Initiate and influence legislation, governmental programs, national health policy, and international health policy.
e. Support systematic study, evaluation, and research in nursing.
f. Serve as the central agency for the collection, anal-

---

*ANA bylaws, Am. Nurse, p. 15, Nov.-Dec. 1982.

ysis, and dissemination of information relevant to nursing.

g. Promote and protect the economic and general welfare of nurses.

h. Provide leadership in national and international nursing.

i. Provide for the professional development of nurses.

j. Conduct an affirmative action program.

k. Ensure a collective bargaining program for nurses.

l. Provide services to constituent state nurses' associations.

m. Maintain communication with members through official publications.

n. Assume an active role as consumer advocate.

o. Represent and speak for the nursing profession with allied health groups, national and international organizations, governmental bodies, and the public.

The biennium of 1982 to 1984 became transition years to effect the changes in the national and state organizations.

The American Journal of Nursing is the official publication of the ANA.* It offers much in the way of information about association activities as well as clinical nursing subjects. *The American Nurse* is received by ANA members as the official means of communication with members regarding association activities.

American Nurses' Foundation

To further promote nursing service and the art of nursing, the ANA founded the American Nurses' Foundation (ANF) in 1955 as its research unit.

The ANF sponsors, conducts, and stimulates research, provides research consultant services, and disseminates research information. General research areas have been nursing procedures, the effects on nursing resulting from changing patterns of patient care, the effects of administrative organization on patient care, nursing needs of patients, and nursing in different categories of illness.

Research is a vital component of any profession.

---

*Headquarters: 2420 Pershing Rd., Kansas City, Mo. 64108.

Independent and collective research is necessary if the nursing profession is to grow and become a distinctive contributor to the health care of our nation. With the addition of the ANA Commission for Nursing Research, the profession has geared itself to the fulfillment of its responsibilities and accountability to nursing and the health needs of the nation.

The ANF is supported primarily through public funds, and although nurses do not join as members, they can support the ANF* by contributing money, by helping to determine research, and by either offering to participate in a research survey or suggesting areas in which research is needed. Through the ANF, nurses can achieve goal 1 of the ANA stated in 1958, which has to do with determining and stimulating research in nursing.

International Council of Nurses

The International Council of Nurses (ICN)† was founded in 1899 in Boston, Massachusetts. It is a federation of international nursing organizations. Its purpose is to provide:

a medium through which [inter]national nurses' associations may share their common interests by working together to develop the contribution of nursing to the promotion of the health of people and the care of the sick. Objectives are: to assist national nurses associations to improve the standards of nursing and the competence of nurses; to promote the development of strong national nurses associations; to serve as the authoritative voice for nurses and nursing internationally; to assist national nurses associations to improve the status of nurses.‡

In 1973 the ICN formally adopted a code for nurses—Ethical Concepts Applied to Nursing. The code speaks to nurses and people, nurses and practice, nurses and society, nurses and co-workers, and nurses and the profession. It identifies the re-

---

*2420 Pershing Rd., Kansas City, Mo. 64108.
†Headquarters: PO Box 42, Ch-1211 Geneva 20, Switzerland.
‡Yakes, N., and Akey, D.: Encyclopedia of associations, ed. 13, vol. 1, National Organizations of the U.S., Section 8, Health and medical organizations, Detroit, 1979, Gale Research Co.

sponsibility of the nurse as being fourfold: to promote health, to prevent illness, to restore health, and to alleviate suffering.

Membership in the ICN is automatic with payment of ANA dues. A small percentage of the ANA dues is paid to the ICN for membership.

Conventions for the ICN are held every 4 years. The ANA is allotted a given number of delegates according to its number of members. However, every nurse can attend the ICN convention.

The ICN has the privilege of being known as the oldest continuously functioning international council. This organization continued its activities throughout the war years and tried to maintain interest in the work of the ICN. The idea for the international organization originated with an English nurse, Ethel Gordon Fenwick. As of 1977 there were 88 nations represented in the ICN. The official publication is *International Review,* published bymonthly.

National League for Nursing

The NLN* was founded in 1952. Its major purpose at that time was, and continues to be, to promote the improvement of nursing service and nursing education so that nursing needs of society might be met. One of the forerunners of the NLN was the National League of Nursing Education, organized in 1893 under the original title of American Society of Superintendents of Training Schools for Nurses of the United States and Canada. This name was changed to the National League of Nursing Education in 1912. Until 1943 membership in this organization was limited to professional nurses interested in nursing education. After 1943 membership was opened to lay members.

The second organization to become a member of the NLN was the National Organization for Public Health Nursing, which was organized in 1912. Its membership had always included interested lay citizens as well as professional nurses.

The third organization was that of the Associa-

tion of Collegiate Schools of Nursing, which was formed in 1932 and was particularly interested in developing nursing education on a professional and collegiate level. Membership was open principally to those programs that had accreditation and were offering college degrees in nursing.

The fourth organization was the Joint Committee on Practical Nurses and Auxiliary Workers in Nursing Service, organized in the early 1940s. This organization had representation from professional nursing organizations. Their principal responsibility was to study the training program for practical nurses and aides.

The fifth group was the Joint Committee on Careers, organized in 1948 to promote the career of nursing.

The sixth group, the National Committee for the Improvement of Nursing Services, was organized in 1948 and included representation from general education, dentistry, social science, industry, labor and other areas. It was oriented toward improvement of care of patients.

The seventh organization, the National Nursing Accreditation Service, was established in 1949. The purpose of this organization was to accredit schools of nursing and to improve the accrediting procedures.

By the end of the 10-year study, which began in 1942, these seven organizations, and committees were ready to band together under the name of National League for Nursing. Its membership included anyone interested in the promotion of nursing, such as professional nurses, practical nurses, nurse aides, administrators, bankers, and teachers.

It offered several kinds of membership, including individual membership and agency membership. An individual may join this organization by paying individual dues. There is also agency membership, which provides membership for educational programs, hospitals, convalescent homes, public health agencies, and public schools.

In the last 30 years the NLN has had its share of growing problems. However, in 1958 when the question was raised as to whether or not there

---

*Headquarters: 10 Columbus Circle, New York, N.Y. 10019.

should be one organization, the NLN's officers and Board of Directors also formed a committee to study its organizational structure and function. These functions were reaffirmed and restated at the 1963 biennial convention. The study committee continued to work toward a new mechanism with which to implement the functions adequately.

The organizational structure of the NLN includes the Division of Individual Members, which forms the Council on Community Planning for Nursing, and the Division of Agency Members, which forms the following councils: Associate Degree Programs, Baccalaureate and Higher Degree Programs, Diploma Programs, Practical Nursing Programs, and Hospital and Related Institutional Nursing Services. In addition, there is the Assembly of Constituent Leagues. Constituent leagues are formed on a local, state, or regional basis to provide local organized effort for the improvement of nursing.

The officers of the NLN can be either nurses or nonnurses. When the organization was first formed, it was believed that the office of president of the organization must always be held by a nurse. However, in 1963 the bylaws were changed to allow a nonnurse to be president of the national organization. In 1979 the first nonnurse president was elected, Matthew McNulty. All members have the opportunity of voting for the officers. This ruling is different from that in the ANA, in which all voting is done by the House of Delegates.

Each of the councils has standing committees, executive committees, and nominating committees. The executive committee of each council is composed of members from that council who have the responsibility of acting as the officers and board of directors of the division, working closely with the staff and with the members of that particular council.

The functions of the NLN are stated in its bylaws and include the development of standards for quality nursing education and nursing service to meet the nursing needs of the people. The NLN works with the ANA in the recruitment of students. In the beginning (1952) the NLN was responsible for the careers program; however, in 1967 this became a joint responsibility of the NLN, which recruits for all kinds of nursing programs, and the ANA, which assumes the major share of nurse recruitment for professional schools. The NLN provides lists of state-approved schools of nursing and programs that have NLN accreditation.

Another service is accreditation of professional and practical nursing schools. Accreditation on the national level is voluntary. It is desirable for a program to strive for national accreditation, since it does provide higher standards for a school. Each of the councils in the division of education must have its own staff to do the accrediting. The work involved requires not only paid staff but also persons from the various schools to help participate in the accreditation service. In addition to surveying of schools, there is consultation help for faculties to seek out assistance in the areas that are giving them the most concern.

At the 1974 ANA convention, one of the priorities for 1974 and 1975 was the system of accreditation of continuing education. This issue brought into focus the suggested need for the ANA to be responsible for implementing the standards for education as well as for enunciating what those standards should be. It should be remembered, however, that the task of accrediting nursing education programs was delegated to the NLN in 1952. The NLN has fulfilled its commitment to improve nursing education through voluntary accreditation. Since June 1974, ANA and NLN have been examining the accreditation process. In January 1975 the first accreditation conference was held in Denver. The purpose of the conference was to prepare a proposal for studying the feasibility of accreditation of basic and graduate education by the ANA. An outgrowth of this study was the credentialing study. This is discussed fully in Chapter 5.

The councils of associate degree, baccalaureate and higher degree, diploma, and practical nursing programs for the NLN Department of Education launched an all-out support of the NLN's mission of accreditation and the validity of that organization retaining the responsibilities for the process of accreditation.

The Test Construction Service develops and scores eight different kinds of examinations for students and graduate nurses. These include tests for selection of students for schools of professional and practical nursing, scholastic achievement of professional and practical nurse students while in the school, and admission of graduate professional nurses within educational programs.

The services of the NLN are many. A wide variety of publications in all phases of nursing is offered. The official magazine until 1978 was *Nursing Outlook,* published by the American Journal of Nursing Company. Members received *N.L.N. News* quarterly until June 1980, when the new official magazine *Nursing and Health Care* was introduced with the July-August 1980 issue.

The NLN is financed partly by dues, but the majority of the funds are obtained through contributions from organizations. It helps to defray costs by charging nominal fees for meetings, special conferences, conventions, and institutes.

In order that NLN can be understood, it is necessary to emphasize its unique nature. Its unique nature lies in the broad aspects of community service involving nonnurse members and all levels of nurse practitioners.

The functions proposed in January 1966 to the board of directors included defining nursing needs of society, fostering programs designed to meet these needs, and offering services in the form of studies, evaluations, consultations, interpretations, publications, test services, accreditation, and a mechanism through which individual citizens and allied organizations may meet the nursing needs of society.

The NLN worked steadily from 1969 to 1971 to foster a changed image for itself and to promote increased involvement on the part of the community-minded citizens. To this end, the Council on Community Planning had been heard and in 1975 has become a very active part of the NLN.

In 1981 a resolution was passed to provide avenues to facilitate greater communication between and among the councils on education. The NLN board of directors appointed a task force to study the structure of the organization. In addition, the board had a marketing study done to determine what services provided to members and agencies were ongoing as well as some future goals of the organization.

The task force on structure reported to the NLN board in 1984. The report of the taskforce was accepted and forwarded to the committee on long-term goals for further study.

SPECIAL INTEREST ORGANIZATIONS OF PROFESSIONAL NURSES
American Red Cross

The American Red Cross was formed in 1882 through the efforts of Clara Barton. The nursing program began enrolling nurses in 1905. This service did not gain stature until 1909 when Jane Delano was appointed head of the National Nursing Service Committee. The purpose of nurses enrolling in Red Cross originally was to serve in war and disasters. These functions have been broadened as the need for the Red Cross Nursing Service has increased.

The objectives for the Nurse Enrollment Program are as follows*:

To maintain a roster of nurses for disaster and for other local and national emergencies.

To provide a channel through which registered professional nurses and student nurses may participate in Red Cross activities and to make available well prepared nurses for community service.

To develop an understanding of the national and international aspects of the Red Cross and the function of the American Red Cross in international affairs.

To develop and maintain appropriate chapter organization that will provide opportunities for nurses to learn new skills for service to the community and that will

*American National Red Cross: Red Cross nurse enrollment, Washington, D.C., July 1963, The Red Cross, pp. 3, 4, 6.

keep up their interest in the Red Cross through recognition of services performed. . . .

Eligibility—registered professional nurses

Any registered professional nurse whose interest in the philosophy and programs of the Red Cross and whose sincerity of purpose and desire to become a member of the Red Cross nursing organization are evident may enroll as a Red Cross nurse, providing she meets the basic qualifications and is willing to prepare herself in a program of her interest.

As a part of the nurse's preparation, she is required to give from 20 to 30 hours of Red Cross service, either in addition to or in connection with the activity for which she is being prepared. Following the prescribed orientations to the Red Cross the nurse may require the number of hours by volunteering in different types of chapter activities; e.g., participating in the fund campaign, serving at first aid stations, and giving talks to student nurses. . . .

The qualifications for professional nurse enrollment are:

Registration in some state in the United States following the nurse's graduation from a state-accredited school of nursing. (Nurses from other countries are required to be registered in some state in the United States.)

Current registration in the state where the applicant will serve, if registration is required by law for the type of Red Cross activity in which the nurse is engaged.

Satisfactory personal, professional, and educational qualifications and state of health consistent with the activity in which she plans to participate.

Any graduate from a state-approved school of nursing may apply to be a member of the Red Cross Nursing Service. The services a graduate can participate in are teaching home nursing, mother-baby classes, fitness for the future, or projects that would use skills in nursing and would offer better services to the community.

On being accepted into the Red Cross Nursing Services, the nurse receives the official Red Cross badge. A number and a badge are assigned to the graduate for life, or until such time as the badge is returned to the Red Cross. In the event of death, the pin is either buried with the graduate or returned to the Red Cross for the disposition of the number.

Students in schools of nursing also may volunteer their services. A student may participate in disaster nursing programs, Red Cross training programs in civil defense, instruction in care of the sick and injured, and mother-baby classes and function under supervision in disaster operations. There are many ways for students to volunteer their time and become active citizens while learning nursing.

American Association of Occupational Health Nurses

The American Association of Industrial Nurses* was founded in 1942. In the 1970s the name of the organization was changed to American Association of Occupational Health Nurses. Registered professional nurses employed by business and industrial firms, nurse educators, nurse editors, nurse writers, and others interested in industrial nursing may become members of this association. The purpose of the organization is to improve community health by bettering nursing service to management and employees.

This is one of the associations that chose not to band with either the ANA or the NLN. The decision was based on the needs and differences found within the function of the organization for industrial nurses. In addition to belonging to the American Association of Industrial Nurses, an industrial nurse may also want to be a member of the Forum on Occupational Health through the ANA.

American Association of Nurse Anesthetists

The American Association of Nurse Anesthetists† was founded in 1931. Active RNs who have taken a 24-month course in administration of anesthetics and passed a qualifying examination can become members of the association. Its purpose is to advance the art and science of anesthesiology

---

*Headquarters: 575 Lexington Ave., New York, N.Y. 10022.
†Headquarters: Suite 929, 111 E. Wacker Dr., Chicago, Ill. 60601.

and to develop educational standards and techniques.

The American Association of Nurse Anesthetists was given encouragement and assistance through the American Hospital Association to develop an accreditation program for schools of nurse anesthetists. This was accomplished and put into effect in January 1952.

In 1984 the association endorsed baccalaureate education in nursing as the minimum entry into a nurse anesthetist program.

Association of Operating Room Nurses

The Association of Operating Room Nurses* was founded in 1957. Registered professional nurses engaged in operating room nursing on supervisory, teaching, or staff levels may become members. The aim of the association is to improve standards of operating room nursing care through increased understanding, knowledge, and skills of personnel engaged in operating room nursing. The organization's program fosters leadership qualities in member nurses. The organization studies existing practices and new developments in operating room nursing and education.

This organization was founded after the reorganization of the ANA and the NLN in 1952. Once again, a group of practitioners did not believe that their needs were being met in either national organization and determined to band together. An operating room nurse may choose to join this organization to gain more knowledge of this area of nursing. A national congress is held each year.

American Association of Colleges of Nursing

The American Association of Colleges of Nursing† was formed in May 1969 as a means of promoting and improving higher education for professional nursing in the public service. The objective adopted by the association in October 1969 was to study and take knowledgeable positions on issues and problems relevant to higher nursing education as they influence delivery of quality nursing and health service. Membership is restricted to programs offering baccalaureate and higher degrees. The head of the program is the official representative to this organization.

National Black Nurses' Association, Inc.

In September 1972 the National Black Nurses' Association* was incorporated. The objectives of the organization are the following†:

1. Define and determine nursing care for black consumers by acting as their advocates
2. Act as change agent in restructuring existing institutions and/or helping to establish institutions to suit the needs of black people
3. Serve as the national nursing body to influence legislation and policies that affect black people and work cooperatively and collaboratively with other health workers to this end
4. Conduct, analyze, and publish research to increase the body of knowledge about health care and health care of blacks
5. Compile and maintain a national directory of black nurses to assist with the dissemination of information regarding black nurses and nursing on national and local levels by the use of all media
6. Set standards and guidelines for quality education of black nurses on all levels by providing consultation to nursing faculties and by monitoring for proper utilization and placement of black nurses
7. Recruit, counsel, and assist black persons interested in nursing to insure a constant procession of blacks into the field
8. Be the vehicle for unification of black nurses of varied age groups, educational levels, and geograph-

*Headquarters: 10170 E. Mississippi Ave., Denver, Colo. 80231.
†Headquarters: 11 Dupont Circle N.W., Suite 430, Washington, D.C. 20036.

*Headquarters: 425 Ohio Bldg. 175 S. Main St., Akron, Ohio 44308.
†Smith, G.R.: From invisibility to blackness: the study of the National Black Nurses' Association, Nurs. Outlook 23:225, April 1975.

ic location to insure continuity of our common heritage

9. Collaborate with other black groups to compile archives relative to the historical, current, and future activities of black nurses

10. Provide the impetus and means for black nurses to write and publish individually or collaboratively

Membership is open to all RNs, LPNs, and nursing students.

Other nursing organizations

Over the past 10 years, other specialty nursing organizations have formed to fill specific needs of a group of practitioners. Some of these organizations are the Association of Pediatric Oncology Nurses; Association of Rehabilitation Nurses; Association For The Care of Children in Hospitals; Gay Nurses' Alliance; Alpha Tau Delta National Fraternity for Professional Nurses; American Indian/Alaska Native Nurses' Association, Inc.; National Association of Spanish Speaking–Spanish Surnamed Nurses; N-CAP (Nurses' Coalition for Action in Politics); Nurses' Christian Fellowship; and National Association of Physician's Nurses (NAPN). Nurses involved in these specialties may become members. Each of the organizations serves as a means of discussing common problems as well as promoting continuing education of the specialty.

In an effort to work together, the ANA called together the presidents or chairmen of these groups in 1972 to discuss how a coalition could be formed to foster the ideals of nursing. It was agreed among them that it was important to communicate and enunciate clearly the purpose of each organization. To this end each organization will host a joint meeting of all organizations during the years to aid a cooperative relationship and provide unified support for nursing. Subsequently, the Federation of Specialty Nursing Organizations was formed in 1973. The federation is made up of 18 specialty nursing organizations and the ANA. This group is not a policy-making organization but provides a basis for cooperation and collaboration.

ALUMNI ASSOCIATIONS

The primary function of an alumni association is to foster high ideals for the school of nursing from which its members have graduated. It provides an opportunity for the graduate to socialize with a group of people with whom he or she is closely associated. Whatever the function of this organization, its members have a responsibility as alumni to the school of nursing to help it chart its course for the future and to offer suggestions about how the program might be improved and how standards and traditions might be maintained.

RELATED ORGANIZATIONS
American Hospital Association

The American Hospital Association was founded in 1898. It is dedicated to promoting public welfare through the provision of better hospital care for all people. It carries out research and educational projects in such areas as hospital facilities and design, epidemiology, and community relations.

Nurses can be members of this organization through personal membership. Nurses with personal membership include those persons associated with institutional or contracting organizations.

Two other membership categories directly involving nursing are type VIII for hospital schools of nursing and the American Society for Nursing Service Administrators. Type VIII membership exists to assist schools of nursing in improving and gaining national accreditation and, in addition, to support the need for hospital programs. The membership was founded in 1967 in response to the ANA's 1965 position in regard to education and to resolution 5 passed by the NLN in 1965. The American Society for Nursing Service Administrators was organized in 1968. Membership includes RNs active in the field of nursing service administration and nurses responsible for the management of the department of nursing in health care institutions. Its purpose is to ''advance effective administration of nursing service in health care institutions by providing a medium for interchange of ideas and dissemination of information and materials relative to nursing service administration and by conducting educational programs to strengthen nursing service administration.''*

There are many kinds of conferences open to nurses to assist them in improving the practice of nursing. Conventions held annually are open to all nurses. The American Hospital Association, the ANA, and the NLN have many liaison committees, thereby developing a relationship to improve hospital care through nursing.

American Medical Association

The American Medical Association is a society of physicians that was organized in 1847. Its main activities are scientific, including the evaluation of drugs, foods, and medical equipment, coordination of research, and investigation of medical quackery. It has been largely responsible for improving standards of medical education in the United States. It actively supports worthy health legislation and serves as liaison between Congress, various federal agencies, and the medical profession. Its Judicial Council determines questions relating to the profession's medical ethics.

The association is a nonprofit, self-supporting organization of U.S. physicians in practice. Its membership includes women physicians, who were first admitted in 1876. Nurses cannot be members of this organization, but they do participate in conferences and provide input on the changes in nursing.

World Health Organization

The World Health Organization (WHO) came into being on April 7, 1948, on the basis of a constitution signed in New York on July 22, 1946. An interim commission functioned during the intervening period. The functions of WHO are the eradication of epidemic, endemic, and other diseases; the improvement of nutrition, housing, sanitation, and other aspects of environmental hygiene; the improvement of maternal and child health; and research in the field of private and public health.

Although individual nurses do not belong to WHO, there are many leaders in nursing who have participated in its programs. Such leaders include Ruth Sleeper and Marion Sheahan. These are nurses who have met with others involved in the health of the world.

American Public Health Association

The American Public Health Association was founded in 1872. It is the professional organization of federal, state, and local health officers, personnel of national voluntary health agencies, and industrial health workers. The organization maintains a vocational counseling and placement service.

This organization offers activities for nurses as well as for all other persons working in the health field. These provide a supplement to the activities in either the ANA or the NLN.

Nurses' Association of the American College of Obstetricians and Gynecologists

In August 1968 the Nurses' Association of the American College of Obstetricians and Gynecologists* was formed for nurses interested in obstetrics and gynecology. Its purpose is to promote the highest standards of obstetrical, gynecological, and neonatal nursing practice, education and research. It publishes the *Journal of Obstetric, Gynecological and Neonatal Nursing*.

Junior College Association

The Junior College Association has taken an active part in understanding and interpreting the associate degree program in nursing. Support for these programs began early in the development of 2-year nursing education programs. Conferences

---

*Yakes, N., and Akey, D.: Encyclopedia of associations, ed. 13, vol. 1, National Organizations of the U.S., Section 8, Health and medical organizations, Detroit, 1979, Gale Research Co.

---

*Headquarters: Suite 2700, 1 E. Wacker Dr., Chicago, Ill. 60601.

have been held yearly with faculties of nursing programs and administrators of colleges in order to understand and promote nursing education in the junior college system.

Other organizations

In addition to thinking about joining organizations that deal directly with nursing, the hospital field, or the medical field, nurses should consider belonging to other types of organizations that are community centered—organizations that would place the nurse in contact with persons in other professions who would help the nurse use professional talent in a way different from actual nursing practice. There are many kinds of organizations in local communities that are looking for the person who wants outside activities.

Organizations for men are Rotary, Kiwanis, Lions Club, and chambers of commerce. Many others are available. For women there are Ladies of Rotary, Ladies of Kiwanians, Seroptomists, Altrusa, the Junior League, and business-professional women's organizations. These are the places where citizens meet new friends, share ideas, and help in promoting the interests of the community at large. It is not wise to belong only to professional organizations. It is an obligation to belong to professional organizations, but belonging to other organizations is determined by one's own needs and desires to fulfill the obligations one has as a citizen.

SUMMARY

The practice of professional nursing is an art and science. It is a way of life requiring the nurse to adhere to standards and a code of ethics and to continue the quest for new knowledge. It is contributing to a client's welfare through the delivery of nursing care.

Participation in the professional organization of ANA is one way a nurse can demonstrate commitment to professional nursing. The ANA is designed to assist the individual nurse by setting standards of education, service, economic and general welfare, and research. The NLN provides an opportunity for nurses and nonnurses to join together in promoting nursing in all its aspects to improve nursing care to meet the needs of society. Specialty organizations are available for the nurse to foster high standards for that specialty. Nurses are encouraged to join other organizations such as the American Hospital Association and community organizations that may not be health related.

Discussion questions

1. Discuss the difference between profession and professional.
2. Discuss the six basic elements that define a profession.
3. Discuss the characteristics common to professionals.
4. Discuss the rationale for a nurse to belong to the A.N.A.
5. Discuss the difference between a professional and nonprofessional organization.

SUGGESTED READINGS

Academy of Nursing admits 33 fellows, Am. Nurse **7:**3, 14, Oct. 17, 1975.

American National Red Cross: American Red Cross nursing services, Washington, D.C., Aug. 1967, The Red Cross.

Arnold, V.: The past: way to the future, Int. Nurs. Rev. **21:**68-76, April 1974.

Arnold, V.: Years of growth in international services to nursing, Int. Nurs. Rev. **21:**96-106, April 1974.

Bridges, D.C.: The importance of professional organization—national and international, Int. Nurs. Rec. **8:**5, Jan.-Feb. 1961.

Buscaglia, L.: The way of the bull, Thorofare, N.J., 1973, Charles B. Slack, Inc.

Dagsland, H.: A profession and its leadership, Int. Nurs. Rev. **28:**114-115, July-Aug. 1981.

Divided we fall (editorial), Nurs. Outlook **22:**159, March 1974.

Flanagan, L.: One strong voice, the story of the American Nurses' Association, Kansas City, Mo., 1976, American Nurses' Association.

Forster, M.: What ICU means to me, Int. Nurs. Rev. **24:**74, May 1977.

Haynes, I.: N.L.N. at ten, Nurs. Outlook **10:**372, June 1962.

ICN '77, Am. J. Nurs. **77:**1303-1310, Aug. 1977.

Johnston, S.C.: The use of the Rines model in differentiating professional and technical practice, Nurs. Health Care **3**(7):374-379, 1982.

Kluge, E.: Nursing: vocation or profession, Can. Nurse **78:**34-36, Feb. 1982.

LaMonica, E.L., and Siegel, F.F.: A professional organization that helps all of us, J. Nurs. Admin. **9:**16-18, May 1979.

Leone, L.P.: The league idea at work for nursing, Nurs. Outlook **11:**251, April 1963.

Lewis, E.: How it all came about (editorial), Nurs. Outlook **25:**96-97, Feb. 1977.

Merton, R.K.: Dilemmas of democracy in the voluntary associations, Am. J. Nurs. **66:**1055, May 1966.

Messages from three presidents: Nurs. Outlook **10:**378, June 1962.

Milner, I., and Shae, E.: A.N.A. and affirmative action, Am. J. Nurs. **73:**1738, 1973.

Nichols, B.: Rebuttal A.N.A.: A multipurpose, representative professional association, J. Nurs. Admin. **9:**19-21, May 1979.

NLN Convention, 1979: Nurs. Outlook **28:**398-405, June 1979.

Powell, F.: Changing A.N.A. to meet changing needs. I and II, Am. J. Nurs. **64:**111, 113, March and April 1964.

O'Reilly, D.: Toward autonomy of the nursing profession, Nurs. Leadership **5:**18-22, Sept. 1982.

Schrader, E.: Should federation be a nursing superorganization (editorial), A.O.R.N.J. **21:**759-60, April 1975.

Stuart, G.W.: How professionalized is nursing? Image **13**(1):18-23, 1981.

Styles, M.M.: On nursing: toward a new endowment, St. Louis, 1982, The C.V. Mosby Co.

Styles, M., and Wilson, H.S.: The third resolution, Nurs. Outlook **28:**42-44, Jan. 1979.

Walsh, M.E.: N.L.N. faces the seventies (editorial), Nurs. Outlook **18:**27, March 1970.

CHAPTER 14
Legal aspects of nursing and licensure

OBJECTIVE: On completion of this chapter, the student of nursing will have an understanding of how the law influences nurses and nursing practice.

The primary thrust of this chapter is to provide an understanding of how the law influences the practice of nursing. It is the function of the law to constantly define and redefine individual and societal rights and obligations and to balance the conflicting interests of personal freedom and public welfare. In this regard, changes in the law would constantly modify the sphere of acceptable practice within which the nurse must function. The content here is basic, somewhat simplistic, and meant to be foundational. A comprehensive source of information on this whole area is *Legal Accountability in the Nursing Process.**

Every student of professional nursing has a personal and ethical responsibility to be aware of state licensing laws and other facets of the law as it affects practice. There is a difference between one's ethical or moral responsibility and legal responsibility. Ethics refers to the science of moral duty involving ideal human character and moral principles, quality, or practice. Since ethical conduct stems from the person's own religious beliefs and standards of conduct taught throughout childhood, the individual nurse is governed by an individual ethical code, the professional code for nurses, as well as the affirmation duties the law imposes.

The nurse, in addition to knowing statutory law and being aware of the common law, should know the contents of the professional code for nurses, as set forth by the American Nurses' Association (ANA). Although the code is not enforceable by the ANA, it does provide guidelines for the professional nurse to follow (see Chapter 13).

FUNCTION OF LAW IN SOCIETY*

Laws have developed over the centuries to balance the rights of the individual with the needs of society as a whole, to correct inequities, to punish forbidden acts. Laws arose in part from the religious teachings of right and wrong. They respond to changes in customs, acknowledge and incorporate advancements of technology, promote changes that may benefit society, and redefine minimum standards of behavior in light of these changes. Laws should be viewed as a positive force that provides a foundation for the everyday orderly transaction of human affairs.

Laws enacted through the legislative process are called statutes. They define the obligation of the citizen to act in a particular manner, for example, to follow the speed limits or be sanctioned. The criminal laws are mostly statutory. These define which acts, intentionally done or where intent is presumed, are forbidden and what punishment can be rendered for the commission of such acts.

---

*Murchison, I.A., Nichols, T.S., and Hanson, R.: St. Louis, 1978, The C.V. Mosby Co.

*Material on pp. 212-219 contributed by Shirley Mowdood, R.N., B.S.N., J.D., Attorney at Law, Akron, Ohio.

Decisions arising out of the judicial process are called the common law. Judges, when hearing a case or controversy, determine what law applies to the facts and what the law allows or condemns. Judges act to define or construe statutes; when their meaning is ambiguous, they apply earlier common law decisions to the facts. When a jury is present during a trial, it is the finder of facts; otherwise a judge acts as the finder of facts as well as finder of the law. The law to be applied in civil actions, particularly negligence actions, comes from earlier common law decisions dealing with similar fact situations as well as from statutes. When no similar fact situations have been ruled on, reasoning from analogous situations is used, or a precedent is said to be established.

To illustrate the difference between the types of rights and responsibilities a citizen may have, all citizens have a right to the use of the highways or public roads provided they are properly licensed as required by statute. This right, however, carries the obligation to know and obey the speed limits and other traffic laws and regulations and to drive with reasonable care for the safety of all other users of the road. When one violates a traffic law and is cited for speeding, the law provides that a fine may be imposed or a license suspended. The driver's intention is irrelevant. When one uses a motor vehicle intentionally or recklessly to injure another, a criminal charge may be brought by the state that could result in a jail sentence. When one unintentionally harms another's person or property by the negligent use of a motor vehicle, the individual who was harmed may bring a civil action for money damages.

Criminal prosecution is not concerned with compensation to the injured party. It is an action by the state for the disruption of the peace and tranquility of society as a whole. Traffic regulations define the minimum standards by which all citizens are bound. A civil action, on the other hand, is concerned with compensating the injured individual with money damages. This is an attempt to make the injured party whole again, although money, clearly, cannot compensate someone completely for loss of a bodily function or loss of another person.

Nurses are subject to the law in the same way. Each state legislature has enacted a nurse practice act that defines who can practice nursing and what responsibilities it entails. Failure to comply with statutory requirements may result in the suspension of the nurse's license to practice by the administrative agency charged with the duty of regulating nursing practice. If a nurse violates a criminal statute, as, for example, in an assault, the state will seek to bring criminal charges against that nurse separately from any action of the administrative body. Here the state must usually prove beyond a reasonable doubt that the nurse *intentionally* injured another individual; however, if an action is grossly negligent it may rise to the level of criminal negligence, as in negligent homicide, and intention is not required for penalty to be applied. If the nurse unintentionally injures an individual for whose care the nurse is charged, that patient may bring a civil action in negligence for damages. A different burden of proof is required. This shall be discussed more fully later. The individual can also bring a civil action for money damages where the nurse intentionally harmed him or her.

Although the actions of the administrative agency, such as a state board of nursing, are granted a presumption of constitutionality, constitutional safeguards—for example, due process, notice and a hearing, lack of arbitrariness, clarity, reasonableness and equal protection—must be met. Lack of fundamental fairness may be charged by one who wishes to challenge a finding of the administrative agency when there is no basis for the finding of the agency relative to the conduct it is charged with regulating.

THE NEGLIGENCE CAUSE OF ACTION

When one breaches the standard of care by doing an act or failing to act when there is a legal duty to do so, that individual can be liable in damages for any injury resulting. It is not sufficient that there is injury, no matter how grievous, but there must be a direct relationship between the act or omission complained of and the injury caused. A legal duty, once determined to be present, is breached by an act or omission that does not conform to the prevailing standard of care. The standard of care is determined by establishing how another nurse, in the same or similar circumstances, would have acted.

Negligence does not exist in the abstract but, rather, becomes a legal issue when the requisite facts and circumstances are put into evidence in a controversy between individuals. To sue and win in a negligence cause of action, the person suing must prove by a preponderance of the evidence *each and every one* of the following elements, which were indicated earlier and are explained more fully here:

1. A legal duty to the individual existed.
2. The legal duty was breached by the failure to conform to the standard of care by an act or omission.
3. A close causal connection was proved between the act or omission and the resulting injury, and it was foreseeable that such act or omission could cause injury.
4. The individual was actually harmed.

These elements are elaborated in the following cases, which exemplify situations which nurses may encounter and in which it is assumed that a former patient is suing:

A nurse has a legal duty to exercise reasonable care to see that no unnecessary harm comes to the patient under the nurse's care. Example, the nurse must use reasonable care in the administration of drugs. The nurse has a legal duty to administer the correct drug in the proper amount at the times ordered by the appropriate means according to the order of the physician and in conjunction with the nurse's knowledge of pharmacology and the individual being treated. Further, the nurse has a duty to be aware of possible drug reactions and to act reasonably should one occur.

A charge of negligence does not arise because a patient had a drug reaction that was not foreseeable. However, if in the course of care of the patient, the nurse administers the wrong drug or fails to be aware of the reaction or respond reasonably to it, the nurse has failed in that duty to exercise reasonable care to see that no unnecessary harm came to the patient.*

The nurse must act reasonably, or the nurse's actions must conform to how other reasonable nurses in the same or similar situations would have acted. Example: If an industrial nurse treated a patient who sustained a puncture wound, the standard of care would be to probe the wound for foreign bodies that could reasonably be present. It would also require that if such foreign bodies could be deeply imbedded in a wound, the patient would be referred to a physician. Further, it would be unreasonable for a nurse to fail to refer to a physician any condition that the nurse was not competent to treat. In such a situation the nurse could be said to have acted unreasonably if the nurse failed to probe the wound and refer the patient to a physician. In so doing, the nurse failed to conform to the standard of care established.† In a trial the standard would be established through testimony of other nurses who were equally qualified as the defendant nurse or by an expert in the field.

For a long time the standard of care was determined by the "locality rule" (i.e., what nurses in the same or similar locality would have done). Today the locality rule has been abrogated because a national standard for nursing education and practice has developed.

It must be proved that there was a direct causal connection between the act or omission and the resulting injury and that it was foreseeable that such act or omission would cause injury. Example: A patient sustained a broken left leg and was seen by a physician who ordered that the circulation of

---

*Budgen vs. *Harbour View Hospital,* Nov. 5c. 2, 2DLR 388 "1947."
†*Cooper* vs. *National Motor Bearing Co.,* 136 Cal App. 2d, 299, 288 p. 2d 581, "1955."

the left foot be carefully monitored. Between 11 PM and 6 AM, there were no notations by the nurse that the foot was examined. At 6 AM the nurse noticed that the left foot was cold and dusky. The failure of the nurse to note the condition of the foot during the night or to inform the physician of the condition lead to the eventual amputation of the leg. The nurse should have known that the damage from ischemia becomes irreversible in a matter of hours. Therefore the nurse's failure to observe and inform was a direct proximate cause of the subsequent amputation, and it was foreseeable that such an injury could result if constant observations were not made and reported.*

The patient was actually harmed. There are many times where incidents occur or mistakes are made. For the patient to become a successful claimant, the mistake must cause injury. A medication error that does not increase a patient's pain or suffering or alter the disease process probably causes no actionable harm to the patient.

In the examples just given the nurses were found negligent. In the first example the nurse supplied the physician with the wrong medication (epinephrine instead of novocaine) during a minor surgical procedure with the resultant death of the patient. In the second example an industrial nurse failed to probe a puncture wound for a foreign object and failed to direct the patient to a physician after the wound did not heal properly. This patient subsequently developed skin cancer, found to be attributable to these acts. In the third example a youth had to have his leg amputated at the knee joint as a result of irreversible ischemia. In each of the cases, all the criteria of negligence discussed were satisfied.

DOCTRINE OF RES IPSA LOQUITUR

There is one other way in which an individual may prevail in a lawsuit alleging that an injury occurred as a result of someone's acts or omissions,

---

Collins vs. Westlake Community Hospital, 57 Ill. 2d, 388, 312 N.E. 2d, 614, ''1974.''

without proving all the elements required in a negligence action. This is through use of the legal doctrine of res ipsa loquitur, that is, ''the thing speaks for itself.'' This doctrine permits the plaintiff to allege and prove only the following:

1. But for the negligence of someone, the injury would not have occurred.
2. Whatever or whoever caused the injury was under the direction and control of the individual named as defendant.
3. The individual plaintiff in no way caused or contributed to the injury (contributory negligence as a defense is discussed later).

An example of such a case would be that of a comatose patient who, as a part of the prescribed treatment, was to receive hot water bottles to the extremities. Two hours after the hot water bottle was applied, a nurse discovered a large reddened and blistered area on the extremity where the hot water bottle has been. In a lawsuit the patient's case would be proved if the above circumstances were shown to be true. The individual need not prove what standard of care applied or that it had been breached nor that injury was foreseeable. Obviously, the comatose individual in this situation could not have contributed to the injury. The individual charged with the negligence now has the burden to prove that the burn did not occur through his or her negligence. This cause of action, because it allows such a powerful inference of negligence, is severely limited to those cases in which the three criteria listed are precisely met. The courts have decided as a policy decision that in instances in which it would be impossible for the plaintiff to establish the who, what, when, and where of the case but the plaintiff can establish the above factors, the defendant must then prove that injury did not occur because of his or her negligence.

ALLOCATION OF LOSS

Vicarious liability is the legal doctrine which provides that a party without any wrongful or negligent conduct of his or her own may be responsible for the acts of another. Since normally individuals are responsible for their own acts and their consequences, this legal doctrine, to be understood, must be viewed as a policy decision made by the courts and legislatures. The purpose is to allocate the risks of loss (damages) to the one who can best bear them, the one on whose behalf the acts were performed.

One type of vicarious liability is respondeat superior. When it is applied, the losses caused by the wrongful acts of the servant, which were done while the servant was conducting the master's business, are placed on the master because the master is better able to bear the loss or redistribute the losses through price and rate increases and through insurance. Additionally, it was for the master's benefit that the servant was engaged in the acts that caused the injury. In a hospital situation the nurse is the servant and the master is the hospital.

One group of employees must bear the burden of their acts directly and may not rely on the doctrine of respondeat superior to allocate the damages: independent contractors. An independent contractor can be identified by looking at the amount of control the employer has over the mode and manner of the work to be done. Employees of a hospital, whether resident physicians, nurses, or maintenance persons, all fall within that group over which the hospital has control and for which the hospital must respond in damages if they negligently harm a patient. Attending physicians and private duty nurses are usually viewed as independent contractors, since the hospital does not have control over the manner in which their work is done.

Even though the nurse is an employee of the hospital, this does not mean that the negligent nurse may not individually be sued. The nurse who is charged with negligence may be sued and a money judgment taken against the nurse if the charge is proved. The hospital, as employer, is also legally responsible for the wrongful acts and must also respond in damages so that the injured party is made whole. All nurses employed by hospitals, especially if the hospital is self-insured, should have a clear understanding of their individual exposure to liability under this doctrine. When a nurse is working directly under the supervision and control of a physician, the physician may be vicariously liable for the nurse's negligence, but this does not relieve the nurse from individual liability.

There is a new species of negligence action that deals with the liability of the institution for corporate wrongdoing. It is also important to note that the employer, that is, the hospital, aside from its vicarious liability, is the one in the best position to know who is competent or qualified to perform the work required and to provide the personnel necessary. Particularly in the hospital situation, only the employer can make decisions about staffing, the ratio of staff and patients, qualifications, kinds of personnel, available equipment, specialty units, and availability of physicians or house staff to maintain quality care. The nurse has little input into such quality control decisions that directly affect patient care. The hospital itself is liable for losses to patients as a result of its negligence as the employer, in addition to its liability for negligent acts of its servants, the nurses. The law has recognized that the hospital, while holding itself out as a provider of quality care, owes a duty to the patient to ensure that adequate care is provided. In a recent case, the plaintiff used as evidence of the standard of care to which the hospital should be held the *Standards for Hospital Accreditation of the Joint Commission in Accreditation,* to which the hospital had applied. The court took the view that the hospital was more than a building of brick and stone and that it had a duty independent of that of the physician to monitor the care that the patients receive. The standards for hospital accreditation, state licensing regulations, and hospital's bylaws demonstrate that the medical profession and other responsible authorities regarded as both desirable and feasible a hospital's assumption of certain responsibilities for the care of the patient. This view of hospital liability now provides the injured party with another source from which to recover damages.*

The liability of the hospital for failure to provide equipment in good working order has long been established and is a type of strict liability. That is, if the equipment is offered for use on the patient and it malfunctions, even though not being used negligently, and the patient is injured thereby, the hospital is liable for those injuries without a showing of negligence.

DETERMINATION OF DAMAGES

Once negligence has been proved, damages are awarded to compensate the injured individual. Compensated items include medical and hospital expenses, loss of wages, pain and suffering, anticipated cost of future treatment, humiliation or anguish for disfiguring scar or injury, permanent disability, and loss of future income. Plaintiffs are compensated on an individual basis, since it is not the injury itself that is compensated but the effect of that injury on the particular person. A broken leg, for example, that heals improperly due to negligence will result in a larger award of damages to a ballet dancer than to a sedentary individual.

Punitive (or exemplary) damages are awarded to the injured party to punish the wrongdoer and are not awarded in the typical negligence action. Punitive damages may be awarded, however, where an act was done intentionally or the negligent acts were so recklessly done as to constitute a total disregard of the consequences.

DEFENSES

Every individual injured by the acts of another has a right to bring a lawsuit to determine fault, and, if fault is proved, to be awarded compensation for the injury. This person is called the plaintiff. The individual alleged to have caused the wrong, the defendant, also has the right to raise whatever

---

Darling vs. *Charleston Community Memorial Hospital*, 33 Ill. 3d 326, 211 N.E. 2d 253, ''1966.''

defenses are available. The trier of the facts, usually a jury, will not find in favor of the plaintiff until the trier is convinced that the plaintiff has proved by a preponderance of the evidence each and every element of the charge of negligence. The defendant in a lawsuit should never forget that it is the plaintiff's duty to prove his or her case. However, once the plaintiff has put in enough evidence to do so, the defense must then present its case to attempt to disprove or disclaim the plaintiff's evidence. If the trier of facts finds that the evidence is about equal, pro and con, then the defendant wins, for the plaintiff must prove its case by the greater weight of the evidence. This differs from a criminal case, in which the burden of proof necessary to convict is that amount of evidence that convinces the jury beyond a reasonable doubt.

STATUTE OF LIMITATIONS

In most states an action for negligence against a nurse must be brought within 2 to 3 years from the date the act or occurrence complained of occurred. An exception may be where the act complained of is not discoverable for a longer period of time, as, for example, a hemostat in a surgical site. The time may then be lengthened to 2 to 3 years from the time the plaintiff knew or should have known that something was wrong. If the plaintiff fails to file the lawsuit within the time allotted by statute, the plaintiff may not then file at all and is said to be barred by the statute of limitations.

CONTRIBUTORY OR COMPARATIVE NEGLIGENCE

When a plaintiff by his or her actions contributes to the injury complained of, the plaintiff may be limited or barred from recovery. In the hot water bottle example, if the patient had not been comatose, the patient would have complained that the bottle was too hot, since one has a duty to use ordinary care for oneself. If a patient who as a practical joke gets into another patient's bed, identifies himself as the other patient, receives the second patient's medication, and is injured thereby—although the nurse should have checked the patient's identification band—the patient certainly contributed to the injury by misconduct. Many states by statute or common law have laws requiring that the plaintiff be completely free from contributory negligence. Other states have laws requiring that when an individual may have contributed to the injury, the plaintiff may only recover whatever proportionate amount of damages were caused by the defendant. In either event, then, if the individual's act actively contributed to the injuries received, this is a partial or complete defense.

EMERGENCY EXCEPTION

Although a life-threatening situation is not uncommon in hospitals, when a bona fide emergency exists, the law does not require juries or a trier of facts to look back with 20/20 hindsight to determine what ought to have been done. The chief question will be the reasonableness of what action was taken in light of the fact and circumstances and the courses of action available at the time of the emergency. A nurse who acts reasonably given the circumstances of the time of an emergency will not be found guilty of negligence.

CONFIDENTIALITY

The nurse has an affirmative duty to protect the patient's privacy and to safeguard information that comes to the nurse through contact with the patient. That is, the nurse should not divulge any information given in the course of nurse-patient relationship unless first the patient agrees. This patient-nurse privilege of confidentiality, however, is upheld only in a few states. Where this privilege is upheld, the nurse may not be compelled in court or otherwise to reveal the confidences. Once, however, the patient becomes a plaintiff in a lawsuit, charging the nurse with negligence, the patient

waives that privilege and the nurse is released from that obligation of silence.

Patients have rights to personal privacy to which all health care personnel must be sensitive and which must be protected. They also have rights with respect to privacy of medical records and unauthorized photography. Only the patient, or the personal representative so authorized, may waive these rights. A waiver must be in writing, and the consent must meet the requirements of informed consent; that is, the patient must be clearly informed of the use to which said picture or records will be put. One common example of such a waiver is one to the insurance carrier of the patient giving the insuror the right to review all medical records. Another example especially in large teaching hospitals (where a waiver is needed but not always obtained) is one granting use of patients' records at medical grand rounds.

The nurse, as employee of the hospital, should recognize the hospital's policy toward protecting these legal rights of patients and act accordingly.

FUTURE TRENDS

Plaintiffs determine whom to sue on the basis of, in part, the ability to collect a judgment of damages. Whether to sue a nurse is primarily determined by the nurse's mode of employment. It is true that nurses may be sued individually, but, practically speaking, plaintiffs elect to sue the employer when the doctrine of respondeat superior applies. At the present time, if a nurse was working within the scope of employment when the negligence occurred, the employer *must* respond in damages. The next question is whether the employer will elect to sue the nurse to recover whatever damages were paid to the plaintiff. This can be a matter of contract or of policy. Nurses should require clarification of this issue in writing at the time of employment. The nurse may then elect to carry individual liability insurance. Clearly, if the acts or omission complained of by the plaintiff were outside the nurse's employment (e.g., unauthorized practice of medicine), the nurse would be the primary target of the suit.

Nurses who are employed as well as independent practitioners should carry individual liability insurance. Once all nurses are perceived to have insurance coverage, they may succeed in becoming target defendants. The courts or legislators could make a policy decision that nurses must stand to answer in damage for any or all negligence. Nurses must understand the ramification of such a policy change. They should work through their state and national organization to present their views on such a policy change. It would require that hospitals accept and use nursing input into staffing decisions. Nurses must decline to be ''floated'' to cover areas where they are unqualified, unprepared, or nonoriented. Nurses should use peer review or other comparable means to police their own procedures and promote a standard of practice based on the standards of care to which they would answer legally.

CONTRACTS

A knowledge of the general rules of contract law is useful to the nurse in various situations. Whether a person is an employee or independent contractor determines rights to workmen's compensation, protection from liability suits, and other benefits.

A contract is an agreement between two or more persons. It implies mutual promises enforceable by law. A contract may be an oral agreement or a written document. Legally, to be enforceable, a contract must include the offer of one or more parties, and the acceptance of the offer by the other party; both parties must have the legal capacity to contract; the contract must be for a lawful purpose, and the value of services or monies involved must be stated.

When accepting an offer of employment, the nurse contracts or promises to perform various services for the employer. The contract obligates the nurse to work on behalf of and in the manner dictated by the employer. The employing agency promises to pay a certain salary and offers certain benefits. The employer is obligated to provide safe working conditions and equipment for the nurse to use.

Contracts may be made by two parties face to face. They also can be made by a third party acting as an agent for one of the parties, as, for example, when a registry secures a private duty nurse for a patient. The patient and nurse do not agree face to face regarding the terms of employment, but the registry has overall terms of employment that are accepted.

A contract may state how both parties involved may dissolve the agreement. A contract may be dissolved by mutual consent or by failure of one of the parties to fulfill a promise or promises. The law recognizes it to be a duty to fulfill mutual promises in a contract. When that duty is not performed by either party, the contract is breached, giving the parties certain legal recourses.

AUTOPSIES

In most states before an autopsy can be performed, legal consent must be obtained from the next of kin. This should be the closest relative of the deceased. It is important that the autopsy slip be read by the family so that they will be aware of what will happen. It is also important that the physician seeking the consent give the patient's family some understanding of what will occur during an autopsy. There may be limitations placed on the autopsy, for example, an examination of the head might not be allowed; therefore this exclusion would have to be placed on the autopsy sheet. Generally speaking, the nurse does not ask for the autopsy. This is usually the physician's responsibility. However, it may be the nurse's responsibility to sign along with the physician the slip witnessing the signature of the relative. This the nurse should do only after having been with the physician and the relative during the discussion of the need for the autopsy so that the nurse could testify if necessary that the family gave a voluntary, informed consent.

LICENSURE
Historical aspects

The ANA began in 1896 as a general society of graduate nurses called the Nurses' Associated Alumnae of the United States and Canada. In 1911 the original name was changed to the American Nurses' Association. From the time of the inception of the organization in 1896, the members saw the need for legislation that would set standards. The ANA continues to assume responsibility for legislation that affects nursing.

North Carolina was the first state to pass a law to license nurses. The attempt to pass such legislation was opposed, but a law to license nurses was enacted in March 1903. New Jersey and New York also enacted licensing laws in April 1903, and in quick sucession four other states passed their first laws. However, it was not until 1952 that all states and territories had a nurse practice act. Throughout the years, to amend existing laws and pass new laws, nurses through organized effort interpreted to the public and to legislators the need for legislation to ensure safe nursing care for the public.

Nursing is the only profession that began with permissive licensing laws. Practice of professional nursing was not protected. Under a permissive law, individuals may practice nursing as long as they do not use protected titles such as "registered nurse." Permissive laws do not protect the public.

Mandatory licensure protects the title of registered nurse, defines the practice of nursing, and states the educational requirements of the nurse. New York in 1938 was the first state to pass a mandatory law, although it was not put into effect until 1947. Mandatory licensure means it is illegal to practice nursing for compensation without a license. As of 1980 all states and territories have mandatory nurse practice acts except Texas, which continues to have a permissive nurse practice act. The Texas Board, however, states that licensure is expected of all RNs. Employers of all RNs do require licensure as a condition of employment.

The ANA in the 1950s published a manual entitled *Principles of Legislation Relating to the Practice of Nursing*. The manual set forth a model law for state nurses' associations to follow when preparing legislation relating to the practice of nursing. This was a model for a mandatory law. The definition of the practice of nursing included in the early licensing laws had been developed over a period of years by the ANA with the advice of attorneys and well-qualified nurses.

This definition served as the one used by most states and was considered acceptable until the 1970s, at which time many states enacted new state practice acts to redefine nursing. The issue during this period was to more clearly define nursing as an independent profession. New York, in 1971, was the first state to enact a new law that provided for the use of "nursing diagnosis." The New York law also provided for independent practice as a part of the nurse's role. California, Idaho, Washington, Colorado, and other states quickly followed with similar definitions of nursing.

The entire issue of licensure became one of question. Should there be licensure? Should there be more than one type of licensure for RNs? Should licensure be required for all health workers? What is the purpose of licensure—protection of the public or prestige of the worker?

Hershey* maintained in 1968 that licensure was no longer in the interest of the public but merely served to protect the status and economic position of the licensee. He further indicated that as other health workers seek licensure, it becomes even more unwieldy and meaningless.

However, the recommendations for licensure in the Lysaught report (1970) were:

(1) all remaining states, without mandatory licensure laws for registered nurses, immediately adopt appropriate regulations to this effect, (2) all state licensure laws for nursing be revised to require periodic review of the individual's qualifications for practice as a condition for licensure renewal, (3) the language of licensing laws in

*Hershey, N.: Lawyer holds licensure not in public interest, Am. J. Nurs. **68**:1408, July 1968.

Legal aspects of nursing and licensure   **221**

nursing and medicine be couched in flexible terms to permit role evaluation in accord with the emergency features of health service, (4) in view of the emergence of advanced levels of clinical practice in nursing; a single license be retained for the registered nurse, and advanced levels of nursing practice be recognized through: designation by approved bodies of such purposes, presumably the Academy of Nursing; state licensing standards for health service units, qualifications for personnel policies for appointments, promotions and compensation.*

As the basis of licensure has been questioned, one alternative presented has been institutional licensure. The idea was promulgated because of the number of health workers, licensed and unlicensed, working in hospitals. Each health occupation classification was seeking licensure, which meant that if laws were enacted for each occupation, flexibility in the use of personnel would disappear. Because of this situation, the American Hospital Association asked for a national moratorium on licensing of new personnel in 1971. During the 1970s much time was spent discussing individual versus institutional licensure. Institutional licensure is licensure of the hospital, which then can utilize the health worker, including the nurse, in any position that is needed at the moment. Although workers would have specific responsibilities, if a need arose, the worker would move from one role to another without violating a specific licensure act.

In 1973 the ANA House of Delegates reaffirmed its support of individual nurse licensure as one means of assuring the public that nursing practitioners possess the basic knowledge and skills to enter the profession and voiced opposition to institutional licensure. The ANA assumed the position that nursing is a discipline with a specific body of knowledge and should be protected by laws that define nursing and who should practice nursing. Whether individual or institutional licensure is the valid approach, the most important issue is to as-

sure that the public receives nursing care only from competent practitioners.

In 1981 the ANA published a new manual entitled *The Nursing Practice Act: Suggested State Legislation*. In this document two definitions of nursing were suggested to be used in revised nurse practice acts. They are as follows:

The practice of nursing means the performance for compensation of professional services requiring substantial specialized knowledge of the biological, physical, behavioral, psychological, and sociological sciences and of nursing theory as the basis for assessment, diagnosis, planning, intervention, and evaluation in the promotion and maintenance of health; the casefinding and management of illness, injury, or infirmity; the restoration of optimum function; or the achievement of a dignified death. Nursing practice includes but is not limited to administration, teaching, counseling, supervision, delegation, and evaluation of practice and execution of the medical regimen, *including the administration of medications and treatments prescribed by any person authorized by state law to prescribe*. Each registered nurse is directly accountable and responsible to the consumer for the quality of nursing care rendered.

The practice of practical nursing means the performance for compensation of technical services requiring basic knowledge of the biological, physical, behavioral, psychological, and sociological sciences and of nursing procedures. These services are performed under the supervision of a registered nurse and utilize standardized procedures leading to predictable outcomes in the observation and care of the ill, injured, and infirm; in the maintenance of health; in action to safeguard life and health; and *in the administration of medications and treatments prescribed by any person authorized by state law to prescribe*.*

The following year, 1982, the Council of State Boards of Nursing published their manual entitled *The Model Nursing Practice Act*. They defined the practice of nursing, the registered nurse, and the practical nurse. These definitions are as follows†:

---

*National Commission for the Study of Nursing and Nursing Education, Jerome P. Lysaught, director: An abstract for action. Copyright by McGraw-Hill, Inc. Used by permission of McGraw-Hill Book Co., pp. 141-144.

*The nursing practice act: suggested state legislation, Kansas City, Kan., 1981, American Nurses' Association, p. 6.
†The model nursing practice act, Chicago, 1982, Council of State Boards of Nursing, pp. 2-3.

The "Practice of Nursing" means assisting individuals or groups to maintain or attain optimal health throughout the life process by assessing their health status, establishing a diagnosis, planning and implementing a strategy of care to accomplish defined goals, and evaluating responses to care and treatment.

"Registered Nurse" means a person who practices professional nursing by:

a. Assessing the health status of individuals and groups;
b. Establishing a nursing diagnosis;
c. Establishing goals to meet identified health care needs;
d. Planning a strategy of care;
e. Prescribing nursing interventions to implement the strategy of care;
f. Implementing the strategy of care;
g. Authorizing nursing interventions that may be performed by others and that do not conflict with this Act;
h. Maintaining safe and effective nursing care rendered directly or indirectly;
i. Evaluating responses to interventions;
j. Teaching the theory and practice of nursing;
k. Managing the practice of nursing; and
l. Collaborating with other health professionals in the management of health care.

"Licensed Practical Nurse" means a person who practices nursing by:

a. Contributing to the assessment of the health status of individuals and groups;
b. Participating in the development and modification of the strategy of care;
c. Implementing the appropriate aspects of the strategy of care as defined by the Board;
d. Maintaining safe and effective nursing care rendered directly or indirectly;
e. Participating in the evaluation of responses to interventions; and
f. Delegating nursing interventions that may be performed by others and that do not conflict with this Act.

The Licensed Practical Nurse functions at the direction of the Registered Nurse, licensed physician, or licensed dentist in the performance of activities delegated by that health care professional.

It is one thing to be licensed at the beginning of practice but it is another to maintain competency throughout a lifetime practice. Therefore state laws are being changed to include the provision that nurses show evidence of competence as part of their annual or biennial renewal. California was the first state to enact such a law; in 1975 it became a requirement for all professional nurses to show evidence of continuing their education. However, by 1981 there were efforts to repeal the mandate.

As of 1981, 13 states had enacted legislation to require continuing education as a requirement for renewal of licensure. In some instances states were requiring evidence of continued competency of practice by requiring the licensee to show proof of having practiced nursing in the period of renewal. For example, a nurse had to work 90 days every year to maintain a license as well as attend continuing education courses.

Colorado set aside its first (1979) mandate until 1982 when it was once again approved. Discussion is now in progress to determine if mandating continued education really does help the nurse in maintaining competency. The value of programs offered has received much attention. Chapter 16 discusses continuing education in depth.

Sunset legislation

Sunset legislation was first introduced in Colorado in 1976 with Alabama, Florida, and Louisiana following suit. By 1981, 35 states had enacted such legislation. Sunset legislation provides the avenue for an evaluation process to occur in determining if state agencies should continue to be in existence.

Built into the law is a cyclic review of every state agency. Sunset occurs if no evaluation is done or if on examination the state agency no longer serves in the public interest. The agency can be abolished, altered, or remain. For an agency to continue, legislative action must occur. If no action is taken, the sun is allowed to set on the agency.

Colorado and New Hampshire were among the first states to apply sunset legislation to boards of nursing. Other states, such as Florida and Texas, have gone through the process. On sunset, Colorado and New Hampshire found themselves without state boards of nursing with which to regulate the practice of nursing or approve nursing education programs. Coalitions of nurses quickly formed in order to have the boards reinstated. In order to do this, major changes occurred in each of the nurse practice acts.

All states that have sunset legislation need to be aware of the date their board is scheduled for review. Self-evaluation studies need to be accomplished, and nurses and the public served need to be aware of the board's activities and how well the board meets and discharges their obligations.

In New Hampshire, for example, the sunset commission determined that ''unregulated nursing would not frequently result in major, irreparable harm to the health and safety (of the public.''* The rationale was that for the most part state regulation was not an effective means for the discipline of poor practice.

Sunset legislation is an effective way for state government to monitor all agencies supported by state funds. Particularly as state economic pressures are brought to bear on the efficiency or effectiveness of state government, it has become imperative for state boards of nursing to maintain vigilance on why they exist. Boards of nursing and nurse practice acts exist for the protection of the public and not for the vested interest of the profession.

STATE BOARD OF NURSING

A state board is an administrative agency created by the adoption of a licensing law by the state legislature. The creation of a state board has as its primary purposes the protection and the safeguarding of the public. Requirements for licensure, renewal of licenses, powers of suspension or revocation of licensure, and approval of schools of nursing are established for the welfare of the public. These requirements do have a beneficial aspect for nurses in reserving the practice of nursing or use of the title for those who are properly licensed.

A state board of nursing may be an autonomous agency of state government responsible directly to the governor of the state, or it may be a department of the state government. The board possesses such legal power as is delegated to it by the legislature.

Boards may vary in numbers of members. In the past it was recommended by the ANA that all board members be professional nurses. Selden* believes that boards of nursing entirely composed of professional nurses are archaic. He suggests that unless there are other interests on the board, the public's welfare is not being served and that only the profession of nursing is being protected. As the new laws of the 1970s were enacted, consumers were included as board members to assure that the vested interest of nurses was not dominating the board of nursing. (Consumers are persons who are not members of any of the health care professions.) Most state laws speak to the qualifications for board membership and length of term of office. Board members are appointed by the governer.

The board has three basic functions: licensing of qualified applicants, adjudication of the practice of nursing, and approval of basic nursing education programs. The board in most states is authorized to carry out the following functions:

1. Adopt and, from time to time, revise such rules and regulations not consistent with the law as may be necessary to enable it to carry into effect the provisions of this act.
2. Prescribe standards and approve curricula for educational programs preparing persons for licensure under this act.
3. Provide for surveys of such programs at such times as it may deem necessary.
4. Approve such programs as meet the requirements of the act and of the board.
5. Deny or withdraw approval from educational programs for failures to meet prescribed standards.

*Thomas, C.: Sunset: how and when, Nurse Practitioner 7(4):10-11, 1982.

*Selden, W.K.: Licensing boards are archaic, Am. J. Nurs. **70:**124, Jan. 1970.

6. Examine, license, and renew the licenses of duly qualified applicants.
7. Develop and enforce standards for continuing competency of licensees continuing or returning to practice.
8. Conduct hearings concerning charges calling for discipline of a licensee or revocation of a license.
9. Issue subpoenas, compel the attendance of witnesses, and administer oaths to persons giving testimony at hearings.
10. Cause the prosecution of all persons violating this act and to incur such necessary expenses therefor.
11. Keep a record of all its proceedings.
12. Make an annual report to the governor.

Decisions made by the board must be based on what is the best protection of the public. The board promulgates rules and regulations and makes decisions that will meet the ever-changing needs of society so long as they are within the scope of the law and legislatively delegated powers. The board, after analysis of the law and definition, may also issue opinions in the form of position statements.

To enforce the law, each state board is assisted through the state's attorney general's office. The attorney general's office represents state agencies and boards and on request advises the board informally or in public opinions on legal matters or interpretations of the law (the difference being that official or public opinions are open to the public, whereas other opinions offered as legal adviser are confidential because they are lawyer-client communication).

In 1947 the state boards of nursing requested that the ANA form a committee. The special Committee of State Boards of Nursing was formed, which later became the Council on State Boards of Nursing. It was composed of one professional nurse employee from each state board. The committee made it possible to conduct a more detailed study of specific problems inherent in the implementation of nurse practice acts. Through activities of the committee, boards of nursing were informed of problems and decisions to be made such as how to handle licensure, giving the licensing examination, and drug abuse by nurses.

The Council of State Boards of Nursing voted to become an independent organization in 1978. The organization became known as the National Council of State Boards, Inc. Member states financially support the organization through dues. Each state has two voting representatives. The organization identified its functions to include the development of a statutory definition of nursing practice and standards of nursing education and practice.

The model practice acts prepared by ANA and the National Council of State Boards provide what each believe should appear in a nurse practice act. Rationale for each section appears in the documents. Students and graduates need to familiarize themselves with the two documents so that when state laws are revised they can be informed as to what is considered appropriate contents of an act.

Licensure by examination

State boards of nursing are required by law to provide an examination by which the graduate can qualify to practice nursing. Early board examinations consisted of essay-type questions with a practical examination in a classroom setting. This approach was acceptable until the number of graduates grew to such proportions that it was no longer practical. Individual states had different standards, which caused difficulty when a graduate wanted to move from state to state.

In 1944 state boards united to provide a national examination that would accommodate the larger number of graduates, provide an easier and faster means of scoring the examination, and facilitate movement from one state to another. The National Test Pool has been used since then. The examination became a paper and pencil test in the five major clinical areas: medical nursing, surgical nursing, nursing of children, obstetrical nursing, and psychiatric nursing.

The pattern for the examination remained fairly constant; however, in 1982 the National Council of State Boards Inc. changed the format. Instead of having five parts, as discussed earlier, the examination was prepared as a single one. The content was an integration of all major nursing content. The examination tests minimum knowledge surrounding nursing practice problems. The student needs to integrate the content of physical, social, and behavioral sciences along with pathology, pharmacology, nutrition, and nursing process. The examination is taken over a 2-day period. On receipt of the results the student receives one score and a determination of failure or passing. If failure occurs, the student receives a diagnostic profile giving clues as to where he or she did poorly. In retaking the test, the student takes the entire examination again.

Licensure by endorsement

Licensure by examination usually occurs in the state where the graduate was educated. Licensure by endorsement occurs when movement from the original state of licensure is made. Endorsement verifies the graduate having taken the examination and having graduated from an approved school of nursing.

Licensure by renewal

Renewal of the license varies from state to state; however, annual or biennial renewal is usually required. The nurse is notified to renew a reasonable time before renewal is necessary. Failure to renew a license results in a lapsed license. The law reads that a board may, but does not have to, reinstate a lapsed license. The responsibility to renew rests with the nurse. Often the board may impose an additional fee for reinstatement of a lapsed license.

NURSE PRACTICE ACTS

The state board of nursing is held responsible for administering the nurse practice act to safeguard the public. In recent years state boards of nursing have had increased numbers of cases that involve the individual nurse's practice of nursing. The public and the profession have become increasingly aware of and concerned about the behavior of the individual nurse. Particular areas of concern are negligence, addiction to drugs or alcohol, poor emotional health, and lack of regard for statutory laws.

The decision to revoke or suspend a license is made in the light of facts presented to the board at a hearing. The degree of seriousness of the offense will depend on the issues involved. No decision is made without consideration of all implications for the individual involved and the public. At any time that a nurse is undergoing possible license revocation, legal counsel should be retained.

After a license is revoked, a nurse may appeal to the civil courts for reversal of the board's decision. If in the future the nurse can produce evidence of having been rehabilitated, a license may be reinstated by taking the National Test Pool.

APPROVAL OF SCHOOLS

Boards of nursing at periodic intervals visit schools of nursing for the purpose of approval. Data are collected regarding the total program, and a report is prepared for the board. The board reviews the report at a board meeting and votes on whether to continue approval. The board is concerned with the quality of nursing education. Regulations or standards are written by boards and used to evaluate the programs of schools of nursing. Between survey visits, consultation visits are made. One must graduate from a state-approved school to write a state board examination or be licensed.

SUMMARY

Legislation that is enacted for nurses and nursing is often enacted for the good of the public. The nurse practice act is primarily for the public's protection and not the nurse's protection. The nurse practice act gives the definition of nursing, the requirements a nurse must have to practice nursing, and what must be done to retain the license to practice nursing. Nurses are first licensed by examination and can practice in another state by endorsement. A license is kept up-to-date according to the renewal act of every state. There are two types of licensure laws—mandatory and permissive. The permissive licensure law protects the title only; the mandatory one defines nursing and protects the use of the title. Nurses can be sued for negligence and malpractice. They are held responsible for their own acts, whether they be acts of commission or omission. The ANA and each state association conduct a very active legislative program. It is the professional organization's responsibility to work for laws that will assist the practitioner and the public. Nurses should be aware of the changes in laws both as citizens and as professional individuals.

Discussion questions

1. Discuss the function of law in society and how it relates to the individual nurse and nursing as a profession.
2. Discuss how the standards of practice outlined by the ANA relate to nurses' adherence to your state's nurse practice act.
3. Discuss your state's nurse practice act, the board of nursing function, and the individual nurse's responsibility to maintain an active license.
4. Discuss the difference between permissive and mandatory licensure and how each is or would be enforced.
5. Discuss sunset legislation as it relates to the state in which you reside.

SUGGESTED READINGS

Agree, B.C.: The threat of institutional licensure, Am. J. Nurs. **73:**1758, Oct. 1973.

Creighton, H.: Law every nurse should know, ed. 3, Philadelphia, 1975, W.B. Saunders Co.

Grobe, S.J.: Sunset laws, Am. J. Nurs. **181:**1355-1359, July 1981.

Hershey, N.: Lawyer holds licensure not in public interest, Am. J. Nurs. **68:**1408, July 1968.

Hershey, N.: Licensing revocation, the board of nursing and the court, Am. J. Nurs. **69:**567, March 1969.

Mancini, M.: Death with dignity: are living wills an answer? Am. J. Nurs. **78:**2133, Dec. 1978.

Mancini, M.: Documenting clinical records, Am. J. Nurs. **78:**1556, Sept. 1978.

Mancini, M.: Consent to treatment: what does it entail, Am. J. Nurs. **79:**1139, June 1979.

Mancini, M.: Proving negligence in nursing practice, Am. J. Nurs. **79:**337, Feb. 1979.

Murchison, I.A., and Nichols, T.S.: Legal foundations of nursing practice, New York, 1970, Macmillan Inc.

Murchison, I.A., Nichols, T.S., and Hanson, R.: Legal accountability in the nursing process, St. Louis, 1978, The C.V. Mosby Co.

National Commission for the Study of Nursing and Nursing Education, Jerome P. Lysaught, director: An abstract for action, New York, 1970, McGraw-Hill Book Co.

Rothman, D.A., and Rothman, N.L.: The professional nurse and the law, Boston, 1977, Little, Brown & Co.

Sarner, H.: The nurse and the law, Philadelphia, 1968, W.B. Saunders Co.

Schmidt, M.S.: Why a separate organization for State Boards? Am. J. Nurs. **80:**725, 1980.

Selden, W.K.: Licensing boards are archaic, Am. J. Nurs. **70:**124, Jan. 1970.

Seldon, W.K.: A new licensing exam for nurses, Am. J. Nurs. **80:**723, April 1980.

Shindel, J., and Snyder, M.E.: Legal restraints on restraint, Am. J. Nurs. **81:**393-394, Feb. 1981.

Thomas, C.: Sunset: how and when, Nurse Practitioner **7**(4):10, 1982.

Thomas, C.: Sunset: what and why, Nurse Practitioner **7**(3(:10, 1982.

Thomas, C.: Role evaluation as legislation, Nurse Practitioner **8**(3):9-12, 1983.

Trandel-Korencheck, D., and Trandel-Korencheck, K.: Current legal issues facing nursing practice, Nurs. Admin. Q. **5**(1):37-42, 1980.

Trandel-Korencheck, D. and Trandel-Korencheck, K.: State nursing laws, Nurse Practitioner **5**(6):39-42, 1980.

Trandel-Korencheck, D., and Trandel-Korencheck, K.: Conflicting loyalties of the nurse, Nurs. Admin. Q. **6**(2):63-66, 1982.

Trandel-Korencheck, D., and Trandel-Korencheck, K.: Patients' rights and the preservation of human dignity, Nurs. Admin. Q. **6**(4):83-86, 1982.

Trandel-Korencheck, D., and Trandel-Korencheck, K.: Malpractice and preventive risk management, Nurs. Admin. Q. **3:**75-80, Spring 1983.

CHAPTER 15
Opportunities in nursing

OBJECTIVE: On completion of this chapter, the student of nursing will have knowledge about opportunities available on graduation, be familiar with the requisites for a position, and understand self-goals for entry into the profession of nursing.

As the student pursues various clinical learning experiences, each area of nursing will be considered as a possible field of practice. Often the experience one receives while a student will influence the selection of a specific division of nursing practice after graduation. Many students have identified for themselves before entering school which field of nursing they will pursue as graduates.

It is not unusual for the student to vacillate from one clinical experience to another in trying to determine the area of nursing in which to practice. Nor is it unusual for the student to be unclear at the time of graduation just what his or her long-term future in nursing and professional and personal career goals will be.

However, it is necessary to have knowledge about the opportunities available in order that a personal assessment and self-goals can be made for entry into the profession of nursing.

The purpose of this chapter is to provide information on selecting the beginning position, career planning, areas of nursing practice, and employment responsibilities.

SELF-ASSESSMENT

Before graduation the student needs to begin doing a self-assessment. This process involves the student's evaluation of self-knowledge, such as manual skills, temperament, communication skills, spirituality, role position preference, and cognitive skills. This is a time to be honest and critically look at self.

A self-assessment will provide a better understanding about what the student is like and what might be considered some short- and long-term goals and will set the stage for selecting the first position.

Self-knowledge needs to be explored. The student needs to be as aware of self as one becomes aware of patient or client needs. What behaviors or skills are the most predominant; what areas of cognitive or manual skills might be considered strengths or weaknesses; what values might be considered a particular strength for one area of practice and a weakness for another; what are the most predictable behaviors and which ones are unpredictable; and what level of development is sufficient to accept the entry position to the practice of nursing?

The assessment needs to be done over time and as thoroughly as if doing a term paper, case presentation, or demonstrating one's skill on the most complex nursing problem. Utilizing peers and faculty will provide the student with the objectivity needed. Doing a written assessment provides the student with a document that prepares the way for the eventual interview. The document will assist the student in knowing how to respond to questions as well as what to ask the interviewer.

An outcome of the self-assessment is the determination of what immediate goals need to be pursued in order to prepare whatever career and personal goals are for the future. For example, the student wishes to work in a critical care unit. The assessment may show the student to have the wrong temperament or lack of manual skills. If the wrong temperament, the student needs to rethink a career goal; if manual skills, the student may have to insert a short-term career goal in order to prepare for the long-term goal.

SELECTING A BEGINNING POSITION IN NURSING

In selecting an area of nursing practice, the prospective nurse should be aware of the realities to be faced. An analysis of the following aspects of employment is helpful: the need for nurses in the area of practice desired, the expectations of the employer, the nurse's own expectations, the qualifications needed, the salary, the opportunity for advancement, and the ultimate goals of the practitioner.

The first position the nurse takes should be selected with care. There are many openings for every nurse graduated. The supply of professional nurses does not begin to fill the need. Throughout the United States there is a maldistribution of registered nurses. Once the nurse was limited to hospital nursing, but today the nurse can select one of the following: hospital nursing, military nursing, office nursing, occupational health nursing, school nursing, public health nursing, community mental health nursing, nursing education, nursing service administration, independent practice, nursing research, nurse recruitment, or nurse politician. Nurses can be found in various kinds of agencies—public, private, or volunteer.

The employer will expect the graduate to perform with competency, to be loyal, to fulfill responsibilities, and to be accountable as a nurse and a person. The nurse should be able to expect from an employer personnel policies that provide an equitable remuneration for services received. Employment conditions should be such that the nurse

can perform nursing care humanistically and with professional autonomy.

A career in nursing can either be planned or be moved into without regard to future goals. At 18 years of age, very few students of nursing know their ultimate goal in nursing. Students only know that they want to be nurses to help people. As the student progresses, this concept begins to change and should take on greater depth of meaning as the career becomes directed. For example, in progressing from student to employee, the nurse may decide to be a teacher of nursing students. To qualify for an instructor's position, the nurse needs a master's degree in nursing. Therefore the graduate of any program of nursing will need further education. Since some schools also require nursing service experience before the appointment as a faculty member, the young graduate might need experience in nursing as well as further education.

The goals of the beginning nurse will change as experience and maturity are gained. As goals change, the nurse will need to reexamine qualifications and ability to perform in the chosen field.

The first position will be somewhat frightening, but so will every new position. As the graduate moves from one place to another, new adjustments will be made. What Miller said in 1962 is equally appropos today:

It is reported that the first and fourth years in a position are the most critical. In the first year, the crucial factor was found to be the kind of introduction to the work situation the employee received. In the fourth year, it was boredom—the job no longer challenged, had become routinized and, therefore, uninteresting. . . . .

The first year . . . is most vital, however. In this year work habits, behavioral and attitude patterns, and work commitments may become fixed, often lasting throughout the person's lifetime.*

There are many ways of learning about available positions. Five of the most common sources are professional periodicals, local newspapers, friends

---

*Reprinted, with permission, from Miller, M.A.: Transition: student to employee, Nurs. Outlook **10:**84, Feb. 1962.

and other nurses, employment agencies, and state nurses' associations.

In recent years the *American Journal of Nursing, R.N. Magazine,* and *Nursing* (current year) have published extensive guides to career opportunities. They are published once a year, usually in the early spring, to provide the student with the most up-to-date information on what is available in the United States. Throughout the year these journals include articles on career planning and career information that will assist students in the self-assessment process.

Senior students can check these sources near the completion of their educational experience. This often provides students with ideas of the area of the country in which they wish to work, as well as with the opportunities open to beginning practitioners.

Other sources of information about available positions are private employment agencies, professional contacts, college placement services, alumni placement services, and nurse registries.

Employment agencies are either governmental or private. When an agency is used to obtain employment, the individual may be charged a fee for the help received in securing a position. Government agencies make no charge; however, private agencies are in business for profit and therefore will charge a percentage of the first week's or month's salary. This charge can be as high as 50% of 1 month's salary. This helps the agency to defray the cost of service. When using an agency, the nurse must be sure to find out if there is a fee for the services rendered and then should determine if securing the position is worth using the agency.

A recent addition in seeking career information and placement is the job fair and the accompanying nurse recruiter. Job fairs are held in major communities throughout the United States. Employers have booths where students can go and see what is available. Nurse recruiters are available to answer questions as well as seek information from students. The nurse recruiter may or may not be a

nurse; however, nurse recruiters are well prepared to know what the specific needs are for the institutions they represent.

A well-prepared resume is a necessary tool with which to secure a position. The resume is a document that describes you, the nurse. It provides data for the employer about accomplishments, positions held, and education received. This document is often called the vita or curriculum vita. The young graduate's resume will have only basic information, but with time the resume becomes a chronological history of the nurse's career. The appearance of the document is very important, since it can often determine who is chosen for the position. The student should begin developing a resume and then keep it updated. This document should contain the following data: name; current address; social security number; formal education, beginning with high school (dates, institutions, locations, and diploma and/or degree); continuing education (credit/no credit), giving dates, sponsor, and location; positions held (dates, institutions, and locations); states in which the nurse is licensed to practice nursing; membership in professional and nonprofessional organizations; honors, awards, scholarships, etc.; nursing and community activities; elected offices and committee appointments; and authorship of articles, textbooks, and major addresses.

The resume can be filed with a college placement service or a similar agency, or it can be kept with one's personal file. For an example of a resume see Fig. 4.

AREAS OF NURSING PRACTICE

Since 1951 the American Nurses' Association (ANA) has concerned itself with standards of nursing practice. The first endeavor was to define functions, standards, and qualifications for general duty nurses, educators, administrators, public health nurses, school nurses, occupational health nurses, and head nurses. These soon became outdated. Instead of standards to define types of nurses in practice, in 1974 the Congress for Nursing Practice

Resumé
Mary Sue Smith
1910 Elm Street
Chicago, Illinois 89110
825-22-6942

Formal Education

    High School: Old Central High School, Chicago, Illinois, 1980, diploma

    Nursing Education: Excellent School of Nursing, Chicago, Illinois, 1985, B.S.N. degree

    Continuing Education: "Monitoring the Woman in Labor," Workshop, Illinois Nurses Association, Feb. 1985, 1.5 CEUs

Positions Held

    University Hospital: Extern, summer 1984, postpartum unit

Licensed to Practice

    Application filed to take National State Board Examination July 1985 in Illinois

Professional Organizations: Does not apply

Honor Societies

    Alpha Omega Chapter of Sigma Theta Tau, 1984

PreProfessional Organizations

    National Student Nurses Association State and School, 1980-1985

Honors

    Dean's List three out of four years at Excellent School of Nursing

Awards

    Presidential Scholar

Scholarships

    The Falor Scholarship

Community Activities

    Participated in teaching mother-baby classes in Red Cross

Fig. 4. Sample resume.

recommended standards of nursing practice in five areas:

1. Medical-surgical nursing practice
2. Community health nursing practice
3. Gerontological nursing practice
4. Maternal-child health nursing practice
5. Psychiatric–mental health nursing practice

Current standards of practice are available from the ANA in every major area of nursing practice and in many specialty areas such as practice of gerontological nursing and critical care.

Positions of nursing are in the categories of clinical nursing, administration, education, or research. These kinds of positions are available in public, private, or volunteer agencies (Table 2).

Although standards have been prepared for major areas of practice, a nurse can specialize in such areas as adult nursing, maternal-child nursing, public health, community mental health, gerontological nursing, or family health nursing. These nursing specialties can be divided further into subspecialties such as coronary care, intensive care, care of the cancer patient, care of the stroke patient, care of the transplant patient, industrial nurse, school nurse practitioner, and independent nurse practitioner. Specialization in any area requires additional education beyond the initial educational experience. The nurse through continuing education can learn new techniques that give additional skill in making decisive judgments regarding specific patients.

Certification can occur in 17 specialties through the ANA. Certification requires the nurse to have experience and additional knowledge and to pass an examination in that specialty area.

Certification in maternal and child care can occur through the Nurses' Association of the College of Obstetrics and Gynecology (NACOG). Information regarding certification and the qualifications needed can be obtained through ANA and NACOG.

For the nurse to become a clinician, a master's degree in nursing is required. Ability to make nursing judgments is necessary; thus the beginning practitioner should expect to need experience and further education before accepting a position in these vital areas of nursing. The majority of nurses assume positions in nursing services, which have the basic objective of meeting the care needs of patients.

Table 2. Agencies employing nurses

Private	Public	Volunteer
Hospital nursing	Military nursing—Army, Navy, Air Force, National Guard	Peace Corps
School nursing		American National Red Cross
Private duty nursing	S.S. Hope	Local Red Cross
Nursing education	Government hospitals	VISTA
Office nursing	Indian Service	Any nursing area of volunteer's choice
Occupational health nursing	U.S. Public Health Service	
Industrial nursing	Veterans' Administration	
Organizational nursing	Boards of health	
Research	Nursing section of Children's Bureau	
Nursing consultants	Public health nursing—city and state	
Group health agencies		
Extended care facilities	Visiting nurse service—city and state	
Zoos		
Independent practice	Health maintenance organization	
	Health and Human Services	

The nurse also may choose to practice nursing in the armed forces. For years, discrimination occurred in the military service for women. On November 8, 1967, President Lyndon B. Johnson signed into law a bill giving equal rights to women in the armed forces. The bill allows women to hold permanent grade up to and including the rank of general. The ANA has long been a supporter of military nursing and has suggested that every RN serve 2 years in one of the military services.

The armed forces have been moving toward making a baccalaureate degree in nursing a requirement for entrance into the services. The army since 1975 has accepted only B.S.N. graduates, and now 93% of the corps is made up of B.S.N. graduates. The navy and air force, as of 1979, still accepted graduates from all three registered nurse programs. However, the baccalaureate degree will be required in the near future.

Instead of accepting a position in a nursing service, the graduate nurse may enter the field of nursing education. It is estimated that the greatest short-

age in nursing continues to be in leadership positions and nursing education. Many schools are without qualified faculty. The minimum requirement for a nurse educator is a master's degree in nursing. There are many undergraduates who should be stimulated to secure master's and doctoral degrees and join the ranks of nursing educators. (See Fig. 5 to determine what teaching means to you.)

Most nurses will be securing positions with public or private agencies. However, the beginning practitioner might wish to investigate volunteer nursing. One area of need is the Peace Corps. The late President John F. Kennedy created the Peace Corps in March 1961. Its purposes are as follows:

1. To help the peoples of the developing countries in meeting their own needs for trained manpower
2. To help promote a better understanding of the American people on the part of the people served
3. To help promote a better understanding of the

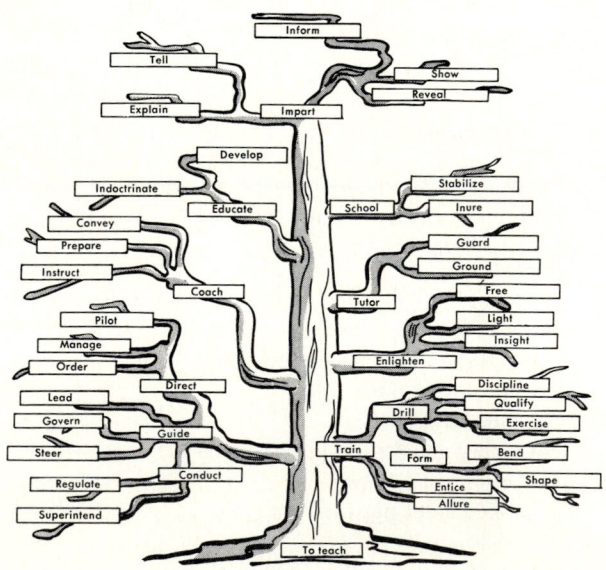

Fig. 5. Functions of a teacher. (From Dunn, P.H.: You too can teach, Salt Lake City, 1962, Bookcraft, Inc.)

people of the developing countries on the part of the American people

Another volunteer service is that of the Red Cross. Volunteer Red Cross nurses teach mother-baby classes, courses in physical fitness, and home nursing classes. They also assist in disasters and emergencies.

CAREER PLANNING

The opportunities in nursing are many. Some are lucrative but difficult to secure without advanced academic degrees. Some jobs are easy to obtain but are not satisfying in the day-to-day activities. Career planning may not occur at the time of graduation. The first ''job'' is often selected on the basis of need and desire. Within 1 year of employment, discontentment often occurs. The reasons given most often are ''I can't practice the way I was taught,'' ''Staffing is terrible,'' ''I am bored.''

A basic question for the female nurse is ''Am I going to combine a career of nursing amd marriage; pursue a career and then marriage, returning to a career in later years; or pursue a career only?'' Male nurses may also face these same issues, but they usually do not ''drop in and out'' of nursing as do female nurses.

Career planning starts with defining one's goals for 5, 10, and 20 years in the future. Plans can be altered as needs change. For example, if further education is a goal, being situated near a university that has a desired program may be the reason to select employment in that area. One may also select employment because of tuition reimbursement. Planning can cause a goal to be achieved rather than remaining a wish.

A significant decision to be made is where one wants to be at a certain point in time and how to get there. One must determine what resources are needed, what characteristics one has to demonstrate, and what type of incremental moves have to be made to achieve the long-term goals. Investigation on the part of the nurse becomes a project of importance. This investigation includes search-

ing the literature on nursing opportunities, talking to nurses who have already achieved the goal desired, and making lists of one's own assets and deficits. Drawing conclusions based on data rather than intuition provides the nurse with a sound basis to direct a career of choice rather than one of serendipity.

CAREER LADDER

The career ladder concept first emerged in the late 1960s but was fairly dormant until the late 1970s. For years, career advancement for nurses meant moving from direct patient care to positions of administration or education. This implied that the only way to utilize advanced degrees and secure more money and greater recognition was through a movement from direct care.

In the 1980s the career ladder concept has taken on new meaning. Career ladder means remaining in the clinical track of nursing and advancing from beginning staff nurse to clinical specialist. Each step requires experience, education, and certification for the next step of the ladder. Clinical nursing is defined as the giving of primary care in a variety of settings. Primary care is defined as the professional assuming direct responsibility and accountability for client care.

I believe there are four career ladders for a nurse to pursue. They are clinical nursing, administration, education, and research. Each of these career ladders has its own distinct requirement for education, experience, and recognition. All four are equally important and require collaboration in order that nursing can move as a united force in achieving quality nurse care.

EMPLOYMENT RESPONSIBILITIES

It is never to early to review opportunities available in nursing and to begin considering where and in what field of nursing to practice. The decision may not be where to go but in what field of nursing to practice.

Looking for and accepting the right position are extremely important. Graduates may decide that the best place is in the hospital or agency where initial educational experiences were achieved. This decision is often made because, first, they are familiar with the nursing care given. Second, they have new knowledge and can contribute to the agency that provided clinical practice.

Others will select positions outside of the domain of the educational setting. It makes no difference where one chooses to practice nursing; what does make a difference is in discerning the right position at the right time. There is no point in selecting a position where failure almost can be predicted. Therefore the selecting of a position becomes the first employment responsibility. Once the position or positions have been determined, the nurse will need to inquire about, apply for, and interview for them. The following hypothetical situation illustrates the procedure of applying for and accepting a position.

A nursing journal has the following advertisement that is of interest to the student: "Staff nurses needed for a 200-bed hospital, midwestern town, near a local college. Cultural opportunities available. Beginning salary $20,000 per year. Personnel policies excellent. Write Director of Nursing Service, Harmony Hospital, 101 14th Avenue, Sioux City, Iowa." The graduate is interested in a relatively small hospital but one that is not so small that guidance and direction would not be available.

The first step for the applicant to take in seeking employment with this hospital is to write to the director of nursing service, giving the following information:

1. Name
2. School from which graduation occurred
3. Date of graduation
4. Licensure information—whether the examination for state licensure has been taken or is in the process of being taken
5. Position for which the inquiry is being made and source from which the information for said position was obtained
6. Reason why information about employment in this area is being sought

The letter should be typewritten if possible, on good-quality white stationery and in proper letter form (Fig. 6). A resume should be included with the introductory letter.

The second step is the letter of application, which will include a cover letter enclosing the application for the staff nurse position. At this time the applicant will ask for a personal interview at the convenience of the director (see Fig. 7).

The third step of employment is the interview. This will be the graduate's first meeting with the director of nursing service. In some instances personnel officers will conduct the initial interview. The impression made in this interview will be a lasting one. Therefore appearance is of great importance.

An anecdote that appeared in the *Saturday Evening Post* some years ago is most appropriate to the subject of appearance. A young man was waiting to be interviewed. It was a hot summer day, and the office did not have air conditioning. There were several other men waiting to be interviewed for this particular job. The time for each interview was lengthy, and as the day wore on, one by one each man took off his coat and loosened his tie, looking rather disheveled. The first young man, however, sat straight in the chair with his coat on and his tie in place. He was the last one to be interviewed and without much question was given the position. The young man asked the interviewer, "Why am I being given the job? What qualities did I have over and above the other men who have been in here?" The interviewer explained, "You are the only one who sat through the heat with his coat and tie on." When the young man returned home and told his wife of the experience, she replied, "But, dear, why didn't you take your coat off? You usually do." He chuckled and said, "Dear, remember—this is the shirt that you ironed only the collar and cuffs and the front of. I was too embarrassed to take my coat off." Although it was through a mere mishap that this man did get the job, it does point out that a well-groomed appearance is essential to a successful interview.

<pre>
                                     1910 Elm Street
                                     Chicago, Illinois 89110
                                     March 27, 1985

Director of Nursing Service
Harmony Hospital
101 14th Avenue
Sioux City, Iowa   51102

Dear Madam:

     I will be graduating from Excellent School of Nursing

in June of 1985. As yet, I have not taken the State Board

Examinations. These will be offered in Illinois on July 10,

1985, for my initial license in Illinois. I will be available

for employment as soon as the results of this examination are

received. I anticipate this to be September 1, 1985.

     Your advertisement which appears in the March issue of

_____, 1985, indicates there is a need for staff nurses.

I am particularly interested in working in the obstetrical area

with maternity patients. I am interested in working in Sioux

City because I have friends living there, and I have been told

what a fine hospital you have.

     I am interested in receiving the following information

regarding the positions you will have available: job description,

personnel policies, philosophy and objectives of the department,

and an application.

     Enclosed please find my resumé.

                                   Sincerely yours,

                                   Mary Sue Smith
                                   Mary Sue Smith
</pre>

Fig. 6. Letter of inquiry.

1910 Elm Street
Chicago, Illinois 89110
April 10, 1985

Miss Susan Young
Director, Nursing Service
Harmony Hospital
101 14th Avenue
Sioux City, Iowa 51102

Dear Miss Young:

Enclosed please find the application for a staff nurse position in obstetrical nursing, beginning September 1, 1985.

In order that we might become acquainted and I might know more about your hospital, I would like to ask for a personal interview sometime during the week of June 15, 1985. I am available Monday through Thursday.

I am looking forward to hearing from you.

Sincerely yours,

Mary Sue Smith

Mary Sue Smith

Fig. 7. Letter of application.

In preparing for the interview, be organized in thought as well as in physical presence. On a card write the questions down that need to be asked. Be prepared to ask the following: what is the philosophy and model of nursing practice at the institution; what autonomy does the professional nurse have; what are the staff development opportunities; what is the length of orientation; are there preceptors or internships; what "reality shock" measures are there to assist in the transition from student to practitioner; and what are the economic benefits?

Prepare for the interview physically and emotionally in order that the presence displayed is one of self-assurance and a feeling of well-being.

It is important to be at the director's office at least 5 minutes before the appointed time. The applicant should not arrive too early but should not be late.

During the interview the director of nursing service is allowed to ask the questions. The applicant should not turn the tide of the interview by interviewing the director. When the director asks if there are questions is the appropriate time to ask questions.

The questions the director will ask will be about the graduate as an individual and why the graduate thinks himself or herself qualified for the position. The nurse should not undersell himself or herself during the interview but should be confident in ability. The graduate should not be overbearing but speak freely about what he or she believes are personal qualifications for accepting the position being offered. The graduate should be prepared to state his or her philosophy of nursing. The interview may last 10 minutes or an hour, depending on the nature of the position, how much the director wishes to know about the nurse, and how much the nurse wishes to know about the position.

Following are the reasons for having an interview:

1. For the prospective employee to see the institution and talk about the position being sought
2. For the director of nursing to have the op-

portunity of seeing the nurse and determining if the nurse qualifies for the position

3. For the nurse and the director to have the opportunity of knowing each other before employment
4. For the nurse and the director to have the opportunity of asking questions regarding this employment

The close of the interview will be indicated by the director of nursing service, who will probably say "Thank you for coming in. We will get in touch with you." When this has been said, the graduate should not continue with the interview, since such a statement indicates that the director has completed the interview. When leaving, the applicant should thank the director for the time spent and should indicate whether he or she wishes to hear positively from the director. If, at the time, the nurse believes that the job is not suitable, this is the time to say so. However, it might be easier to say this in a letter.

In the third letter the nurse will thank the director for the time spent in the interview and will state whether interested in the position. After having been offered a position he or she wishes to accept, the nurse will write a letter of acceptance (Fig. 8).

Some institutions require that employees sign contracts. However, this has not been a common practice in nursing. A contract is a document prepared by the institution, giving such information as work and personnel policies. It is signed by the employee and the employer as an agreement of employment. Usually a letter of acceptance and a letter from the director indicating the terms of employment are considered a contract.

Accepting a position, whether or not a contract is signed, constitutes an agreement that should not be broken unless some unavoidable problem arises. In agreeing to work, one owes the agency the courtesy of fulfilling that agreement. If the graduate finds it impossible to honor the agreement, the employer should be notified in writing immediately. The director will have made plans for the nurse's coming; many people will be disappointed. To ac-

1910 Elm Street
Chicago, Illinois 89110
June 23, 1985

Miss Susan Young
Director, Nursing Service
Harmony Hospital
101 14th Avenue
Sioux City, Iowa 51102

Dear Miss Young:

    I am pleased to accept the position of staff nurse in the
obstetrical department.

    I will be at Harmony Hospital on September 1, 1985, at
8:00 A.M.

    I am looking forward to a profitable association with you
and the staff.

                    Sincerely yours,

                    Mary Sue Smith

                    Mary Sue Smith

Fig. 8. Letter of acceptance of position.

cept a position and fail to appear mars the nurse's employment record.

The responsibilities of the nurse include being loyal, dependable, honest, and accountable. Loyalty to an employer is a sincere desire to fulfill the functions that have been agreed on. For the nurse, loyalty means being interested in the institution, the community, and the persons with whom one works. One of the first ways that the nurse can show loyalty to the employer is to refrain from complaining. The nurse seeks out the employment and accepts the position. If the happiness desired is not found in that position, it is the nurse's responsibility to resign and not carry feelings of discontent to other members of the staff.

An example of the situation just described occurred many years ago in my first teaching position when I worked with an extremely fine, intelligent person who held a responsible position and was admired by all those with whom she worked. However, she had been in the position for several years and was becoming dissatisfied with herself and with the job. Almost every morning she would come to work and say, "I'm going to quit." It was not long before I, too, had these feelings, believing the institution was not the best place in which to work, that there were things wrong with it, and that it would be best to quit. However, the person with whom I worked did finally resign, and it was amazing how soon I found that the institution for which I was working was really a fine place; no longer did I feel every morning as if I wanted to quit. The atmosphere and the attitude of the whole department changed. I cite this experience to emphasize that one unhappy person can make other people unhappy. The employee who is unhappy should resign but should not expect other people to assume these same feelings.

The second responsibility to an employer is dependability. Dependability is a virtue that should be possessed by everyone. For the nurse it means that she will be at the proper place when expected.

It takes all staff members working together to provide exquisite nursing care. There will be times when the employee or a member of the family is ill or when death of a relative or a close friend prevents the nurse from meeting obligations. The nurse should call and explain the situation as soon as he or she knows that there is a need to be away. If the employee is not a frequent offender, other members of the staff will be most understanding and will work twice as hard, knowing that when they are away the nurse will do the same for them.

Personnel policies will include provision for days off, holiday time, vacation time, and sick leave for a purpose. Days off, holiday time, and vacation time are to be used by the employee for renewing energy and the capacity to accomplish nursing practice with utmost skill. The nurse may not always get the time off just when desired, but this is no excuse to stay away. Planning ahead will help both the nurse and teammates to have the time they want when they want it. The employee who stays away without regard to co-workers cannot expect much goodwill to exist.

Sick leave is granted as an insurance policy. Leave without loss of pay is available when the employee needs it. Just because the policy reads "1 day of sick leave per month" does not mean that the day should be used indiscriminately. In most institutions the policy goes on to read "accumulative to 'x' number of days." If 1 day per month is used for minor illnesses, sick leave will never accumulate, nor will the employee have days available if serious illness occurs. The nurse who calls in sick just to have the day off is not dependable. The dependable employee is considerate of others, and others can count on him or her. One of the greatest rewards nurses enjoy is knowing they can depend on each other to be at work when needed.

The third responsibility is honesty. Being honest to yourself, the employer, co-workers, and patients is a virtue not to be missed. The nurse has to live with himself or herself and therefore should obey the creed "to thine own self be true." A dishonest person is not liked, is not trusted, and soon becomes a lonely, selfish individual. It is a matter of not only knowing right from wrong but also doing the right thing.

Being honest with co-workers and patients is the nurse's ethical responsibility. No one likes to be given untrue information. When there is faith in others, much more can be accomplished. All human beings err. To err and to not set the record straight is unforgivable. Errors do occur in nursing. They are more serious when they involve patients. As soon as an error has been discovered, the nurse must tell all concerned, making sure that the patient has not been harmed. If the error has caused injury to the patient, it is important to rectify the error and provide nursing emergency measures. An error also can be cause for a lawsuit.

Patients do not like to be told untruths. If the truth cannot be said, it is best to say nothing. Patients also expect nurses to keep their word. If the nurse promises to do something for a patient, the nurse should do it or explain why it cannot be done but should never let the patient down by ignoring the request. Nurses do not like for someone to break a promise, so why should a patient not resent such behavior?

The fourth responsibility of the nurse is to be accountable. All through the nursing education experience, principles of care have been learned. It is up to the graduate to put these principles into daily practice. Each graduate should know what comprises good nursing care and thus be accountable for putting it into practice. Accountability is the ultimate of a professional.

Accountability to the patient or client and to oneself is a mandate in practicing nursing. Being accountable is a form of evaluation. It can be measured by one's productivity and how patients respond to one's nursing practice. In assessing accountability, nurses need to determine to whom they are accountable, for what, how accountability will be manifested, how performance will be monitored, how levels of accountability will be assessed, and whether accountability will be controlled and regulated. Accountability becomes a commitment to professional nursing by remaining open to new learning experiences and knowledge, unconditional accuracy and integrity, and a continued search for truth.

As one functions in nursing, changes in policy, procedures, and facilities will occur. How nurses meet these changes will depend on their own knowledge of the situation, their own personal involvement with the change, who instituted the change, the extent of the change, the new skills that may have to be learned, and how much they were involved in proposing the change. The tendency to resist change is a natural phenomenon. As change is proposed and one recognizes the feelings of resistance, one needs to identify the reason for it: by asking why the change is necessary, what problem exists that creates a need for the change, how the change can make the situation better, when it would be best to change, under what circumstances the change needs to occur, and where the change should occur. By examining one's own feelings about change, resistance to it can be identified, understood, and modified.

Changes need to occur in nursing and the health care system. Therefore, as a professional, one needs to know whether a specific change promotes the welfare of the nurse, nursing, and the clients being served. The nurse needs to be a part of change either by promoting change or effecting change suggested by others. Change is incremental, meaning that it occurs in small steps, and only after many years does one see the actual change. For example, nurse leaders began in the early 1900s to effect a change in nursing education, and it has taken 75 years to actually see the majority of nurses educated in the system of higher education. Chapter 3 helps the reader to visualize the resistance to change and understand what it means to cope with change when it affects one as an individual.

RESIGNING FROM A POSITION

There are many reasons why an individual might desire to resign from a position. Once the decision to resign has been made, the nurse should go to the director of nursing service and discuss the mat-

1021 Blair Street
Sioux City, Iowa 51102
October 2, 1986

Miss Susan Young
Director, Nursing Service
Harmony Hospital
101 14th Avenue
Sioux City, Iowa 51102

Dear Miss Young:

Following our conversation of September 30, 1986, I am

submitting my letter of resignation.

As we discussed, I now feel it is time for me to continue on

in my educational endeavors. I have applied to and been accepted

into the University of Minnesota for further graduate work.

My last day of employment will be October 13, 1986. I will

have been here a little over one year and would like to request

terminal vacation.

It has been a pleasure working here as a first year graduate

nurse. I have learned a great deal and feel this knowledge will

be profitable to me in future experience.

At this time I would like to ask if I might submit your name

to be used as a reference when desiring further employment.

My very best wishes to you and your staff.

Sincerely yours,

Mary Sue Smith

Mary Sue Smith

Fig. 9. Letter of resignation.

ter. When discussing the resignation with the director, the employee should be as honest as possible but should always leave the door open for a possible return, since there may be a time when the nurse would like to again assume a position at that institution. Also, the nurse will want to secure a recommendation from the employer. If the resignation is because of problems existing within the hospital or agency, it is important to discuss this with the director of nursing service. The director may not be able to correct them for the one who is resigning but certainly can help to correct them for those coming after or those who are still employed. It is desirable to be honest with the director but in a manner that is not quarrelsome or argumentative and is helpful to others.

The letter of resignation follows the verbal announcement. The letter of resignation should include the reason for leaving, location of the new position, date of termination, and, if vacation time is due, whether it is to be terminal. In addition to this, the nurse should ask permission to submit the director's name for further recommendations (Fig. 9).

ANA ECONOMIC SECURITY PROGRAM

The ANA has an active program that deals with the economic and general welfare of the individual. In 1946 this program was accepted by the membership. From 1946 until 1966 there was a standing committee who had the responsibility to establish standards for the economic and general welfare of the nurse. When the organization changed its structure, this committee became the Commission on Economic and General Welfare (E & GW) with the following responsibilities*:

a. Establish the scope of the association's responsibility for the welfare of nurses.
b. Develop general economic standards for the profession and devise methods for gaining their acceptance and implementation through appropriate channels.

c. Establish committees for each of the major occupational areas in nursing. These committees shall identify, study, and advise on the concerns of nurses in their respective occupational settings.
d. Develop basic principles of desirable employment conditions of nurses and promote the use thereof in places of employment.
e. Study and evaluate the economics of health care.
f. Study and evaluate the economics of nursing in the various occupational settings.
g. Initiate research and studies related to the economic position of the nursing profession.
h. Develop and implement a program of economic education.
i. Formulate policy and recommend action related to federal and state legislation in the field of economics and general welfare of nurses.
j. Advise and assist constituent associations in the development of their programs in economic and general welfare.
k. Evaluate developments and trends in health care practices and the general economy for their social and economic implications for nurses.

The ANA functions in a supportive role to state nurses' associations by giving both technical and financial assistance. The ANA also monitors and responds to changes in federal legislation, rules, and regulations. Individual nurses can receive legal assistance through the E & GW program.

Since 1970 the philosophy of the E & GW program has been the following*:

• Belief in the profession's responsibility to work for the common good of society
• Belief in the profession's responsibility to develop and implement standards of practice
• Belief in the profession's responsibility for the welfare of its practitioners
• Belief in the right of individual nurses to participate fully in the determination of all matters relevant to the profession of nursing
• Belief in the responsibility of the professional association to represent nurses in their employment setting

*American Nurses' Association: Bylaws, New York, 1970, The Association, p. 25.

*American Nurses' Association Commission on Economic and General Welfare, Kansas City, Mo., 1975.

Each state will have its own way of achieving an economic and a general welfare program. The importance of collective bargaining is in providing a method whereby nurses in either a local or a state organization can receive needed assistance through an organized manner.

For 22 years the ANA had a "no strike" clause as a national policy. In June 1968 the House of Delegates set this policy aside because it was not enforceable and was inconsistent with what some states were doing. Instead, the ANA supports each state in whatever action it deems right and consistent for that state, its laws, and its policies.

Through the Economic Security Program nurses have achieved a number of benefits, foremost of which are better personnel policies having to do with hours of work, vacation policies, sick leave, accurate job descriptions, and better salaries.

Until 1966 there had never been a national effort to set a minimum salary for nurses. At the ANA convention in 1966, the House of Delegates went on record to accept and implement a minimum salary of $6500. In 1968 the effort was for $7500 for nurses with diplomas or associate degrees and $8500 for those with baccalaureate degrees, thus beginning the practice of recognizing the different programs. At no other time has the association voted to have a national minimum salary.

Throughout the years the E & GW Program has been controversial; however, the ANA has continued to reaffirm its position in supporting the need for collective bargaining. The issues in the 1980s are more complex and far more difficult to solve. Although personnel policies still are a part of the negotiation, the issue most germane is the right for nurses to make decisions regarding where they practice.

Graduate nurses need to be aware of the political ramifications of this complex issue, which ultimately affects their welfare in the practice of nursing, and take an active part in directing their own destinies, not leaving these decisions for others to make. Chapter 10 discusses collective bargaining in nursing.

SUMMARY

On graduating or before graduating, the student will be looking for a position. The position should be suited to the student's basic educational preparation and should be in a nursing service area. The graduate has responsibilities in gaining and maintaining employment. These are submitting an application, being interviewed, accepting the position, being loyal and accountable to the employer, and giving the employer the services agreed on. In selecting a position, the nurse will need to examine personal goals hoped to be achieved in a nursing career. The position selected should meet the nurse's present qualifications and ability to function in the area and to maintain and help elevate the standards set forth by those persons already serving. It is the responsibility of the individual nurse to participate in decisions that affect the nurse's welfare. It will be necessary for the nurse to continue professional education, both formally and informally, to meet the demands and changes of nursing.

Discussion questions

1. Discuss the need for and what questions to explore in developing a self-assessment document.
2. Discuss what should be looked for in selecting the first position in nursing.
3. Discuss the variety of opportunities available and the need for career planning.
4. Discuss career planning in relation to four tracks in the career ladder: clinical nursing, administration, education, and research.
5. Discuss the concepts of accountability and autonomy for the professional nurse.

SUGGESTED READINGS

The AJN guide, New York, American Journal of Nursing.
Balint, J., et al.: Job opportunities for master's prepared nurses, Nurs. Outlook **31**(2):109-114, 1983.
Beason, C.: Nursing's labor relations crisis, R.N., pp. 21-33, Feb. 1979.
Connelly, C.E., et al.: To strike or not to strike, Sup. Nurse, p. 52, Jan. 1979.
Crooks, E.: Nurses' associations and collective bargaining: wave of the past? R.N., pp. 83-88, April 1979.

Emerson, W.: The American Nurses' Association and collective bargaining, Imprint, p. 55, April 1977.

Emerson, W.L.: Appropriate bargaining limits for health care professional employees, J. Nurs. Adm., pp. 10-15, Sept. 1979.

Fahey, P.L.: A small-town nurse is still a nurse and a lot more, R.N., pp. 60-61, May 1979.

Fay, M.: The challenge of O.R. nursing, Nurs. '77, pp. 98-100, Oct. 1977.

Godfrey, M.A.: Nurses' salaries today, Nurs. '77, pp. 81-97, June 1977.

Joel, M.: Adult nurse practitioner: one of the most satisfying nursing roles, Nurs. '79, pp. 92-95, Jan. 1979.

Masson, V.N.: International nursing: what is it and who does it? Am. J. Nurs., pp. 1242-1245, July 1979.

Morrow, K.: Specialize in general nursing on an overnight unit, Nurs. '79, pp. 122-126, May 1979.

News: Sierra Vista ruling supports SNA's; NLRB revokes earlier decision, Am. J. Nurs., pp. 1054-1055, June 1979.

Robinson, A.: Career choice by life style—the better way, Imprint, pp. 28-91, Oct. 1979.

Stanley, L.: Expanded role nursing hits the hospitals, R.N., pp. 55-59, Oct. 1979.

Storlie, F.: Do you want to specialize in CCU nursing? Nurs. '78, pp. 71-73, Jan. 1979.

Wiley, L.: Job interviews: oh boy! are they important, Nurs. '77, pp. 65-69, Aug. 1977.

Williamson, L.: Future prospects, Nurs. '77, pp. 50-51, Feb. 10, 1977.

Youmans, P.M.: The developmental pediatric nurse practitioner, Nurs. '79, pp. 115-116, Nov. 1979.

CHAPTER 16

Continuing education

VIRGINIA NEWBERN

OBJECTIVE: On completion of this chapter, the student of nursing will appreciate the need for continuing his or her education and become a lifelong learner.

As the half-life of knowledge continues to diminish and as the cry for accountability becomes formalized, the very survival of a profession may depend on the ability of its members to document competency, currency, and credibility. Continuing education is one method to meet those needs.

The construct of continuing education has many facets. This chapter provides a historical perspective, definitions, and an introduction to the concept of continuing professional education, as well as the current state of continuing education and a forecast of future trends.

HISTORICAL PERSPECTIVE

Learning has always been an intrinsic part of the ''need to know,'' which enables human beings to survive, to cope, and to move toward self-actualization. Most of human learning has been acquired by doing; much of it has been through independent efforts or trial and error. More formal, structured efforts at continuing education are relatively new, with a direct relationship between these efforts and the rate of change in knowledge that society has experienced in the past 2 centuries. Beginning with the advent of the industrial revolution the available knowledge base has grown geometrically, precipitating an ever-accelerating rate of change and a consequent need for systematized, sequential resources for continuing education. These learning needs now encompass the range of human experience and the full span of human life since knowledge and experiences acquired in youth and young adulthood cannot be counted on to be useful in middle and old age.

Education in the colonies

Higher education was initiated in the United States with the establishment of Harvard University in Massachusetts in 1636 and the College of William and Mary in Virginia in 1693. Informal continuing education was through the efforts of printers, who provided such adult reading matter as newspapers and religious and political tracts. Group discussion of these materials did much to foster the sense of community that was a large factor in the success of the colonies in winning independence from Great Britain.

Inception of formal adult education

Denmark was the first nation to formally underwrite adult education, establishing evening classes in 1814. Adult education did not gain a formal foothold in the United States until the last decades of the nineteenth century. The Morrill Act of 1862 established land grant colleges, one for each state. Land grant colleges were charged with updating the knowledge and competencies of farmers, and each became more commonly known as the agricultural college or university of its state. Over the years this charge has been expanded to include a wide variety of subjects. The Cooperative Extension Service, which evolved before World War I, was the basis for many of the present continuing education programs.

Through the 1920s and 1930s the scope of the adult education movement widened. Adult basic education courses prepared many immigrants for American citizenship. Night school courses taught basic skills such as typing and automotive repair. The first courses in leisure living evolved. Educators began to believe in adults as learners and to recognize their need for opportunities to increase their knowledge. In 1926 these educators formed the American Association for Adult Education. In 1951 the name was changed to the Adult Education Association of the United States (AEA), this organization provided an umbrella for adult educators with widely divergent interests, concerns, and needs. This tradition was continued with the consolidation of AEA and the National Association for Public Continuing and Adult Education (NAPCAE) into a new organization, the American Association for Adult and Continuing Education (AAACE), during the years 1982 and 1983. AAACE, like AEA before it, functions as the professional organization for adult educators.

Continuing education in nursing

Although Florence Nightingale espoused the concept of continued learning, nurse educators before World War II did little to foster the spirit of continuing education. Nursing education, then primarily hospital based, was not education as we know it today but training aimed at the accomplishment of specific skills and tasks. For most nurses graduation meant the end of the educational process with the exception of some incidental learning. Relicensure requirements based solely on payment of a fee reinforced such thinking.

A few nurses did attend postgraduate courses to enhance their knowledge and skills in a selected area of clinical practice or, more often, to obtain clinical experience that was not provided in their original preparation in such areas as communicable diseases and psychiatric nursing. These courses were, like the basic education, usually hospital based and varied widely in length and quality. Nurses who did attend such postgraduate courses were often chosen to fill supervisory and other leadership positions. The system did not allow them to function as role models for the nurses at the bedside, so a natural opportunity to provide ongoing learning was lost. Nevertheless, for many years these postgraduate courses offered the only formal means by which nurses could obtain additional education.

Short-term (1- and 2-day) educational experiences were given beginning in the 1920s. Many of these were presented by the National League for Nursing Education and were open only to nurse educators. Most were offered in large metropolitan areas or university centers and so were unavailable to many nurses across the country.

In-service education has existed in a primitive form in nursing for many years. Often it took the form of an apprenticeship, with the older nurse taking the new practitioner "under her wing" until the latter demonstrated the ability to do the tasks. Through the years, procedure books have been used to reinforce learning and to orient new nursing staff to the accepted practices of a given institution. Physicians who enjoyed teaching delivered lectures to nursing staffs on new knowledge and skills. Many of the first nurses to staff coronary care units learned the related pathophysiology, pharmacology, and skills, such as reading monitors, from internists and cardiologists who had spearheaded the development of such units.

The post–World War II era intensified the need for in-service education. The population was increasingly mobile; no longer could administrators count on a staff that had grown up within the institution. Changes in nursing education ended the use of students as the primary source of labor. The rapid development of medical technology mandated staff who understood its uses and abuses. The concomitant proliferation of new and exotic drugs necessitated in-depth knowledge of pharmacology and drug management. Other examples abound; at this writing the use of a computer as a nursing tool may be primary.

Yet even today many in-service programs consist of little more than orientation for new staff plus demonstration of new gadgets, machines, or drugs, with the teaching being provided by company sales people. Past practice has been, all too often, to tack the in-service educator function onto the job description of already busy supervisors, assistant directors, and others. The result, in the main, has been that the function was largely ignored or, like Topsy, "just grew." Fortunately, however, with the implementation of the Joint Commission on Accreditation of Hospitals (JCAH) standards, which include criteria for staff development, the picture has changed. Many large institutions now have excellent staff development departments with well-qualified instructors. Smaller institutions purchase the services for staff development from larger institutions.

Early university involvement

By the 1920s a few universities were offering postgraduate nursing courses, workshops, and institutes, both credit and noncredit. Some of these evolved from the needs of medical centers associated with the sponsoring university. With the exception of the schools of public health, higher education, however, paid only cursory and sporadic attention to the educational needs of nurses until 1959, when federal funds became available for nursing education.

In 1955 the University of Wisconsin allocated a faculty position for development of continuing education in nursing. Two years later the Western Council on Higher Education for Nursing (WCHEN) was established, and that body has addressed continuing education needs since. The Southern Regional Educational Board (SREB), established in 1948, has attempted to address the ongoing educational needs of nurses throughout its history.

In the autumn of 1969 nurses throughout the country concerned with the issue of continuing education met in Williamsburg, Virginia, under the sponsorship of the school of nursing of the Medical College of Virginia (MCV), now a division of Virginia Commonwealth University, Richmond. This meeting was the genesis for the annual meetings of continuing educators in nursing. After the establishment of the Continuing Education (CE) Council of the American Nurses' Association (ANA), these annual meetings were jointly sponsored by the CE Council and a school or college of nursing through 1980. By the 1980s the Continuing Education Council had come of age and now represented not only university-based continuing nurse educators but also staff development directors and entrepreneurs. The efforts begun in Williamsburg had come to fruition.

Role of the American Nurses' Association

The ANA, increasingly concerned about standards of nursing practice, issued a statement, "Avenues for Continued Learning," in 1967. In 1970 the organization established a new position, coordinator of continuing education. The following year the ANA board of directors appointed a task force to study the question of mandatory continuing education requirements for licensure and relicensure. The Council of Continuing Education for Nursing was established in 1972 and subsumed under the Commission of Nursing Education of the ANA. At this writing the council has a membership of about 400 persons from across the United States. The council provides a mechanism whereby its members can share concerns, problems, and solutions and build networks to support each other in their efforts. The annual meetings are attended by continuing nurse educators from education, service, and private business, as well as entrepreneurs from outside the profession.

The council is charged with the advancement of

continuing education in nursing. To that end it develops standards and monitors the progress of continuing nursing education. It provides consultation to the National Accreditation Board (NAB) of ANA regarding the accreditation process for continuing nursing education programs and offerings. The council speaks to the continuing education of the individual nurse and works to promote the acceptance of continuing education at an organizational and fiscal level on a par with other educational efforts, including nurse faculty prepared at the graduate level.

DEFINITIONS

It is imperative to understand meanings in order to understand concepts, ideas, processes, and problems. The following definitions are helpful in coming to grips with the concept of continuing education:

adult education Learning experiences that address the needs of the adult learner; they may be directed toward making up earlier educational deficits (adult basic education), enhancing leisure hours (informal or nonformal education), or supplying new skills and competencies or enhancing old ones (formal, nonformal, or recurrent education).

contact hour Time span of 50 minutes.

continuing education Formal, or more commonly nonformal, learning experiences developed to meet the needs of the adult learner. In nursing, continuing education has been defined as ''planned learning experiences designed to promote the development of knowledge, skills, and attitudes for the enhancement of nursing practice, thus improving health care to the public.''*

continuing education unit (CEU) Ten 50-minute contact hours of participation in a planned continuing education experience under responsible sponsorship, capable direction, and qualified instruction.

continuing professional education Planned learning experience, both credit and noncredit, presented to reinforce or enhance the skills, knowledge, and competency of professionals in their own fields, in related disciplines, and in areas germane to their own field (e.g., management, computers, labors relations).

formal education Organized schooling involving established groups and speficied teachers.

informal education ''The truly lifelong process whereby each individual acquires values, skills, and knowledge from daily experience and the educative influences and resources in his or her environment—from family and friends, from work and play, from the marketplace, the library, and mass media.''*

in-service education Planned instructional or training programs provided by an employing agency in the work setting and designed to increase competence in a specific role; in-service education is one aspect of staff development.

lifelong learning Purposeful learning activities, occurring throughout the life span and engaged in both within and without formal academic systems.

nonformal education ''Any organized educational activity outside the established formal system—whether operated separately or as an important feature of some broader activity that is intended to serve identifiable learning clienteles and learning objectives.''*

orientation Planned instructional experience provided by a given agency to acquaint new employees with its policies, procedures, and parameters.

recurrent education A continuation of the educational cycle that allows for the use of educational resources to meet the learning needs of the adult as those needs relate to relevancy, competency, and self-actualization.

staff development Formal and nonformal learing experiences, provided or subsidized by a given agency, to reinforce or enhance the employee's knowledge and skills (may take place on site or in another institution; instruction provided by agency staff or by outside content specialists).

MANDATORY CONTINUING EDUCATION

With the recognition of the knowledge explosion of the 1960s, the need for systematic continued learning began to be documented. At that time the half-life of knowledge was estimated at 5 years; as of 1978, that estimate was reduced to 2 to 2½ years! As the "expiration date" for knowledge has been pushed forward, mandatory continuing education as a valid remedy has been legislated. Two types of legislation have been utilized:

1. *Enabling* The state board of nursing of a given state is granted the authority to require continuing education for license "if" and "when" the board deems this necessary.

---

*Revised definition approved by the Council on Continuing Education for Nursing at the Biennial Convention of the American Nurses' Association, Honolulu, Hawaii, June 1978.

*Harmon, D.: Recurrent and nonformal education: a definitional prelude. In Expanding recurrent and nonformal education, San Francisco, 1976, Jossey-Bass, Inc., Publishers, pp. 1-7.

2. *Directive* The state board of nursing is directed to require evidence of continuing education from nurses seeking relicensure and is given the authority to set up the requisite rules and regulations for this process.

California was the first state (1974) to direct mandatory continuing education. Kansas, Florida, Minnesota, New Mexico, Iowa, Kentucky, Massachusetts, Iowa, and Nebraska have followed suit. Kansas was the first state to implement its legislation, followed within hours by California (July 1, 1978).

Oregon, South Dakota, Louisiana, and Colorado enacted enabling legislation for mandatory continuing education in the years between 1970 and 1978. Some states (e.g., Oregon and Georgia) require evidence of continued learning for any RN who has not practiced within 5 years.

A number of states mandate continuing education for nurse practitioners. Included are Alaska, Idaho, Mississippi, New Hampshire, and Oregon.

Some questions and concerns

Given that professional nurses are motivated to engage in continuing education activities and that institutions are motivated to encourage such involvement, what difference does it make? Can learning, as demonstrated by behavior change, be documented? Are the results worth the time, money, energy, and commitment invested?

There are no easy, simple answers. It is not just a question of whether learning can, in fact, be mandated. Involved are such variables as sanction to use new learning and opportunities to apply, modify, transfer, and manipulate new learning so that it truly becomes integrated.

How effective for learning, then, are "one-shot deals": 1- or 2-day workshops, conferences, and seminars? How does the continuing education client evaluate such programs: how can a program's objectives be judged, as well as the depth and scope of its content, and are they congruent with the client's needs?

A number of recent studies have addressed concerns related to mandatory continuing education.

Gaston and Pucci looked at mandatory continuing education in Kansas and found that consumers had become more sophisticated and selective. They identified such problems as cafeteria-style offerings, the difficulty in getting to an offering in a rural state, no methodology for measuring learning over time or effect on practice, and the need for a complete statewide calendar.*

Schoen surveyed Illinois nurses regarding their perceptions of the worth of continuing education and the value of mandatory continuing education. Respondents overwhelmingly perceived continuing education as beneficial but were evenly divided in their support of mandatory continuing education.†

A report of the study that precipitated the move toward mandatory continuing education in Indiana documents that "the least educated nurse, functioning in a single nurse situation and providing the most direct nursing care, was least likely to attend continuing education activities."‡

So the vote is still out on the value of mandatory continuing education, and the pace of implementation has slowed considerably. Obviously there is a need for controlled studies to validate the value of mandatory continuing education, along with creative efforts to develop alternatives for facilitating lifelong learning.

STATE OF CONTINUING EDUCATION

Continuing education in nursing, as in other professions and disciplines, grew rapidly in the 1970s as the relationship between lifelong learning and competency became increasingly apparent. Such rapid growth always entails a risk of disarray, lack of standardization, scarcity of competent workers in the field, and threat to the comfort of

*Gaston, S., and Pucci, J.: Mandatory continuing education in Kansas three years later, J. Contin. Education Nurs., pp. 15-17, March-April 1982.
†Schoen, D.: The views of Illinois nurses toward requiring continuing education for licensure, J. Contin. Education Nurs., pp. 28-37, Jan.-Feb. 1982.
‡Puetz, B.: Legislating a continuing education requirement for licensure renewal, J. Contin. Education Nurs., p. 10, Jan-Feb. 1983.

the status quo. All these risks became actualities for continuing education in nursing. As continuing nurse educators entered the 1980s, with those problems still unresolved, they encountered a diminishing national economy and a national policy based on competition. Suddenly the task has become to make extremely scarce dollars stretch and stretch *while continuing to provide quality programing*. Cost effectiveness and productivity are now the overriding concerns. Therefore each of the problems listed above will be discussed within the context of financing.

Disarray

Debate continues as to what learning can legitimately be considered "continuing" and how such learning can be measured. ANA's definition of continuing education is broad enough to fit many modalities of learning within these parameters. The measure of fit is then determined by how well those modalities "promote the development of knowledge, skills, and attitudes. . . ." Both in-service education and staff development can fit within these parameters. So, too, can courses taken for credit, as well as self-directed learning, which can be for credit or noncredit.

The question of measurement is inextricably interwoven with the type of educational effort. Measurement also depends on who's measuring and by what standards. Measurement of learning will be addressed in the discussion on standards.

But the fiercest debate concerns who will provide that continuing learning and collect scarce dollars. The 1983 annual meeting of the CE Council was titled "The Business of Continuing Education," and sessions were devoted to marketing, budgeting, and the like. The meeting theme was an accurate reflection of how continuing nursing education is increasingly perceived, not only by entrepreneurs but also by nurses in education and service.

That this is true is manifest by the number of continuing education programs in schools and colleges of nursing that have been abolished or downgraded to a minimum effort or been given a man-

date to become self-supporting. In a 1980 survey of collegiate continuing education programs Sparks found that although only 15.2% were self-supporting, 60.2% were expected to become so.[*]

With regard to service, staff development programs across the country have lost positions. Many are contracting with outsiders for specific needs; many are marketing their programs to the nursing community in an attempt to generate direct funds.

Both education and service continuing education suffer from the lack of foresight regarding funding displayed by many planners when the continuing education programs were implemented. Sparks found that only 10.8% of collegiate programs had hard money as a source of support while 33% depended at least in part on grant (soft) money. Buisson found, in an informal survey, that staff development programs are for the most part funded indirectly; that is, their budgets are part of other budgets.[†] Thus in too many instances, continuing education programs in education and service have no sound fiscal base from which to operate.

Standardization

As continuing education activities "grew like Topsy" in the early 1970s, the need for some form of standardization, some valid mode for measurement, became increasingly apparent. To that end ANA's Council on Continuing Education established an ad hoc committee to study the question of accreditation and to make recommendations. In 1975 these efforts came to fruition with the establishment of a voluntary national accreditation mechanism. The contact hour was recommended as the basic unit of measurement; inherent in this recommendation is equation of continuing education activities for nurses with traditional education activities within academe. The continuing education unit (CEU) became the common standard unit

---

[*]Sparks, P.M.: An organizational analysis of collegiate CE programs, Update, p. 7, July 1983.
[†]Buisson, C.J.: Contracting, New York, 1983, National Nursing Network.

of measure. The CEU has been defined as "ten contact hours of participation in an organized continuing education experience under responsible sponsorship, capable direction, and qualified instruction."

Continuing education providers can now seek approval for each offering, or they may seek accreditation as a provider or an accrediting agent. In the latter case two routes are open: accreditation from their state nurses' association or through the appropriate regional accrediting committee of ANA. The process for acquiring such accreditation is much like that for receiving National League for Nursing (NLN) accreditation for basic educational programs in nursing.

At this writing, NAB is proposing major changes in the accreditation process that will ease the path of private business and entrepreneurs to acquire status as accredited providers of continuing education for nurses. Although the membership of the CE Council expressed a number of reservations to the proposed changes, the issue will be decided by the House of Delegates at ANA's biennial convention in New Orleans in June 1984. If the revised standards are approved, the ramifications for continuing education may be great. It is difficult now to forecast how these changes will affect the cost of continuing education for the average participant. It is not difficult to forecast problems with the quality of offerings since there is no mechanism for ongoing monitoring of quality control.

Credentials of continuing education

As the thrust for continuing education grew, the function of the continuing, or in-service/staff development, educator was in all too many instances simply appended to someone's position description. Usually these "victims" had no interest, education, skills, or experience in adult education, and they already had a full-time job. It is little wonder that their efforts were often haphazard, ill planned, and ill executed and sometimes no more than orientation sessions or presentations by salespeople of new products. In-service programs have

become, to many nurses, either something to be avoided or a way to get off the unit for a specified period of time.

Continuing education efforts within higher education have not always fared better. Again, the continuing education function was often appended to a full-time instructor's load. Noncredit education has traditionally been suspect within the ivory towers; it has not had, and does not now enjoy, either status or funding in the usual manner of a university. Perhaps for this reason some schools and colleges of nursing have refused this function and others have been eager to give it up when budgets got tighter.

However, the pool of adult learners will not diminish in the forseeable future. Nor will the demands for accountability, for currency, and for competency in practice lessen. That means that nurses will have to continue to learn, and it also means that someone will have to do the teaching.

Health care agencies, for their own well-being, will have to provide some of that learning. Private enterprise may provide much of it, as will colleges and universities. As the number of young students diminished, academe belatedly discovered adult learners, the reason for being of continuing education. It may be that most of the continuing education based on academe will come to be credit offerings, in the mode of traditional extension offerings, simply because credit offerings make a better fit and because they are more cost effective.

If that occurs, then the credentials of continuing education offered by higher education will be impeccable. Still, some workable form of evaluation, whether as a part of accreditation or some other process will have to be implemented for noncredit continuing education, and one of the measures of effectiveness is sure to be the ratio of cost to outcome.

Competent workers

One of the functions of the Council on Continuing Education for Nursing, as delineated in the rules for operation, is to "promote the establishment of graduate programs for the preparation of nurses in staff development and continuing education positions." The pace has been slow. A few tracks in continuing education have been included in master's programs in nursing, for example, at Indiana University. The University of California has initiated a master's level continuing education specialist program; it is not housed within nursing. Master's and doctoral programs in adult/continuing education are available across the country; most are within the domain of schools and colleges of education. This slow pace will probably continue in the foreseeable future as fewer new graduate programs or tracks within extant programs are funded.

Still, there are some continuing educators who would like to see the Standards for Continuing Education specify that the director of an accredited program must hold a master's degree in nursing. This will probably not occur until additional graduate programs are available and probably should not occur at all until graduate nursing curricula contain content relevant for continuing education practice preparation.*

Threat to the status quo

Nurses have been accused of being "doers, not writers." Since most of the nurses presently practicing were initiated into the profession through what was essentially an apprentice system, they may also be said to be "doers, not thinkers." That is, many nurses still consider trial and error as their favorite mode of learning, still see tasks and skills as the heart of nursing practice, and tend to problem solve only within the context of the particular situation at hand. My research validates these assumptions for the population studied. The study found that the involved nurses, graduates of associate degree, diploma, and baccalaureate programs, had great difficulty in using process in content areas addressed.*

According to my research, continuing education may seem, for those nurses who have difficulty in processing information so that it is readily transferable to new domains and different situations, "unnecessary, expensive, not related to nursing, a waste of time." Further, as noted above, mandatory continuing education presents a real threat to relicensure or reciprocal licensure in those states requiring it.

The current emphasis on belt tightening and cost control will probably reinforce those negative values and attitudes toward continuing education. Nurses holding those values and attitudes will not want to spend their own money for continuing education fees. Agencies have cut their budgets for outside staff development significantly. This usually means that administration decides what the nurse needs, not the nurse. The nurse's need to know may never be filled. The implications for professional practice are significant.

Continuing professional education

Drucker has described continuing professional education as "the fastest growing part of our educational system" and "the true growth industry in the United States."† As more than half the states move toward some form of mandatory continuing education as a prerequisite to professional relicensure and as the pool of high school students decreases, his words gain credence. Entrepreneurs in continuing education abound, as a glance at mail delivered to any health care agency on any day of the week will attest.

---

*Welch, D.: The real issues behind providing CE in nursing, J. Contin. Education Nurs., pp. 17-21, May-June 1980.

*Newbern, V.: A study of the perceptions of currently practicing nurses of their competency to deal with mentally retarded clients, unpublished doctoral dissertation, Denton, Texas, 1978, North Texas State University.
†Drucker, P.: Managing for results, New York, 1964, Harper & Row, Publishers, Inc., p. 95; and Drucker, P.: The age of discontinuity, New York, 1969, Harper & Row, Publishers, Inc., p. 321.

Concern for continuing education is not the sole province of nursing or the health professions. Houle, who may be considered one of the fathers of modern adult education, has addressed continuing education from the definition of a profession and the characteristics that distinguish a professional. He says:

These characteristics, such as increased competence in solving problems, are related to the entire life career of the individual practitioner and to the status of the occupation to which he or she belongs. Therefore, a lifetime of learning is required to establish, maintain, or elevate the level of accomplishment suggested by each of these characteristics.*

Morris, with tongue in cheek, has expressed the view that college degrees, like credit cards, should have an expiration date.† Although Morris offers this strategy as a way to make colleges and universities cost effective, his idea may not be so fanciful if the diminishing half-life of knowledge is considered.

On a less lofty level, the literature increasingly addresses problems associated with the postindustrial, high-technology era in which we live. Wright, for example, speaks to adult education's role in retraining adults.‡

Thus, regardless of the number of levels finally assigned to nursing, the need for continuing learning will not abate.

PREDICTIONS FOR THE FUTURE

Any prediction of the future of continuing education must be predicated on the course of nursing as a whole. That course will be determined, in large measure, by whether nursing is able to establish itself as an autonomous discipline, both responsible and accountable for its members and their practice, and reaches the goal of full professionalism. If nursing remains a vocation with external controls, predictions regarding continuing education are simple: practicing nurses will do what they are told to do.

Predictions also must be considered within the context of the state of the nation. The best guess must be that we must finally come to terms with the knowledge that all resources are finite, that more is not necessarily better, and that we must make do or do without. So the predictions listed below reflect both creativity and austerity (i.e., survival in a cost-conscious world) and are based on the assumption that nurses at all levels will control their own practice:

1. Nurses, as professionals, will take responsibility (including financial responsibility) for their own continued learning.
2. Nurses, as professionals and as responsible adults, will demand programing that meets their learning needs, schedules, learning styles, and fiscal resources.
3. Nurses will join with other practicing professionals in interdisciplinary learning activities.
4. Continuing learning will be done, in large measure, through the use of the computer, telecommunications, or some combination.
5. The use of preceptors or mentors will become an important facet of continuing education for practice.
6. Continuing education sponsored by institutions of higher education will concentrate on credit offerings.
7. Much continuing education will be done by contracting.
8. Mandatory continuing education will be on hold while efforts are made to develop alternative measures to ensure continuing learning.
9. A new specialty, continuing educator, will evolve in master's education in nursing.

---

*Houle, C.: Continuing learning in the professions, San Francisco, 1980, Jossey-Bass, Inc., Publishers, p. 10.
†Morris, D.: Point of view, The Chronicle of Higher Education, p. 64, Aug. 31, 1983.
‡Wright, J.: Retraining the adult workforce, Lifelong Learning, pp. 20-24, Oct. 1983.

10. The constitutionality of mandatory continuing education will be challenged in the courts; following precedent set in suits involving mandatory public education, mandatory continuing education will stand "for the public weal."

These predictions fit well with the pragmatic outlook of most nurses as well as the philosophical view of the adult learner, expressed by Chene, that autonomy of the adult learner is related not only to independence and the need to know, but also to an awareness of the process of learning and existing norms as well as ability to make critical judgments.* So a further prediction might be that nurses will become more sophisticated in their choice of learning offerings and increasingly more self-directed in achieving that learning—and continuing education will have to keep pace.

SUMMARY

Learning has always been an intrinsic part of the "need to know." Continuing education as a means of meeting the need to know has been on the American scene since the early 1920s; however, the impetus for professional nursing has only been in the last 15 years.

There are many approaches to securing continuing education, such as formal course work, workshops, seminars, and staff development programs. Legislation for mandating continuing education has occurred in several states. The issue of quality and change of nursing practice has become one of concern. Disarray has occurred within the system of continuing education.

Questions of who should offer, control, or pay for continuing education are uppermost in this era of cost containment.

Some predictions for the future are made, based on finite resources and the infinite reaches of human creativity. They may be summarized as foreseeing

nurses becoming increasingly more responsible for fulfilling their need to know and in selecting creative, pragmatic ways to meet that responsibility.

If this occurs, then the student of today will find excellent role models to emulate as (1) he or she moves from student to graduate and (2) the full importance of continuing education to competency, to good patient care, and to a sense of self as a practitioner of nursing begins to be realized. Only then will the truism that graduation from a nursing program is just the beginning of lifelong learning become real to the new practitioner of nursing.

Discussion questions

1. Discuss the historical basis for continuing education as it relates to the enterprise of professional continuing education.
2. Discuss the efficacy of mandatory or voluntary continuing education.
3. Discuss the difference between a formal course of study and continuing education.
4. Discuss the problems surrounding continuing education.
5. Identify for yourself the need for lifelong learning and how you will measure the difference in your practice of nursing.

SUGGESTED READINGS
Texts

Alford, H.: Power and conflict in continuing education, Belmont, Calif., 1980, Wadsworth, Inc.

Bell, D.: The role of education in facilitating adaptation to technological change: an analytical framework and review of the literature, Santa Monica, Calif., 1976, Rand.

Carnegie Commission on Higher Education: Toward a learning society, New York, 1973, McGraw-Hill Book Co.

Clark, C.: The nurse as continuing educator, New York, 1979, Springer Publishing Co.

Cooper, S.: Continuing nursing education, ed. 2, New York, 1979, McGraw-Hill Book Co.

Darkenwald, G., and Larson, G.: Reaching hard-to-reach adults, San Francisco, 1980, Jossey-Bass, Inc., Publishers.

Dunkel, P.: Curriculum for educators in health care institutions, Chicago, 1978, Hospital Research and Educational Trust.

Harmon, D.: Expanding relevant and non-formal education, San Francisco, 1976, Jossey-Bass, Inc., Publishers.

Harrington, F.: The future of adult education, San Francisco, 1977, Jossey-Bass, Inc., Publishers.

---

*Chene, A.: The concept of autonomy in adult education: a philosophical discussion, Adult Education Q., pp. 38-47, Fall 1983.

Hesburgh, T.M., et al.: Patterns for lifelong learning, San Francisco, 1974, Jossey-Bass, Inc., Publishers.

Houle, C.: The design of education, San Francisco, 1974, Jossey-Bass, Inc., Publishers.

Houle, C.: Continuing learning in the professions, San Francisco, 1980, Jossey-Bass, Inc., Publishers.

Jensen, G.: Adult education: outlines of an emerging field of university study, Washington, D.C., 1964, Adult Education Association of the U.S.A.

Knapper, C.: Expanding learning through new communication technologies, San Francisco, 1982, Jossey-Bass, Inc., Publishers.

Knowles, M.: The adult education movement in the United States, New York, 1962, Holt, Rinehart & Winston, Inc.

Knox, A.: Adult development and learning, San Francisco, 1977, Jossey-Bass, Inc., Publishers.

Le Breton, P.: The assessment and development of professionals: theory and practice, Seattle, 1976, University of Washington.

O'Toole, J.: Work, learning, and the American future, San Francisco, 1977, Jossey-Bass, Inc., Publishers.

Rezler, A., and Stevens, B.: The nurse evaluator in education and service, New York, 1978, McGraw-Hill Book Co.

Shortell, S.: A framework for continuing education for the health professions, Ann Arbor, Mich., 1978, Health Administration Press School of Public Health.

Smith, R., et al.: Handbook for adult education, New York, 1970, Macmillan, Inc.

Starpoli, C., and Waltz, C.: Developing and evaluating educational programs for health care providers, Philadelphia, 1978, F.A. Davis Co.

Vermilye, D.: Relating work and education, San Francisco, 1977, Jossey-Bass, Inc., Publishers.

Journal articles

Bunning, R.: Patient teaching implications for university based adult educators, Adult Education 28:121-126, Winter 1977.

Buttedahl, P.: Communications technology and adult education, Lifelong Learning, pp. 4-6, June 1983.

Camin, L.: Survival first, Update, p. 12, Sept. 1982.

Comfort, R.: Higher adult education programming—a model, Adult Leadership, pp. 6-8, May 1974.

Cooper, L.: Make way for recurrent education, Adult Leadership 25:137-139, Jan. 1977.

Cooper, S.: Continuing education, yesterday and today, Nurse Educator, pp. 25-29, Jan.-Feb. 1978.

DeMott, B.: The thrills and chills of lifelong learning, Change, pp. 53-55, April 1978.

Dubin, S., and Okun, M.: Implications of learning theories for adult education, Adult Education, pp. 3-19, Fall 1973.

Forni, P.: Continuing education vs. continuing competence, J. Nurs. Adm., p. 34, Nov.-Dec. 1975.

Kasl, E., and Anderson, R.: Understanding program costs and finance, Lifelong Learning, pp. 12-14, Sept. 1983.

Killian, J., and Killian, R.: Computer competency: tailoring inservice to professional needs, Lifelong Learning, pp. 21-25, Sept. 1983.

Mikulecky, L., and Winchester, D.: Job literacy and job performance among nurses at varying employment levels, Adult Education Q., pp. 10-15, Fall 1983.

Rivera, W.: Professional life planning: a self directed approach, Lifelong Learning, pp. 10-13, Jan. 1983.

Roberts, H.: Goals, objectives and functions in adult education, Adult Education, p. 123, Winter 1976.

Rockhill, K.: Mandatory continuing education for professionals: issues and trends, Adult Education, pp. 106-116, Winter 1983.

Special issue: accreditation and continuing education in nursing, J. Contin Education Nurs., March-April 1983.

Spikes, F.: A multidimensional planning model for continuing nursing education, Lifelong Learning, pp. 4-8, Feb. 1978.

Talbot, G.: Keys for successful budgeting, J. Contin. Education Nurs., pp. 8-11, May-June 1983.

Wiley, K.: Effects of a self-directed learning project and preference for structure on self-directed learning readiness, Nurs. Res., pp. 181-185, May-June 1983.

CHAPTER 17

Dynamic nursing

"Life truly lived is a risky business, and if one puts up too many fences against risk, one ends by shutting out life itself."
Kenneth S. Davis

OBJECTIVE: On completion of this chapter, the student of nursing will have the author's thoughts about the profession of nursing as a dynamic force in one's professional life.

The profession of nursing is perhaps the most dynamic profession a person can enter. The concepts of nursing have stood the test of time, from Florence Nightingale to today's theorists: Rogers, Roy, Newman, Orem, and others.

Throughout the text the student has studied the history of nursing as it relates to many issues. No issue could be studied without touching on another. All of the issues have become interwoven; thus none are simple, all are complex.

In a few short years we will move from the twentieth century to the twenty-first. We already are near the end of the industrial age and well along in the technical age. Nursing is forging ahead in meeting the demands of technology in one's personal and professional life, while still struggling through the industrial model of solving nursing's professionhood.

It has often been said that there is nothing new under the sun, only refinement and advancement.

Caring is the oldest concept of nursing. It is indeed the very essence of being. Knowing about human beings and what we believe is one of the newer concepts. What we believe about technology and its use in nursing is unclear.

The technological age has brought to health care the machinery to save lives, to maintain life, and to change life. It has brought ethical issues that are a far cry from those issues of 30 short years ago. In the technological age, where is the humanism or, if you will, the concept of caring?

Caring is a feeling, an attitude; it is an outward demonstration of one being to another. It is a respect of self, colleagues, patients and clients, family, and friends. Often students of nursing have felt completely void of caring because the demands of the technical world have overshadowed the humanism aspect to be integrated and ultimately portrayed when giving care or interacting with others.

One of the dynamic forces that will impinge on the professional life will be restoring the concept of caring in the milieu of the technological age. Just how individual nurses will include this force as a means in nursing will depend on self-worth and respect of others.

The nurse's concept of valuing will be another force to provide guidance in one' professional life. As different approaches to nursing care are explicated, questions of ethical or moral valuing will need to be addressed. How one values self and others is as important as what technique is used to perform nursing care.

Valuing is a part of caring. Thus to me the most viable force to become dynamic is how we in nursing teach and nurture the concept of caring and how each individual nurse includes this concept in the ''care plan'' for individuals and groups of people, whether in an acute care center or in a home health care setting.

Relationships with all health workers, including the physician, are a force to be reckoned with in the late twentieth century. Presently, nurses are at odds with other health workers. Carving out specific roles for each of the disciplines of medicine, nursing, and the myriad of health care workers is a necessity. Increased blurring of roles will and has occurred; thus nurses need to be aware of the dynamics surrounding turf issues. Perhaps it will become necessary to bury definitive roles, such as the hierarchy of physicians, nurses, and others, and to conceptualize each working in concert, as a symphony orchestra, to achieve medical, nursing, and health care.

The issue of education needs to be put to rest. Education is the most dynamic force to be utilized in the professional life. Basic nursing education can never provide the wherewithal to practice nursing. Dynamic nursing is education; it is the means with which to risk changes, to study, and to make decisions about what needs to be done for a specific individual, for families, or for self. Rather than continue the dialogue of who is the better prepared, the dialogue should center around what preparation is needed to meet the needs of patients requiring nursing care. Career goals need to be the determining factor in the education issue. If the goal is clinical nursing, then all academic preparation should lead to the purist in nursing with skills in clinical research; however, if education is the career goal, the academic preparation needs to be a combination of nursing and education.

Formal academic preparation should never end. Continuing education in seminars, workshops, reading, and conferences will maintain and create

the dynamic force in altering oneself and thus changing nursing.

Political and social forces will demand changes in the professional life. Gone are the days to ignore the world around us. A healthy nation needs to be a paramount concept in every political and social action taken. These two focuses will impinge on the professional life as interactions with society occur. It will be vital for every nurse to become involved in society's awakening to changes in the health care system. The individual nurse needs to be acutely aware of the economics of care and how they encroach on nursing care.

An all-RN staff is a goal to be considered as realistic, and yet not all RNs are of the mind set to do the basics of nursing care. A question to be asked is, ''What would happen if there no longer existed a 'let George do it' mentality?'' With RNs performing all the nursing care, I visualize colleague relationships existing rather than a hierarchy of care givers.

The practice of nursing would exude a dynamism among and between colleagues who collaborate with each other in perfecting nursing. The practice arena is the force to provide the nurse with knowledge, attitudes, and skills in order to deliver nursing care to a healthy community, state, or nation.

How society chooses to pay for nursing care will be addressed and solved in the next 5 to 10 years. Fee for service and contracting for nursing services will be considered as modes for solving the economic issue of the industrial model of collective bargaining. As registered nursing takes its rightful place in determining policy of nursing care, a new era in the quest for professionhood will occur.

Dynamic nursing is what a professional life is all about. It is taking an active part in the decisions to be made for self, the society served, and the professional goals of organized nursing. It is being an involved individual in the political, social, and economic forces that change society and ultimately the role a nurse will play.

On graduation and entering the pragmatic world, the new nurse will have a basic background to practice nursing. The experience and further education will add to the zest of nursing.

Combining a career in nursing with a social life and a life as a homemaker will be the most dynamic force to face. Whether man or woman, making the most out of life and all the surrounding opportunities will provide a career in the dynamics of nursing.

As you, the student, accept your role in the practice of nursing either as a direct care giver, educator, administrator, or researcher, you have a heritage on which to build. In 20 years you will be the leaders making policies and setting new goals for the profession of nursing. Only as the quest for new knowledge occurs, will nursing continue to be the dynamic force in health care. Do not be afraid to risk, to change, and to be bold in your dreams for nursing.

Glossary of terms for evolution of theories for nursing

To understand the nature of theories one must also know the language used to describe and discuss theories. The following concepts were selected to help the beginning student to acquire the language of theories by looking at the Greek and Latin derivatives. References used to search for this information included *Webster's New World Dictionary of the American Language*, 1970; *The New Webster's Encyclopedia, Dictionary of the English Language*, 1977; *Webster's New Collegiate Dictionary*, 1978; *Roget's International Thesaurus*, 1978; and the writings of several authors who have written about theory development. Selected concepts have been more extensively defined in Chapter 4.

analogue (Greek *analogia, ana,* according to, and *logos,* ratio or proportion) An agreement or likeness between things in some circumstances or effects, when the things are otherwise entirely different; conformity, parallelism, likeness; implies general differences.

art (Latin *arsis,* a lifting up; *ar,* to join, fit together) Human ability to make things; creativity of humans as distinguished from the world of nature; creative work or its principles; making or doing of things that display form, beauty, and unusual perception; art includes painting, sculpture, architecture, music, literature, drama, the dance; any branch of creative work (*Webster's,* 1970).

assumption (Latin *assiomo,* to take) Taking for granted; a postulate or proposition (without proof); synonymous with supposition.

axiom (Greek, a self-evident truth or proposition) A proposition whose truth is so evident at first sight that no process of reasoning or demonstration can make it plainer; an established principle in some art or science; the starting point for derivations.

concept (Latin *conceptum,* what is conceived, held within) An object conceived by the mind; an abstract idea; a word; product of the imaginative or inventive faculty; a general notion; that which constitutes the meaning of a general term.

conceptual framework Network within which questions, theories, and data fit together; global ideas about the individuals, groups, situations, and events of interest to a discipline.

construct (Latin *construo,* to pile up) Structure to put together parts (concepts) into their proper place and order; to build; to form mentally; more than one concept joined together to convey a meaning.

deduction (Latin *deducere,* to lead down, bring away) Reasoning from a known principle to an unknown, from the general to the specific, or from a premise to a logical conclusion.

empirical (Greek *emperikikos,* experienced) Pertaining to experiments or experience or to a person who relies solely on practical experience rather than on scientific principles.

empirical concept An idea evoked by a concrete object, property, or event; it is verifiable and experienced by the senses.

fact (Latin *factum,* a thing done) Anything done or that has come to pass; something known to exist; a phemomenon that is tangible and can be validated empirically.

generalization (Latin *generalis,* belonging to a genus, a kind) To reduce or bring under a general law, rule, or statement; to bring into relation with a wider circle of facts; to deduce from the consideration of many particulars; to classify particulars under general heads or rules.

hypothesis (Greek *hypo,* under, and *tithemi,* to place) A supposition; something not proved, but assumed for the purpose of argument; a relationship statement that is tested in research.

259

induction (Latin *inducere,* to lead into, bring toward) To draw a general rule or conclusion from particular facts; to infer; to bring about; to cause; to effect; to conclude; a form of reasoning that moves from the specific to the general.

law (Latin *lex,* lay down, legal) A rule of action laid down or prescribed by authority; a theoretical principle deduced from practice or observation; a formal statement of facts invariably observed in natural phenomena.

model (French *modèle,* a little measure) A pattern of something to be made; a form in miniature to be made on a larger scale; a copy in miniature; that by which a thing is to be measured (*Webster's,* 1970).

paradigm (Greek *para,* beside, and *deigma,* example, from *driknumi,* to show) A pattern *(Roget's International Thesarus);* an example; a model.

phenomenon (Greek *phainomai,* appear) An observable fact or event (plural, phenomena).

postulate (Latin *postulo,* demand) A position or supposition of which the truth is demanded or assumed for the purpose of future reasoning; the enunciation of a self-evident problem; a supposition or assumption without proof.

premise (Latin *prae,* before, and *mitto,* I send) To set forth or make known beforehand; to lay down as an antecedent proposition; a proposition laid down as a base of argument.

principle (Latin *principium,* beginning, origin, element) The prime source or element from which anything proceeds; a general truth, a settled rule of action; a law comprehending many subordinate truths; a law on which others are founded or from which others are derived; a governing law of conduct.

proposition (French *proposer,* for a purpose or to pose) To bring forward or offer for consideration, acceptance, or adoption; to form or declare an intention or design; a statement of a truth to be demonstrated or an operation to be performed.

research (French *recercher,* to travel through, survey) Diligent inquiry or examination in seeking facts or principles; laborious or continued search after truth; investigation; to examine anew; careful, systematic, patient study and investigation in some field of knowledge, undertaken to discover or establish factors or principles (*Webster's,* 1970).

science (Latin *scire,* to know, to discern, to distinguish) Systematized knowledge derived from observation, study, and experimentation carried on to determine the nature of principles of what is being studied; a branch of knowledge or study, especially one concerned with establishing and systematizing facts, principles, and methods, as by experiments and hypotheses; the systematized knowledge of nature and the physical world.

system (Greek *systena,* together, to set) An assemblage of things forming a regular and connected whole; a plan or scheme according to which things are connected into a whole; regular method or order; methodical (*Webster's,* 1970); an integrated whole comprised of distinct yet integrated parts.

taxonomy (Greek *taxis,* arrangement, division, and *nomos,* a law) Classification of phenomena according to their natural relationships (*Webster's,* 1978); the science of classification; laws and principles covering the classifying of objects.

theorem A position laid down as an acknowledged truth or established principle; a proposition to be proved by a chain of reasoning and analysis; a rule expressed by symbols or formulae.

theory (Greek *theoreo,* to look, to see or to observe, to view) A philosophical explanation of phenomena; a connected arrangement of facts according to their bearing on some real or hypothetical law or laws; speculation (*Webster's,* 1977); a way of explaining reality, invented for some purpose; an elaborate scheme for explaining, describing, prescribing, or controlling reality.

truth (Anglo Saxon *treówe,* whence, faithful, fixed) Conforming to fact or reality; a truth withstands the test of scientific debate.

variable (Latin, changeable) A factor that influences the occurrence of a phenomenon; an object, event, or property that is changeable or results in variation; variables are empirical indicators that are measurable.

Index

Nightingale, F., 1, 13, 33, 38, 75, 78, 83
  and development of nursing theory, 75-76
  history of nursing and, 42-44
  nursing education and, 42-44
Nightingale era
  nursing education before and during, 40-44
  nursing service in, 12-17
Nile River, culture of, 4
Nonformal education, 248
Nurse(s)
  as actor/reactor, 172
  power, politics and, 166-178
  perspective of, in collective bargaining, 157-160
  rights of, 87-89
Nurse Enrollment Program, 205-206
Nurse Practice Acts, state boards of nursing and, 225
"Nurse politician," 178
Nurse practitioners, 36; *see also* Nursing, practitioner(s)
Nurse Training Act of 1964, 54
Nurses' Associated Alumnae, 49
Nurses' Association of the American College of Obstetrics and
      Gynecology, 209
Nurses' Education Fund, 185
Nurses on Horseback, 19
Nurses, Patients, and Pocketbooks, 51
Nurses for Society in Crisis, 200
Nursing; *see also* Nurse(s); Nursing education; Nursing service
  changing patterns of, 31-39
  collective bargaining in; *see* Collective bargaining in nursing
  contemporary perspectives in; *see* Perspectives, nursing, con-
      temporary
  continuing education in, 246-247
  dynamic, 256-258
  evolution of and trends in, 1-82
  functional, as system of health care delivery, 133
  higher education in, 60-61
  history of, 1-2
  in hospitals, changes in, 34-35
  issues in, 85-97
  legal aspects of, 212-226
    allocation of loss, 215-217
    autopsies, 219
    confidentiality, 218
    contracts, 219
    damages, determination of, 217
    defenses, 217
    emergency exception, 218
    licensure; *see* Licensure, nursing
    negligence, 213-215
      contributory or comparative, 217-218
    res ipsa loquitur, 215
    state boards of nursing, 223-225
    statute of limitations, 217

Nursing—cont'd
  legislative process and, 173-178
  modular primary and primary, as system of health care de-
      livery, 134
  opportunities in
    areas of practice, 229-233
    career, ladder, 233
    Economic Security Program, 242-243
    planning, career, 233
    position, selection of, 228-229
    resignation(s), 240-242
    responsibilities of, 233-240
    self-assessment, 227-228
  primitive, 3-4
  as profession, 163
  professional, 191-211
    alumni associations, 208
    definitions, 191-193
    organizations
      professional, 193-205
      related, 208-210
      special interest, 205-208
  reforms in, 16-17
  research in
    challenge of, 186
    definition, 179-180
    development of proposals, 184-185
    funding, 185
    future of, 185-186
    history of, 182-183
    importance of, 181
    publications related to, 183-184
    types, 180-181
  role of, in government, 171-173
  selection of position in, 228-229
  self-organization of, 19-20
  state boards of, licensure and, 223-225
  support services in, 125-128
  team, as system of health care delivery, 134
  theories of, 67-82
    emergence and development of, 75-76
    evaluation of, 77-78
    nature of, 67-74
    purpose of, 76-77
    status of, 74-75
Nursing administration, as support service, 126
Nursing care
  reimbursement for, 125
  systems for delivery of
    case method, 133-134
    functional, 133
    modular, 134
    primary, 134
    team, 134

Standardization in continuing education, 250-251
State board(s) of nursing, licensure and, 223-225
Statute(s)
    function of in society, 212-213
    of limitations, 217
Staupers, M., 63
Stevens, B.J., 71, 77, 127
Stewart, I.M., 182
Strikes, nurses and, 161-162
Structure
    organizational, as variable in nursing practice, 129-131
    theories and, 72
Studies of nursing education, 51-52
Style(s) of leadership, 140
Styles, M., 92, 191, 192
Suffrage, history of, 167
Sunset legislation, 222-223
Support services in nursing, 125-128
Surgicenters, development of, 27
Swenson, R., 111-114

T

TEFRA, 27, 86, 125
Taft-Hartley Act, 156
Talbott, S.W., 166
Tappen, R.M., 140
Tax Equity and Fiscal Responsibility Act, 27, 86
Taxonomy, theories and, 72
Teachers' College, Columbia University, 50
Team nursing, 34-35
    as system of health care delivery, 134
Technology, nursing and, 256
Teleology, 148
Teutonic Knights, 8
Theory(ies), nursing; *see* Nursing, theories of
Thomas, C., 223
Tigris River, culture of, 4
Toffler, A., 85
Tompkins, F., 194
Tompkins, S., 15
Topeka Board of Education, 86
Total patient system of health care delivery, 133-134
Toward Quality in Nursing, 53, 109
Training, management, as support service in nursing, 127-128
Transplants, organ, as nursing issue, 87
Treece, E.W., 180
Treece, J.W., Jr., 180
Trend(s)
    in nursing, 1-82
    in nursing education, 120-121
Tschudin, M.S., 106
Tuke, W., 10-11

Tuskegee Institute, 62
Twentieth century, nursing service in, 17-28

U

Unification model of organizational structure, 131-132
Uniform, nurse's, early use of, 46
Union(s), nursing, development, 25; *see also* Collective bargaining in nursing
United States Children's Bureau, 19
University(ies), nursing education and, 247
University of Nebraska College of Nursing, 54
Ursulines, 11

V

Vance, C.N., 166
Variables
    influence of, on nursing practice, 129-132
    theories and, 67-68
Vaughn, J.C., 59, 100
Veninga, K., 159
Veninga, R., 159
Veterans' Administration, 183
Virgins, nursing order of, 6
Visiting Nurses, 32
Vocation, versus profession, 192
Vyas, K.C., 6

W

WCHEN, 247
WHO, 209
WICHEN, 182-183
Wagner Act, 156
Wald, L., 15, 33
Walker, L., 76, 80
Walsh, J.J., 7
Washington, B.T., 61
Wasserstrom, R., 149
Welch, D., 252
Wellman, C., 147, 153
Western Council on Higher Education for Nursing, 247
Western Interstate Council of Higher Education for Nursing, 182
Western Journal of Nursing Research, 183
Whall, A., 78
White House Conference on Children and Youth, 19
Whitman, W., 14
Widows, nursing order of, 6
Wilson, F., 64
Women's movement, effect of, on nursing, 167
Work Conference on Graduate Nurse Education, 116
World Health Organization, 209
World War I, nursing service during, 17-19